The Selfish Brain

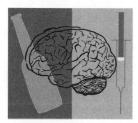

Learning From Addiction

"In his new book, *The Selfish Brain: Learning From Addiction,* Dr. DuPont has linked, for the first time, the rapidly expanding scientific knowledge about addiction and his own intensely personal experiences over more than a quarter of a century of working with addicted people and their families. He extends his useful ideas to the areas of public policy and to the global dimensions of this uniquely human disease. . . .

"This is not a pretty or an easy story, but it is one filled with hope for the future for those individuals, families, communities, and countries ready to confront the real and serious problems of addiction and to find their own unique ways to prevent and overcome these problems. Our country is fortunate to have a man of Dr. DuPont's stature and ability who has dedicated himself to the important cause of the prevention and treatment of addiction."

—Ross Perot

"Dr. DuPont, in this rational and readable book, highlights some of the keys to overcoming chemical dependence for individuals, and for winning the battle against drugs as a nation: honesty, responsibility, hard work, and accountability. As he writes, 'Because an addiction requires dishonesty, honesty is the one-word antidote to all forms of addiction.' I applaud his efforts and this book."

—William J. Bennett
Co-Director, Empower America
Former Director, Office of National Drug Control Policy

"For anyone interested in the shadowy and violent world of illicit drugs and the effects on our children, our homes, our businesses, and our society, Dr. DuPont's book is a must."

—B/Gen Robinson Risner
USAF (Ret)
Organizer and First Director
Texans' War on Drugs

"This is the first book that I've read—and I read every one I get my hands on—that deals with the whole problem of addiction from a historical, cross-cultural, and scientific point of view. It's the first time that the myths of drug use are attacked openly and clearly. . . .

"This book can be used as a tremendous resource for students. Dr. DuPont takes the time to provide all the evidence to support his thesis; furthermore, he analyzes that evidence to make it understandable to the reader."

—Michael K. Mulligan
Headmaster
Thacher School
Ojai, California

The Selfish Brain gives the most comprehensive treatment of chemical dependency I have seen in the last 10 years. It is an essential book for any professional as we approach the year 2000. Dr. DuPont provides us with an interesting narrative of this controversial subject and a thought-provoking, well-researched, detailed, systematic analysis."

—Dan Buie, CAE
President
Texans' War on Drugs

"I found Dr. DuPont's new book intriguing and challenging. As in his previous writings, he successfully draws the reader in. I highly recommend *The Selfish Brain*."

—John T. Schwarzlose
President
Betty Ford Center at Eisenhower

"*The Selfish Brain* is the masterpiece of one of our nation's leaders in addiction medicine. Bob DuPont makes it crystal clear why he is considered to be a masterful psychiatrist, a level-headed national drug policy analyst, and a dedicated foot soldier in the war on drugs. Dr. DuPont can describe the turmoil of the addict, the forces in society, the moral and ethical abyss, the steps in recovery, and the neurobiology of drug seeking in the same sentence with a unique and compelling clarity of style. Rather than a simple follow-up to the ground-breaking *Gateway Drugs*, Dr. DuPont has put together the definitive text that nimbly takes us from the neuron to 12-step recovery meetings and back again. . . .

"This important book on the process and treatment of addiction is an absolute must read for the student or the clinician but also for those with loved ones who are using drugs. . . . From an expert with years of experience from the lab to the White House and to the psychiatrist's office—everyone will find something remarkable, some great insight in accessible terms in *The Selfish Brain*."

—Mark S. Gold, M.D.
Noted antidrug expert
Founder, National Cocaine Hotline
Author, *The Facts About Drugs and Alcohol* and other books

"*The Selfish Brain* clearly articulates issues that I have known and felt but never put into words. What a service for today's parents! This book explains addiction in a clear, easy-to-read manner, consistently supporting the basic role of the family."

—Jean B. Newberry
Board of Directors
National Federation of Parents

"This book will be of enduring help to professionals as well as to recovering people. It will further the debate on how society can seriously address the issue of addiction. The book is particularly adept at calling out the fact that we have not—to date—accepted addiction as a problem and therefore are not fully embracing any possible solutions. This book makes that failure clear and offers suggestions to turn it into an opportunity of great value."

—John Small
Vice-President/Publishing
Parkside Publishing Corporation

"DuPont's writing conveys 'I know a lot about this, and have given it a lot of thought. Here are some ideas I would like you to think about, too.' Reading *The Selfish Brain* is like listening to him in personal conversations about problems that touch us all.

"DuPont's authority is second to none, and his conversational writing style makes even the technical parts of *The Selfish Brain* accessible to any interested reader. The presentation of the factors contributing to 'drug problems' is the best I have read, and the proposal of steps society must take to solve those problems is compelling."

—Harry A. Tiemann, Ph.D.
Professor of Psychology
Chair, Department of Behavioral Sciences
Mesa State College
Grand Junction, Colorado

"Bob DuPont's book, *The Selfish Brain*, is a welcome, innovative, and comprehensive examination of chemical dependency and the problems of drug addiction. The unique nature of this dependency, and the reality of the physiological and psychological cross currents that have caused so much pain and grief for American families, is effectively demonstrated. . . .

"The book is a winner; refreshing, interesting, instructive, and is a must for anyone seriously interested in the field of substance abuse."

—Peter B. Bensinger
Former Administrator
U.S. Drug Enforcement Administration

"Dr. DuPont's book, *The Selfish Brain*, is a thoughtful, thorough, and inspiring book. Having associated with Dr. DuPont for over 15 years, I have witnessed his expertise and dedication to the issue of addiction. As Dr. DuPont eloquently states, 'Addiction is a modern chemical slavery.'"

—Eric A. Voth, M.D., F.A.C.P.
Chairman
International Drug Strategy Institute

"This book is exhaustive and unique as a brilliant blend of science and clinical artistry. I am confident no other work of its kind exists or will in the foreseeable future. It offers glossaries, illustrations, and case histories that form the building blocks of an exciting and worthwhile literary experience. The author's practical appeal is to help all who either have, are affected by, or treat an addictive illness."

—Norman S. Miller, M.D.
Department of Psychiatry
The University of Illinois
at Chicago

"This book is a real contribution to the field. Dr. DuPont takes a bold, sometimes controversial, and consistently comprehensive approach in explaining addictions. In reading this book, one is challenged to take action in small and big ways. He offers ideas and suggestions, from individual commitment to societal action, to change the way we view alcohol and other drug use in society. This is a magnificent combination, rarely seen, of scholarly detail and personal compassion."

—Patricia Owen, Ph.D., M.H.A.
Hazelden
Center City, Minnesota

"This book represents another work by Dr. DuPont on the 'cutting edge' of recovery for addicts and alcoholics. We who are recovering addicts/alcoholics in Narcotics Anonymous and Alcoholics Anonymous applaud this work. This is a must read for anyone who seeks to understand the very nature of the addict. The 12-step fellowships have an author who is 'on target' concerning addiction and alcoholism."

—Stephen W. Ringer, M.S.W., C.A.P.

"*The Selfish Brain* is one of the best books I've ever read about drugs. It is very straightforward, written without compromise and compassionate, but with deep humanity and care for people wasting their lives with drugs."

—Nicolas Lerch, M.D.
Association for the Advancement of Psychological
Understanding of Human Nature (VPM)
Zurich, Switzerland

"Dr. DuPont's book has opened the door for everyone to have a better understanding of the brain and addiction. His emphasis on honesty as an antidote for addiction is excellent."

—Otto Moulton
Committees of Correspondence and
Drug Watch
Danvers, Massachusetts

"Bob DuPont has written yet another landmark book on the subject of drug abuse prevention. He is an expert with the courage to think independently. Every parent, teacher, and business leader should read this book."

—William F. Current
Former Executive Director
American Council for Drug Education

"Dr. DuPont's outstanding book, *The Selfish Brain*, is a major contribution to society's understanding of the addiction problem. His book covers all aspects of chemical dependency, from neurochemical impairment to brain recovery. I was particularly impressed with the section on the 12-step fellowship and the quiet revolution of recovery that is sweeping our nation."

—David E. Smith, M.D.
Founder and Medical Director
Haight Ashbury Free Medical Clinics
President-Elect
American Society of Addiction Medicine

"Sane, balanced, eminently readable: Bob DuPont combines personal honesty, intelligent compassion, and profound insight to offer his readers wisdom as well as knowledge on an important but often too glibly misunderstood topic. This important book will help clear up many confusions even as it deepens its readers' insight and compassion."

—Ernest Kurtz, Ph.D.
Co-Author, *The Spirituality of Imperfection*
Author, *Not-God: A History of Alcoholics Anonymous*
and other books

"*The Selfish Brain* is much more than advice; it gives a broad perspective on drug use that cuts through sloganeering and magical thinking. The reader comes to understand why drugs have been tolerated but are now being rejected. The practical knowledge Dr. DuPont provides will be a welcome gift to anyone concerned about drug abuse."

—David F. Musto, M.D.
Professor of Psychiatry and of the History of Medicine
Yale University School of Medicine

"[Dr. DuPont's] talent with words and his vast experience in the field have been combined to produce a valuable resource for everyone interested in the prevention and treatment of alcohol and drug abuse."

—Donald Ian Macdonald, M.D.
Chairman and CEO, Employee Health Programs
Bethesda, Maryland
Former Director, National Institute on Drug Abuse

The Selfish Brain

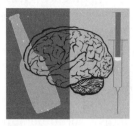

Learning From Addiction

Robert L. DuPont, M.D.

President, Institute for Behavior and Health, Inc.
Rockville, Maryland
Clinical Professor of Psychiatry
Georgetown University School of Medicine
Washington, D.C.

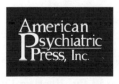

Washington, DC
London, England

Note: The author has worked to ensure that all information in this book concerning drug dosages, schedules, and routes of administration is accurate as of the time of publication and consistent with standards set by the U.S. Food and Drug Administration and the general medical community. As medical research and practice advance, however, therapeutic standards may change. For this reason and because human and mechanical errors sometimes occur, we recommend that readers follow the advice of a physician who is directly involved in their care or the care of a member of their family.

Books published by the American Psychiatric Press, Inc., represent the views and opinions of the individual authors and do not necessarily represent the policies and opinions of the Press or the American Psychiatric Association.

Copyright © 1997 Robert L. DuPont, M.D.
ALL RIGHTS RESERVED
Manufactured in the United States of America on acid-free paper
00   99   98   97   4   3   2   1

American Psychiatric Press, Inc.
1400 K Street, N.W., Washington, DC   20005

Library of Congress Cataloging-in-Publication Data
DuPont, Robert L., 1936–
    The selfish brain : learning from addiction / by Robert L. DuPont.
      p.   cm.
    Includes bibliographical references and index.
    ISBN 0-88048-686-4 (cloth)
    1. Substance abuse.   2. Substance abuse—Treatment.   3. Recovering addicts.   4. Twelve-step groups.   I. Title.
    [DNLM: 1. Substance Dependence—psychology.   2. Substance Dependence—rehabilitation.   WM 270 D938s 1997]
RC564.29.D87   1997
362.29—dc20
DNLM/DLC
for Library of Congress   96-8593
                                                      CIP

British Library Cataloguing in Publication Data
A CIP record is available from the British Library.

For addicted people and their families,
whose courage has inspired this book.

With my gratitude and respect.

*For everyone hoping to help addicted people, including therapists like
me who regularly see the pain of failure to overcome addiction, remember what we are up against: a dreadful, progressive, and potentially
fatal disease. Our failures are our major sources of learning. Our
patients, friends, and families who get well teach us little. When we fail
in our struggles to overcome addiction, despite our best efforts, we are
forced by our pain to grow and to learn. Bless the failures in our lives,
for they are our best teachers.*

*This is a book of hope. Today's failures can always become tomorrow's
successes. Having worked with addicts and their families for over
25 years, I have seen many long-delayed recoveries that are all the more
precious for the high costs that had to be paid to achieve them. I never
give up hope, even in cases that seem the most hopeless. Tomorrow is a
new opportunity for addicted people and their families, as well as for
everyone who cares about them, including their friends, colleagues,
teachers, physicians, and therapists.*

Contents

Section III
Overcoming Addiction

Foreword

A ddiction to alcohol and other drugs is at the heart of many of the world's most difficult human problems, from crime and AIDS to health care costs and highway safety, from decreased productivity to family breakdown. Of all the many causes of these modern dilemmas, the one that is most susceptible to solution is addiction. Addiction, although cunning, baffling, and powerful, has within it the seeds of self-knowledge and a better life for individuals, families, and communities.

Robert L. DuPont, M.D., in his book *The Selfish Brain*, draws on his experience over the past quarter century in helping people learn about addiction. Here is a book that builds on the growing understanding of the biology of addiction to explore addiction in the family and in our communities. This book can help people confronting addiction in their own lives and in their families. It also can help our leaders develop policies to reduce the risks of addiction.

I first met Dr. DuPont in 1975 when he was the White House drug czar for my husband, President Gerald Ford. During my husband's administration, he also held the post of first director of the National Institute on Drug Abuse (NIDA). At that time, the problem of addiction was considered to be concerned primarily with heroin addiction. One of the major achievements of the Ford administration was to curtail the flood of heroin then coming into the United States from Mexico. Another significant accomplishment was the development of a national drug treatment network led by NIDA.

Years later, after confronting my own problems with addiction to alcohol and prescription drugs, I established the Betty Ford Center to help others with addiction. Dr. DuPont's path crossed with mine again when he referred many of his patients to the Betty Ford Center for treatment. Recently, Dr. DuPont has worked with the Betty Ford Center medical staff on a project to help alumni encourage their physicians to recognize addiction in other patients and help them receive effective treatment.

Dr. DuPont possesses unique perspectives on addiction. They range from the most personal, gained through his work as a practicing physician who confronts addiction every day in his patients and their families, to an understanding gained through his national leadership in addiction research and treatment. He has made significant contributions to public policy at the local, national, and international levels. His support of increased public and private funding for treatment is based on the belief that treatment is the best way to help addicted people overcome their denial and start on paths to their own recovery. Addiction treatment is one of the best buys in all of health care. It works to reduce the terrible toll of addiction, not only in economic terms but also in terms of the quality of life for families and communities.

The most important insight in the book may be that Alcoholics Anonymous (AA) and the other 12-step fellowships modeled on AA are the places where most people can find the answers to their questions about addiction. Attending meetings of these fellowships is an essential component in the process undertaken by many addicted people and their families to find lasting recovery. This book can help people in all parts of the world understand addiction and the essential role of 12-step fellowships in overcoming this potentially fatal disease.

As *The Selfish Brain* makes clear, getting well involves far more than stopping the use of alcohol and other drugs. Getting well and staying well means finding better ways to live as individuals, in families, and in communities. Getting well is not about blaming someone else for one's problems, it is about living honest lives filled with loving connections to other people, both inside and outside the 12-step fellowships. That is the good news that this book delivers. It is a hopeful, clear, and important message.

Betty Ford
Chairman
Board of Directors
Betty Ford Center at Eisenhower
Rancho Mirage, California

Acknowledgments

A word of thanks for the people who have worked with me on this book by reviewing and commenting on earlier drafts. Kathryn L. Allen, Alexandria, VA; William J. Bennett, Ph.D., Empower America, Washington, DC; Peter B. Bensinger, Bensinger, DuPont, and Associates, Chicago, IL; Dan Buie, Texans' War on Drugs, Austin, TX; Fred Burford, Council on Drug Abuse, Toronto, Ontario; James F. Callahan, D.P.A., American Society of Addiction Medicine, Chevy Chase, MD; Allan Y. Cohen, Ph.D., Pacific Institute for Research and Evaluation, Rockville, MD; William F. Current, American Council for Drug Education (formerly), Rockville, MD; Betty Ford, Betty Ford Center at Eisenhower, Rancho Mirage, CA; Mark S. Gold, M.D., University of Florida Brain Institute, Gainesville, FL; Enoch Gordis, M.D., National Institute on Alcohol Abuse and Alcoholism, Rockville, MD; Jill Jonnes, Historian, Baltimore, MD; Raymond C. Kubacki, Jr., Psychemedics Corporation, Cambridge, MA; Ernest Kurtz, Ph.D., author, Ann Arbor, MI; Nicolas Lerch, M.D., Association for the Advancement of Psychological Understanding of Human Nature, Zurich, Switzerland; Donald Ian Macdonald, M.D., Employee Health Programs, Bethesda, MD; Edward J. Madara, American Self-Help Clearinghouse, Denville, NJ; Dr. Ma. Elena Medina-Mora, Instituto Mexicano de Psiquiatria, Mexico City, Mexico; Norman S. Miller, M.D., University of Illinois at Chicago, Chicago, IL; Otto Moulton, Committees of Correspondence and Drug Watch, Danvers, MA; Michael Mulligan, Thacher School, Ojai, CA; David F. Musto, M.D., Yale University School of Medicine, New Haven, CT; Katherine Nelson, Bethesda, MD; Thomas R. Neslund, International Commission for the Prevention of Alcoholism and Drug Dependency, Silver Spring, MD; Jean Newberry, National Family Partnership, Corpus Christi, TX; Patricia Owen, Ph.D., M.H.A., Hazelden Foundation, Center City, MN; Ross Perot, The Perot

Group, Dallas, TX; L. Gerald Pond, Radio News and Feature Services, The Church of Jesus Christ of Latter-day Saints, Salt Lake City, UT; Frank Riessman, M.D., National Self-Help Clearinghouse, New York, NY; Stephen W. Ringer, M.S.W., C.A.P., Coral Gables, FL; Brig. Gen. Robinson Risner, USAF (Ret), Austin, TX; Timothy M. Rivinus, M.D., Butler Hospital, Providence, RI; Rita Rumbaugh, Montgomery County Public Schools, Rockville, MD; Robert A. Sammons, Jr., M.D., Ph.D., Mesa Behavioral Medicine Clinic, Inc., Grand Junction, CO; John T. Schwarzlose, Betty Ford Center at Eisenhower; Rancho Mirage, CA; John Small, Parkside Publishing Corporation, Park Ridge, IL; David E. Smith, M.D., Haight Ashbury Free Medical Clinics, San Francisco, CA; Harry A. Tiemann, Ph.D., Mesa State College, Grand Junction, CO; Joyce Tobias, Emilie Gaborne-Dearing, and Patricia Gerlach, Parents' Association to Neutralize Drug and Alcohol Abuse (PANDAA), Annandale, VA; Eric A. Voth, M.D., International Drug Strategy Institute, Topeka, KS; Bonnie B. Wilford, George Washington University, Washington, DC.

An additional word of appreciation to Helen S. DuPont and Sarah Shiraki, Institute for Behavior and Health, Inc., Rockville, MD, for their help in preparing this manuscript.

Special thanks are due to Melissa Andrews and Judy Kramer, my editors, who skillfully and gently helped make this book reasonably literate and readable. Patricia R. Carson, my long-time associate and friend, helped me with my earlier book, *Getting Tough on Gateway Drugs*, and now has provided tremendously valuable assistance in every step of the creation of this book. Without her help, quite literally, there would be no book. My sincere thanks also to Ronald E. McMillen, Carol C. Nadelson, M.D., and Claire Reinburg from the American Psychiatric Press, Inc., for their encouragement and support for this project from start to finish. Martin Lynds, the Project Editor at the American Psychiatric Press, did an impressive job.

Finally, I thank my patients and their family members who have been my teachers about addiction for the past quarter century in my practice of psychiatry. I thank also the many participants in the conferences and workshops I have conducted whose questions and comments have helped me understand what is important and what is not.

Preface

This book focuses on the role of the brain in the disease of addiction. Without the brain's specific interactions with alcohol and other drugs, there can be no addiction. The book is also about how and why people become addicted and how addiction can be prevented and overcome.

This book is written for everyone who desires to learn about addiction to alcohol and other drugs. It is written for people who are concerned about possible addiction in themselves or in a loved one. It is written for students of all ages who want to know more about addiction. This book is for therapists, counselors, educators, and all people concerned about addiction in schools, in workplaces, on the highways, in religious communities, in the criminal justice system, and in health and human service programs. It is also written for people who are interested in learning about the policy issues in addiction, including drug testing and proposals to legalize the currently illegal drugs. Here you will find a unified and comprehensive picture of addiction that ranges from the highly personal to the societal. This book is for interested people in North America and in all parts of the world as the global community is forced to confront the increasing menace of addiction.

You can learn from addiction, whether you are confronting it in your own life, in your family, or in your community. Addiction is a powerful and unforgiving teacher. The word *addiction* is used to describe a group of problems sometimes called *drug addiction* or *alcoholism* and other times referred to more generally as *substance abuse* and *chemical dependence*. All these words describe addiction to brain-rewarding chemicals such as alcohol, marijuana, cocaine, and heroin.

Increasingly, *addiction* is used to describe many pleasure-producing or compulsive behaviors from jogging and television watching

Quick Read—2 Hours or Less

- Read Preface.
- Scan Chapter 1: Addiction to Alcohol and Other Drugs.
- Scan one other chapter of your choice.
- Check out the boxes in each chapter and a few case histories.
- Read Chapter 13: The Future of Addiction.

to gambling and eating disorders. Although these human behaviors share fundamental brain mechanisms with addiction to alcohol and other drugs, to lump such diverse behaviors together is to obscure the unique place of addiction to alcohol and other drugs in the history of human experience and to trivialize the desperate plight of addicted people and of those who care about them.

This is a long book. If you are pressed for time, there are ways to shrink it. Try this 2-hour visit: Read the Preface (which summarizes the book). Scan Chapter 1 (which sets out the context of addiction). Pick one other chapter to scan, then page through the text and read the introductions to the three main sections of the book. Look at the summary boxes, like the one above, and read one or two of the case histories found at the end of each chapter. Finally, settle down with Chapter 13, "The Future of Addiction." Once you have completed this quick trip, continue to read the book at a more leisurely pace as you explore the mysteries of addiction.

The Addicted Brain

Your exploration will take you into the target organ of addiction, the human brain, where addiction produces reward by stimulating the brain's pleasure centers. The brain repeats pleasurable experiences and avoids pain. Automatic brain mechanisms do not think behavior through to its conclusion, and they do not learn from delayed negative outcomes. As long as a behavior produces right-now pleasure, it is repeated, regardless of the long-term consequences. The "selfish brain," like a reckless infant, wants what it wants right now. Drugs turn on the brain's "more, now" button. The highs produced by addictive use of alcohol and other drugs cause serious, often persistent distortions of thinking and actions. They change the brain of the addicted person forever afterward. Addiction causes intoxication and impairment because addictive substances disrupt the functioning of the healthy brain. Addictive drugs harm other parts of the body as well, most often the lungs, heart, and liver. The use of addictive drugs promotes many infectious diseases, from bronchitis to AIDS. The body does not suffer alone. The values, behaviors, and relationships of people with addiction are also harmed by the addicted person's increasing need for destructive pleasure sensations.

Addiction Is Blind

Like people with secret, shameful lovers, addicted people hide their addictions from themselves and from everyone else who might separate them from their lovers. Their behavior continues despite the pain these abusive love affairs produce. Addiction turns love and pleasure, natural processes, into nightmares because of the inescapable long-term negative consequences of the addicted brain's chemical love affair.

Addiction Is Cruel and Unfair

Some people are more vulnerable than others for both biological and environmental reasons. Addiction can afflict anyone, but, similar to most other diseases, it is far more likely to strike some people than others. (This is explained further in the following section, "The Environmental Approach to Addiction.")

Addiction Is as Ancient as Language and as Modern as the Computer

The human brain has been what it is today for the past 100,000 years. It will not change in the next 100,000 years, if the human species lasts that long. In the language of the computer, the brain's hardware is fixed with the vulnerability to addiction hardwired into its structure. Because this vulnerability is inescapable, the best hope for solving the problem of addiction is in the software, the operating instructions that manage the brain's hardware. That means changing human culture to reduce the risk of addiction.

Ideas that influence the risk of addiction are, like addiction itself, not evenly distributed in communities. Some people and families live by antiaddiction ideas, whereas others do not. Some people have values that will not let them use alcohol and other drugs, whereas other people have values that permit or even encourage the use of alcohol and other drugs. Some people live in environments that are relatively free of exposure to alcohol and other drugs, whereas other people are heavily exposed to potentially addicting chemicals. This variability to the risk of addiction makes addiction a highly selective killer of the human spirit and often of the body. Although people can help each other with problems of addiction, the foundation of addiction, like love, is intensely personal. Addicted people and those who care about them have to bear direct responsibility for their own behaviors during every stage of the experience of addiction.

Addiction Is Mysterious and Irrational

Although understanding addiction cannot cure or even prevent it, understanding can change the brain's operating instructions when it comes to alcohol and other drugs. Some experts on addiction believe that people who are not themselves addicted can do little to influence the use of alcohol and other drugs by addicted people. I do not agree with this belief. People who are not addicted can "raise the bottoms" for addicted people. This means creating painful consequences that help addicted people recognize that their lives with alcohol and other drugs are unmanageable. Simply stating that drugs are unhealthy is not a strong enough measure to counter the seduction of addiction for millions of people, especially vulnerable teenagers. Much stronger approaches are needed to prevent and to cure the disease of addiction. Without consequences imposed by others, addicted people are helpless victims of their selfish brains, and most are doomed to fall ever lower, often dying of their illness.

Addictive Drugs Have Always Existed

Studying animal responses to drugs both in natural settings and in the laboratory increases our understanding of addiction. We can learn from the experiences of premodern cultures that used addictive drugs. However, addiction to alcohol and other drugs as we know it today in North America never occurred in any natural animal population or in any premodern human culture. Addiction as a community-wide problem has occurred only in the last one-third of the 20th century because of unique developments in the modern world. These developments include increases in the exposure to different drugs and increases in the potency of drugs and in the ways drugs are taken. Potentially disastrous changes in the values of society have occurred that permit addiction to flourish as never before.

The Environmental Approach to Addiction

The battle to save addicted people, a battle for their hearts and minds, is a battle only they themselves ultimately can wage and win. They are not likely to begin fighting to save themselves until those around them permit the addicts to feel the full force of their harmful choices. This change is called the environmental approach to addiction because it means changing the environment in which decisions to use intoxicating drugs are made every day by millions of individual people. Antiaddiction values increase the ability of individuals, families, and communities to prevent addiction and to intervene forcefully to solve the problems of addiction before they become lethal. Nonaddicted people permit addiction to flourish by ignoring the use of alcohol and other drugs around them and by excusing both the large and small problems that are caused by the use of intoxicating drugs.

Many people see addicts as tyrants because of the often brutal effects of their use of alcohol and other drugs. The inner experience of the addicted person is not that of a willful tyrant; it is the experience of a slave bound to the brain mechanisms of addiction. Addicted people are slaves to their own hooked, selfish brains. They are as much the victims of the disease of addiction as are their family members and others on whom addicts bring so much suffering.

You can take alcohol and other drugs away from addicted people a thousand times, and they will pick up their intoxicants again and again. Once addicts put down their alcohol and other drugs themselves, they can stay clean and sober. The pattern of denial and enabling behavior by those around addicts, often based on misguided compassion, is called *codependence*. The nonaddicted person is an unwitting accomplice in the addict's dependence. By overcoming codependence, nonaddicted people hasten the conversion of addiction into recovery.

Addictive Disease

Because addiction to alcohol and other drugs spreads like a contagious disease, the environmental strategy reduces the chance of infection. Addiction is a complex family and community disease, not merely a relatively simple matter of alcohol and other drugs in the user's brain. Recovery is a lifelong process both for addicts and for those who care about them. For most people, both addicted people and codependents, recovery means participation in one of the 12-step fellowships modeled on Alcoholics Anonymous, a modern miracle. Recovery from addiction means more than stopping alcohol and other drug use. Recovery means finding better ways to live as individuals, in families, and in communities.

Although addiction is more easily prevented than treated, even the most desperate addicts can usually regain control of

Addiction

- Is characterized by an unmanageable life and denial (dishonesty)
- Is a complex, lifelong, incurable family disease

Recovery

- Rests on a foundation of abstinence from alcohol and other drug use
- Means living a healthy, productive, and honest life

their lives through hard work. But this is not always the case. Active addiction is a serious disease that leads inevitably to awesome suffering and sometimes to death. Codependence and addiction, tragically often and sometimes despite the best and most sophisticated efforts, are neither prevented nor treated. The hopeful message of this book needs to be balanced with an unblinking and compassionate recognition of the many failures that continue to occur.

Moral and Medical Dimensions of Addiction

Addiction is a complex biopsychosocial disease, meaning that it has biological, psychological, and social roots. The focus of this book is on the role of the brain in the disease of addiction. The brain's specific interactions with alcohol and other drugs are crucial to addiction. There are psychological roots of addiction, including the tendency of many addicted people to be oriented toward the present rather than toward the future. There are also clear social roots to this disease, including the availability of alcohol and other addicting drugs as well as the social tolerance for their use. There is a deeply spiritual dimension to addiction, as dishonesty and self-centeredness play major roles in the addiction to alcohol and other drugs.

Any disease must have a biological basis, a generally predictable course, and it must not be simply a matter of willful behavior. Diabetes mellitus and pneumonia are diseases rooted in biology with predictable courses, as are asthma and rheumatoid arthritis. Addiction, too, fits this model of disease because addiction to alcohol and other drugs is far deeper and more serious than simple bad behaviors and wrong choices.

Addiction is not an ordinary biological illness, however. There is a moral dimension to addiction that is not present in asthma or pneumonia. Dishonesty is at the heart of addiction. Recovery, or getting well from addiction, has a spiritual dimension that is not present in diabetes mellitus or rheumatoid arthritis. Nevertheless, most serious diseases, like addiction, can have spiritual dimensions, as sufferers and their families often speak of the spiritual growth that occurs when they confront their diseases and learn to live with them.

Unlike a biological disease in which the medical doctor alone plays the leading role, many others make vital contributions to the prevention and treatment of addiction. It is no accident that religion and criminal law have their roles in addiction, as do families and mental health care providers. Unlike pneumonia, recovery from addiction is not a matter of seeing the doctor and taking some pills for a week or so. Addiction is a lifelong disease in which medical treatment plays a potentially important but limited role. One of the most painful lessons of addiction is the limits not only of human knowledge but of love and of efforts to cope with addiction. It is awesomely difficult to recognize and to live with the knowledge that we cannot change other people, even those we love the most. The seemingly unnatural process of dealing realistically with the addiction of a loved one is called *detaching with love*. It means doing what we can to help the addicted person and then honestly admitting our limits. For those addicts and codependents with a more spiritual orientation, recovery means turning one's life over to one's Higher Power and being willing to "let go and let God." Addiction, like other forms of human suffering, has within it the seeds of profound rebirth.

Hard as it is to overcome addiction, it is all the more important to prevent the problem before it takes hold of peoples' lives. There are three circles of prevention based on universal values that protect against addiction. All are rooted in spiritual or religious answers to the question, "How should I live my life?"

The first circle of prevention of addiction is to *live life with honesty,* meaning that when it comes to the use of alcohol and other drugs, we owe honesty to those who care for and about us. This includes our family members and others, from our teachers, employers, and co-workers to our health care professionals and friends. The second circle of prevention is to *live life with gratitude.* We are most likely to lead nonaddicted lives if we feel and express gratitude for the many gifts we have been given in life. The third circle of prevention is to *live life as part of a team,* as part of a community. This means we need to work honestly and gratefully with our families and our communities to fulfill our own potentials and to help others to fulfill theirs. Preventing addiction to alcohol and other drugs is an important part of achieving these potentials as individuals and as communities.

Hope for the Future

Although the use of alcohol and other drugs will grow throughout the world over the next decade, and no community, and few families, will be spared the pain of addiction, this is a book filled with hope for the future. Addiction will continue to grow because of the inescapable vulnerability of the human brain and because of the exposure of increasingly large segments of the world population to alcohol and other drugs in environments that permit and even encourage the use of addicting substances. Precisely because of the growing risk of addiction, it is reassuring to predict that learning from addiction will also grow in individuals, families, communities, and nations.

The cost of not learning from addiction is pain and suffering, which gets worse until the lessons are learned. Once understanding begins, once the rebirth of the spirit begins after the devastation of active addiction, there can be a glorious flowering of the individual human spirit and of the entire community. Rooted in an acceptance of shared vulnerability, of shared imperfection, and in a humble need for each other and for values that transcend immediate, personal pleasure, recovery is the gift of addiction. Recovery from addiction is never a finished project. Recovery is an endless and fragile unfolding that has a firm foundation in the great human traditions of knowledge and faith.

The Structure of This Book

This book is composed of 13 chapters that are divided into three sections. The Preface introduces the book. It is followed by a biographical sketch of the author. Section I sets the problem of addiction in historical context. Section II describes the biology of the brain, the major drugs of abuse, and the experience of addiction. Section III focuses on addiction to alcohol and other drugs, describing practical approaches to both prevention and treatment. These three sections taken together form one comprehensive, integrated picture of the fascinating and frequently deadly disease of addiction to alcohol and other drugs.

I do not want to glamorize the experience of addiction. Addiction is degrading and destructive. But the experience of addiction, whether understood from the inside or from the outside, can teach valuable lessons of wide application. People who are not addicted can learn about addiction without being addicted. People who are addicted need to do whatever is necessary to stop their use of alcohol and other drugs and to regain some measure of control over their unstable lives. Through knowledge they can find help, even though knowledge is helpless against the compulsion of addiction. Once in recovery, knowledge becomes an ally in living a good, addiction-free life.

Features of This Book

This book has several features to help the reader. Each section is introduced with a brief overview that anticipates the chapters to follow. Each chapter is introduced by a sentence that summarizes the message of the chapter. Starting on page 491 is a listing of the commonly abused drugs, what they look like, how they are used, and their popular names. This brief section, titled "Drug Facts," is a quick summary of the drugs of abuse and a review of the more extensive discussion of these drugs in the book. Boxes in the text highlight important ideas and make it easier for the reader to re-member and review major points in the book.

Each chapter ends with a few case histories drawn from my experience. The histories give the reader a chance to apply the ideas in this book to real-life experiences. To protect the identity of my patients, I have changed some facts in each case without changing the basic realities as I understood them when they were written. These case histories also explain how I think about addic-tion and why I came to my views. Finally, the book contains a listing of suggested readings for the further understanding of ad-diction and an index for readers interested in finding specific ref-erences in the text.

This is a book from the heart as well as from the head. I am re-porting my progress in 25 years of learning from addiction. The book gives readers a road map to pursue their own journeys of dis-covery and shares the excitement and optimism I have for this jour-ney. In it I express my sincere respect for those who are living the experience of addiction in their own lives and in the lives of those they love. I have included a diversity of experiences and a diversity of views of addiction that are held by many well-meaning and expe-rienced people.

This book is a time capsule into which I have put an important part of myself. It is my view of the problems of addiction to alco-hol and other drugs from the perspective of the mid-1990s. Like a personal message I am putting into a bottle to be cast off into life's unpredictable seas, it is for the present and the future. I do not know who will find the bottle or where. Most of the people who read the message will never meet me, and I will never meet them. And yet, through the intimate connection of these pages, we be-come close.

About the Author

Robert L. DuPont, M.D., is a practicing psychiatrist who has specialized in the prevention and treatment of addiction to alcohol and other drugs for more than two decades. He was the first director of the National Institute on Drug Abuse (NIDA), serving under Presidents Nixon, Ford, and Carter. Dr. DuPont was also the second director of the White House drug abuse prevention office, a position now known as the drug czar. He is president of a nonprofit research organization, the Institute for Behavior and Health, Inc., and vice president of Bensinger, DuPont, and Associates, Inc., a national consulting firm specializing in the problems of addiction in the workplace. A second major area of professional interest is anxiety disorders such as agoraphobia, panic disorder, and obsessive-compulsive disorder. He was the founding president of the Anxiety Disorders Association of America in 1980.

Dr. DuPont is clinical professor of psychiatry at Georgetown University School of Medicine in Washington, D.C. He received a bachelor's degree from Emory University in 1958 and an M.D. degree from the Harvard Medical School in 1963. He received postgraduate training in psychiatry from the Harvard Medical School and the National Institutes of Health from 1964 to 1968.

Dr. DuPont was born in Toledo, Ohio, and now lives with his wife, Helen, in Chevy Chase, Maryland. He is a fellow of the American Psychiatric Association.

That is the official version of my biography. Many readers want to know nothing more about the author, preferring to let the book speak for itself. Those of you who feel this way are invited to skip to Chapter 1. Other readers want to know the author more personally. For you I offer the following information about me and how I came to write this book. More personal information is important because some of this book can be misinterpreted as political or as reflecting odd personal affiliations. This additional biographical material is offered to answer the questions that may crop up as you read the book.

First, to answer the most obvious question, I am not related to the du Pont family that started the vast chemical company in Wilmington, Delaware. They spell their name with a small *d*, whereas my family, from Toledo, Ohio, uses a capital *D*. My mother taught seventh grade, and my father was a salesman. My father was Robert L. DuPont, so I grew up as "Bob, Jr." Since his death in 1986, I usually do not use "Jr." because with "M.D." tacked on, my name seemed to get lost in terminal abbreviations. For many years my father and my maternal grandfather worked together selling Buckeye Beer, an Ohio brand that vanished in a tidal wave of national brands three decades ago.

My extended family has had its full share of problems with drug abuse and alcoholism. Especially hard hit have been family members born after 1945. A few years ago, a much-loved cousin died as a result of his cocaine and alcohol use despite substantial family efforts to help him. One of my uncles was an early member of Alcoholics Anonymous, which was founded in Akron, Ohio, less than 1 year before my birth.

I am a psychiatrist, having graduated from the Harvard Medical School in 1963, a year after my original classmates. I took time off to travel overland through 20 countries in Africa on a personal adventure. My choice of Africa reflected both my growing up in the South during the breakup of legal segregation after 1954 and my enthusiasm about the emergence of many independent African nations after a century of colonial rule.

When I finished my postgraduate medical training and military service at Harvard and the National Institutes of Health, I went to work in 1968 for the District of Columbia government as a full-time psychiatrist in the Department of Corrections. Inspired by my two heroes, President John F. Kennedy and Dr. Martin Luther King, Jr., I chose public service for my life's work, hoping to use public health techniques to help solve the two serious social problems that most attracted me: crime and drug abuse.

Work in the Nation's Capital

When I went to work for the city government, Washington, D.C., had recently been declared the "crime capital of the nation," leading to an intense bipartisan concern about crime. With a handful of unemployed college students, we tested the urine of all the men admitted to the District of Columbia Jail in August 1969, finding that 45% were positive for recent heroin use. The epidemic of heroin addiction that we identified was a major cause of the city's crime wave. The first mayor of the nation's capital, Walter E. Washington, asked me in 1970 to develop a plan to respond to the problems of heroin and crime in Washington.

With a group of dedicated colleagues, I started the Narcotics Treatment Administration (NTA) as part of the District of Columbia government's Department of Human Resources. That was my introduction to high-profile public service, with frequent testimony before congressional committees and active involvement with the mayor's office and the White House, as well as the electronic and print media. Using the treatment approach to heroin addiction known as methadone maintenance, we helped to cut heroin overdose deaths in Washington from 65 in 1971 to 5 in 1973. The monthly rate of serious crime was cut approximately in half between late 1969 and mid-1973. Major crimes in Washington fell annually from about 80,000 in 1969, at the peak, to under 50,000 in 1973.

The Federal Phase

In June 1973, I moved from the city government to the federal government to head the White House Special Action Office for Drug Abuse Prevention as the nation's second drug czar. A few months later, I became simultaneously the first director of NIDA. Most people considered these jobs a promotion, but I regretted the loss of direct involvement with drug abuse treatment. For me there were as many losses as gains in the move up.

My government career came to an abrupt and involuntary end in 1978 when the new Secretary of Health, Education, and

Welfare decided he wanted his own directors in the three institutes dealing with mental health, alcohol abuse, and drug abuse. I remained active in the drug abuse field in a variety of private roles, including founding, with my wife, the Institute for Behavior and Health, Inc., a nonprofit research organization located just outside Washington, D.C.

My public health interests led me into the new area of workplace drug abuse prevention with the founding in 1982 of Bensinger, DuPont, and Associates, Inc. (BDA), with my friend Peter Bensinger, who had headed the U.S. Drug Enforcement Administration when I headed NIDA. BDA helps employers and employees team up for a drug-free work force. The workplace in the 1980s, like the criminal justice system in the 1960s and public drug abuse treatment in the 1970s, was the center of national drug abuse activity. Drug testing in the workplace became a lightning rod for public debate about drug abuse, as civil commitment had been in the 1960s and methadone treatment had been in the 1970s.

Experiences With Addiction and Anxiety

When I left government service in 1978, I became deeply involved in the study and treatment of the anxiety disorders. These are serious, often crippling illnesses that show up as self-destructive, repetitive behaviors. In addiction and anxiety disorders, strong feelings lead to behaviors that produce positive feelings in the short run and serious personal and family problems in the long run. Addicted people use alcohol and other drugs, whereas people with anxiety disorders commonly avoid experiences that upset them. The treatment of both anxiety disorders and addiction requires learning new ways of understanding the problems and new ways of handling them. Both groups of disorders often are lifelong, involving distortions of thinking and distortions of behaviors.

Successful treatment means living a full, normal life, not eliminating the disordered feelings. Automatic thoughts and behaviors, in the case of both addiction and anxiety disorders, lead ever deeper into harmful patterns of behavior. Recovery is possible but difficult for both addiction and anxiety disorders. For both, misunderstandings of the problems by family and physicians are major barriers to recovery.

For more than 25 years I have had my own practice of general psychiatry, the core of my professional identity. I have a deep respect for my patients and am grateful to them for permitting me to enter into their lives, in some cases briefly and in other cases for decades, as I have attempted to help them and their families. My patients have taught me far more about suffering and hope than any research studies, books, or lectures.

In 1970 I was certified in psychiatry by the American Board of Psychiatry and Neurology, and in 1989 I was certified in addiction medicine by the American Society of Addiction Medicine (ASAM). I value my ASAM membership especially highly because the organization is composed not only of psychiatrists, but of physicians from all specialties who share a professional, and often a deep personal, commitment to the process of recovering from addiction. In 1994 I was certified in Addiction Psychiatry.

Family and Political Life

On the personal side, my wife and I have been married for more than 30 years. We have lived in the same home for more than 25 years. In many ways, we have been raised by two wonderful daughters, who are now grown, married, and living independent lives. Elizabeth is a social worker; Caroline is a physician specializing in psychiatry.

With respect to my politics, I am a lifelong Democrat who has proudly served as White House drug czar under two Republican presidents, Richard Nixon and Gerald Ford. I was director of the National Institute on Drug Abuse under these presidents and under the Democratic president Jimmy Carter.

Although I am liberal in the sense that I am deeply committed to helping people who are suffering, I have developed a conviction that responsibility for each person's life is rooted in that person's choices and values. I now see that rights are linked to responsibilities and that many choices have serious consequences. I have learned to respect the ability of "victims" to help themselves, often by joining others in their efforts, especially when they use practical, experience-based solutions to their serious problems. When victims do this they become survivors and teachers with much to offer.

With respect to marijuana policy—the litmus test of drug politics over the last two decades—I was an enthusiastic supporter of decriminalization of marijuana from 1975 through 1978, a position I now deeply regret. Since that time I have taken strong positions opposing relaxation of legal prohibitions against any illicit drug use, including marijuana. I never supported the legalization of any illegal drug, including marijuana.

My Personal Exposure to Alcohol and Other Drugs

To round out this biographical section, I stopped drinking alcohol in 1978 because of my work with so many people who had alcohol and drug problems. I wanted to raise our daughters to know me as a nondrinker. I am not an alcoholic, although I did drink what I now consider to be too much in my late teens and early twenties. I have never been a member of a 12-step fellowship, such as Alcoholics Anonymous. However, based on my attendance at open meetings and on my work with addicted patients, I consider myself to be a friend of these programs. Both of our daughters have grown up to be like their mother, restrained social drinkers.

With respect to my personal drug use, I tried marijuana a few times while I was a medical student. This became an issue in 1974 when I was asked about my marijuana use in a national press conference. My admission of youthful pot use prompted a brief period of celebrity as talk shows across the country made much of this revelation about a "high official in Washington."

One of my frequent adversaries in public debate, a leader of the marijuana legalization movement, commented to me privately at that time that the press had asked me the wrong question. They should have asked me if I had ever gotten high on pot. The answer to that question would have been "no," since the material I inhaled deeply seemed, as was generally true in that era, to be weak. This pot advocate teased me about what would have happened if I had gotten high and liked the experience.

I never used any other illegal drug and never again used marijuana after the spring of 1962. As one of my drug-abusing patients, a 40-year-old attorney, said to me recently, "You were one of those straight arrows that I never associated with in school." Although I was not as straight as he thought, I did not use illegal drugs as a youth. This said more about the period in which I grew up than it did about my youthful values. No one I knew in the 1950s in Toledo, Denver, or Atlanta, where I grew up, used anything other than alcohol and tobacco.

In mid-1994 I spoke in San Diego, California, at the first-ever meeting of the nation's nine White House drug chiefs. A few weeks later, a patient told me that while she was cooking dinner for her family she heard my voice coming from her living room. She poked her head into the room and saw me on the network evening news show, saying one sentence. Here it is as reported by this patient: "The secret weapon in the war on drugs is the 12-step programs." I thought about that experience for a long time. The modern media knit us together in a remarkably intimate and personal community, a new global village. There was my 15 seconds of fame—and I would have missed it if that patient had not brought it to my attention. But the more I thought about it, the better I felt about that experience. If I were going to pick one single sentence to summarize my 25 years of work with the problem of addiction, I would not have changed even one word. Here, if nowhere else, television news did a great job of both condensing and communicating accurately.

So there you have it, a short summary of my life in the world of alcohol and other drugs and of the major forces that shaped my views. With that out of the way, we can get down to the serious business at hand—learning from addiction.

Section I

Thinking About Addiction

In this section, I introduce the major themes of the book, beginning in Chapter 1 with an overview of addiction. This chapter describes many of the conflicts that make the understanding of addiction difficult. Chapter 2 deals with the history of drug abuse. Chapter 3 looks at the worldwide picture of addiction today.

Some readers will find this introductory material, especially the chapter on the history of addiction, of great interest, whereas others will want to skip to Section II, in which we explore the workings of the addicted brain.

Chapter 1

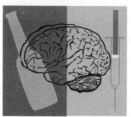

Addiction to Alcohol and Other Drugs

*In this chapter, I discuss many of the controversies
surrounding addiction and explore the roles of biology,
culture, diversity of risk, and values in addiction to alcohol
and other drugs.*

ore than 30 million Americans alive today will experience

addiction to alcohol and other drugs in their lifetimes. Sixteen

percent of Americans, or about one in six, will themselves suffer

from addiction to alcohol and other drugs. Four out of 10 American families are directly affected by addiction. One in every four deaths in the United States today is caused by the use of alcohol, tobacco, and illicit drugs. Addiction is the number one preventable health problem in the United States and throughout the developed nations of the world.

Illegal drug use, excluding alcohol abuse, now costs the nation approximately $67 billion per year. This is an involuntary addiction tax paid by everyone, which comes to about $270 each year for every man, woman, and child in the United States. No part of the nation and few extended families have been spared the deadly, overwhelming, and confusing grip of addiction. Every major social and community institution has been hit by addiction, although many continue to ignore it, treating it as if it were an uncommon problem experienced only by a small number of troubled people. Addiction affects people of all ages and in all walks of life and is an equal opportunity destroyer that places particularly severe burdens on disadvantaged groups and young people.

The Role of Biology

Drugs are chemicals that trick the brain's natural control system. Through this control system, located at the base of the brain in the center of the head, people experience feelings of pleasure and pain. The brain is designed to manage fundamental behaviors such as aggression, feeding, and reproduction.

Communities have learned techniques for managing anger, fear, eating, and sex over thousands of years of cultural evolution, much as individuals learn during their lifetimes how to manage their own feelings. Human behavior is managed by relatively changeable and adaptive cultures even though the brain mechanisms that underlie behavior remain fixed and powerful. Individuals manage behaviors based on their values, experiences, and knowledge. When it comes to behaviors rooted in strong feelings, the family and the community are the principal locations of the hard-won, culturally based behavior management expertise.

When the brain's reward or pleasure centers are stimulated, the brain sends out powerful signals to repeat the pleasure-producing behaviors. With respect to aggression, fear, feeding, and sexuality, the brain is selfish. It simply wants what it wants right now. The brain knows only "more" and "no more" or, in computer language, "on" and "off." The brain directs the person to relieve distress and to promote pleasure. When it comes to many natural pleasures, the brain has built-in protections. It has powerful feedback systems to say "enough" when it comes to natural behaviors, including aggression, feeding, and sex.

These basic, primitive mechanisms, which are common to animals, do not consciously consider future consequences or values. These are genetically determined shut-off systems. Automatic brain mechanisms do not consider other people's feelings or needs or know the importance of delayed gratification. That is why I call this basic pleasure/pain organ *the selfish brain*.

Addiction begins when the brain comes into contact with an addicting substance such as alcohol or other drugs. Without this interaction of the reinforcing chemical and the pleasure centers, there is no addiction. That is why prevention techniques that discourage exposure to addicting drugs, outside rigidly controlled traditional medical and religious contexts, are powerful and effective in preventing addiction to the extent that they can prevent the use of alcohol and other drugs.

People who have never been addicted find the behavior of addicts to be incomprehensible: "Why would anyone pay thousands of dollars every year for a powder to sniff up their noses?" "Why would anyone want to get drunk?" "I cannot imagine wanting to put a needle in my veins five or six times a day, every day of my life." "It is such an awful feeling to have your brain poisoned by alcohol or drugs!"

Compare the drug addict's behavior with the experience of sex. If you take out the pleasurable sensations, it is unbelievable that anyone (or any animal) would engage in such a seemingly bizarre and irrational behavior as sexual intercourse. The explanation for seemingly irrational behaviors (such as drug use and sexual behaviors) can be found in the feelings, including sensations and emotions. The feelings experienced by addicts are intense and compelling. In the end, these feelings, misleadingly called "pleasure" because that word is too mild, take over the whole self

---

How Addiction Works

- Drug addicts fall in love with the good feelings that alcohol and other drugs produce.
- They mistakenly think they can use alcohol and other drugs without harm to themselves or others.
- Addicts stop alcohol and other drug use only when something so painful happens to them as a result of their drug use that they conclude they must stop their use to survive. (This is called "hitting bottom.")

---

of addicts. For this reason, members of Alcoholics Anonymous (AA) call addiction "cunning, baffling, and powerful."

Learning From Animals

Why do otherwise intelligent addicted people repeatedly do things that cause themselves and those they love such pain? The biologically rooted power of addiction can be seen in experiments with laboratory rats that had electrodes placed in the pleasure centers of their brains. When their pleasure centers were stimulated, these rats repeated behaviors controlled by the researchers to get more brain stimulation.

Rats find even mild electric shocks to their feet to be extremely unpleasant. Laboratory rats were placed in a cage that had an electric grid down the middle, which the rats had to cross to get various rewards. The electric shocks to their feet were not strong enough to cause them harm, but they were sufficiently unpleasant to the rats so that they would not cross the electrified grid to have sex or to get food or water. They would die of dehydration and starvation rather than cross that grid. But the rats walked across that electrified grid as if it were not there to get the pleasure centers of their brains stimulated directly.

In other experiments, research scientists gave monkeys cocaine only when the monkeys worked hard enough. The monkeys were also given sex, food, and water as alternative rewards after long periods of deprivation. The researchers measured how much work the monkeys would do to get each of these rewards, all of which produced stimulation of the brain's pleasure centers. The monkeys worked harder for the cocaine than for any other stimulation, including for sex or food. In fact, when the monkeys were permitted to use as much cocaine as they wanted, they used the drug until they died of convulsions and heart failure.

These laboratory experiments with animals make clear that stimulation of the brain's pleasure centers by drugs or by direct electrical stimulation is far more rewarding and controlling of behavior than natural stimulation of these same brain mechanisms, even by food or sex. This same picture is repeated thousands of times a day by addicted humans who put alcohol and other drug use first in their lives. This comparison is not meant to minimize the power of food and sex in controlling human or animal behavior. Clearly, the stimulations of food and sex are often as powerful and sometimes even overwhelming. However, as powerful as food and sex are as stimulators of behavior, they pale in comparison to the potency of addiction to alcohol and other drugs.

With few exceptions, such as a bird occasionally eating a fermented fruit, animals in natural states do not encounter or use alcohol or other drugs. Some students of addiction have discovered that animals in the wild occasionally do encounter plants that have drug effects and that the animals do become intoxicated when they eat these plants. Three conclusions can be reached about these observations of alcohol and drug use in natural populations of animals. First, these natural exposures to intoxicants are distinctly unusual experiences. Second, the experience of intoxication is dangerous for animals (as it is for humans), often leading to the animals becoming victims of predators that they would have avoided if sober. Third, no wild animals have daily access to intoxicating drugs as do human addicts.

A recent experiment shed light on why it is useful to plants to produce intoxicating chemicals. Scientists noticed that the coca bush in South America, containing small concentrations of cocaine, was seldom subject to insect predators, as were other nearby plants. Even young coca leaves rarely show evidence of insect damage. To understand how this worked, botanists sprayed cocaine-containing dust on tender tomato plants before releasing insects known to love tomato plants. After a few minutes of exposure to the plants dusted with cocaine, the insects acted bizarrely and stopped eating, dying within a day or two. The scientists found that the cocaine boosted the effects of the neurotransmitter octopamine in the insects' nerves, hopelessly scrambling their messages. As we see in Chapter 5, cocaine works in human brains by affecting the neurotransmitters norepinephrine and dopamine. This experiment left little doubt as to why wild animals, including insects, generally do not eat coca leaves.

In contrast to animals, it is harder to understand addictive behavior in humans because there are so many complex factors shaping a person's actions. Each act of an individual has many possible explanations. Some observers of human addiction have explained it as a form of slow-motion suicide; as an expression of anger toward spouses or parents; as an economic, racial, political, or ethnic protest; or as an expression of a deep psychological disorder.

The fundamental explanation for addiction is far more simple, as seen in laboratory experiments with addicting drugs. Human addicts use alcohol and other drugs for the same reasons that laboratory animals do, for the brain-reward effects of the substance use. In these animal experiments it is unmistakably clear that the experience of using addicting drugs is more powerful than other rewards and that this behavior does not depend on complex psychological, historical, or economic factors. Addiction to alcohol and other drugs is a universal biological process run amok.

Diversity of Risk of Addiction

Over thousands of years, human beings in all cultures have developed reasonably effective guidelines to deal with pleasure and pain and with associated behaviors. Cultures define when and how aggression, fear, feeding, sexuality, and many more complex but equally important feelings are expressed by human beings living in communities that share many values. Human communities permit and even encourage aggressive behavior in contests and sports, often imposing elaborate rules on the most intensely aggressive behaviors. Exposure to and mastery of fear is managed by common rituals. Culturally based rules are established in human societies for feeding and sexual activity. No human community could exist with unbridled expression of these powerful feelings by each individual community member. The survival of the community itself, as well as the survival of the individuals in the community, depends on the adherence to the community's social contracts governing aggression, fear, feeding, and sex.

Within any community there is a high level of diversity, both cultural and biological. Some people are tall and some are short; some are thin and some are fat; some are quick-tempered and others are calm. Like physical characteristics, habitual behaviors also show great diversity in human (and animal) populations. Some people instinctively court danger and excitement, whereas others strenuously avoid both. Similarly, some people conform to community norms governing pleasure-driven behavior and some do not. Nature has seen to it that biological and cultural diversity is maintained because diverse populations are best able to adapt to changing environments and to exploit changing opportunities. Diversity is as important for adaptations of populations when it comes to values as it is in such physical characteristics as height and weight.

Cultural and characterological diversity means that within any community there are widely different personal values managing the experiences of aggression, fear, feeding, sexuality, and the use of addictive drugs. This diversity translates into diverse risk of addiction to alcohol and other drugs. Some personal values are relatively protective of individuals and the community, and others are less protective when it comes to addiction. Every day we see the consequences of this inescapable diversity of risk of addiction in families, communities, and nations. In a family with three or four children, it is common to see that one child has a drug or alcohol problem whereas the others do not. Similarly, some segments of communities have larger problems with addiction, and others have smaller problems. Age and gender have major effects on the rates of problem behaviors related to the brain, including addiction.

Values and Drug Use in Traditional Cultures

Humans living in relatively homogeneous traditional cultures in all parts of the world did not encounter drugs and had no way of personally controlling alcohol or other drug intoxication, with rare exceptions (see Chapter 2, in which we explore the history of addiction). For these reasons, the brain's hardware in both animals and humans developed without protections from drug-caused risks. Only human beings have developed the capacity to use intoxicating drugs repeatedly, and only in recent times have people learned how to use purified, highly potent brain-stimulating drugs.

Drugs defy the brain's built-in control mechanisms for dangerous behaviors like fear of predators and fear of heights that have developed over millions of years. Traditional values acted to limit exposure to alcohol and drugs as they were experienced in premodern cultures. Traditional values of human societies prohibited the use of intoxicating drugs outside medical and religious ceremonies. Drug use, in all stable premodern cultures, was controlled not by the individual drug user but by the medical or religious leaders of the community.

Early human communities were relatively small, isolated, and culturally homogeneous. The diversity of these communities was limited as the community shared values about the management of aggression, fear, sex, and feeding. Traditional cultures permitted relatively few different roles and little personal choice of behavior. The shared values within these cultures served to inhibit the use of alcohol and other drugs to the extent that there was any exposure to these substances.

Values and Drug Use in Modern Cultures

Since about 1970, a new challenge regarding addiction has emerged as large segments of human populations, especially youth in North America, have been exposed to dozens of addicting drugs, in settings that permit or even encourage drug use. Modern values emphasizing the importance of personal control of one's life and simultaneous increases in the social tolerance for alternative lifestyles have provided a fertile ground for the contemporary drug abuse epidemic. These values have been prominent in North America, especially for youth, in the last three decades.

Modern countries with great cultural diversity have large numbers of people living in complex and interdependent communities. Not only are these modern communities much more diverse with respect to values that determine the risk of addiction, but individuals in them function with far more anonymity and independence than was true in premodern cultures.

Modern communities have many advantages over earlier village-based cultures, permitting, for example, a wider range of lifestyles and greater personal control by each person over his or her own life. However, one result of the new, more diverse, larger, and more anonymous communities is an increased risk of addiction. A major challenge for the future in all parts of the world is to fit effective prevention and treatment for addiction into this modern value system. The challenge is great, as the conflict of values found throughout this book demonstrates.

People are not equally vulnerable to addiction to alcohol and other drugs. Genetic and environmental factors, in particular, heighten vulnerability. People whose parents and other family members are addicts and people who live in environments relatively accepting of alcohol and other drug use are at increased risk of addiction. People who are oriented to immediate reward rather than to delayed gratification, people who are self-centered rather than concerned with the needs of others, people who lack religious values, and people who are impulsive and extroverted are all more at risk of addiction. Relative risk of addiction is affected by many other factors as well, including availability of intoxicating substances, gender, age, drug substance, and route of administration of the drug. For example, addictions to alcohol and other drugs are more common among males and among people ages 15 to 30.

Genetic predisposition to alcoholism and drug addiction is real, important, and increasingly the subject of scientific study. Animal experiments show that some strains of dogs, rats, and other mammals are more likely to drink alcohol than are other strains of the same species. Such heightened vulnerability in animal strains is passed to offspring without regard to life experiences. Careful studies of humans show that the risk of becoming alcoholic is about 15% for the daughters of alcoholics and about 30% for the sons of alcoholics.

Both nonhuman animal studies and human studies show that genetics is not the only factor influencing addiction. The majority of the children of alcoholics or drug addicts do not themselves become alcoholics or drug addicts. Many addicted people do not have parents or siblings who were addicted to alcohol or other drugs. To the extent that addiction is inherited, what is passed on from one generation to the next is the vulnerability to addiction, not the addiction itself. The development of addiction to alcohol and other drugs requires many other forces, including those that are environmental and experiential.

The substance being used affects the risk of addiction. Cocaine and heroin are far more likely to produce addiction than is alcohol, given the same level of use, genetic vulnerability, and social tolerance. Routes of administration are also important in establishing relative risk of addiction. Cocaine is more addictive when smoked or injected than when it is sniffed up the nose. While these factors, and many others, govern relative risk of addiction, all people are vulnerable to addiction. Diversity of risk does not mean that some people are vulnerable to addiction and others are not, but it does mean that some people are relatively more vulnerable than others.

To the extent that people, especially young people, are exposed to nonmedical drug use in relatively permissive environments, the drug problem worsens. Exposure to drugs in settings that are controlled by medical or religious traditions is less risky in terms of addiction. For example, the use of Ritalin (methylphenidate hydrochloride), a stimulant used to treat hyperactivity in children, generally does not lead to addiction. Neither does drinking communion wine in church.

Factors That Raise the Risk of Addiction

Personal

- Having parents or siblings who are addicted to alcohol and other drugs
- Being impulsive and oriented to the present rather than being oriented to delayed gratification
- Having personal values that focus on one's own feelings of pleasure rather than on concern for others, and having no religious or spiritual values
- Being between 12 and 30 years old

Environmental

- Being exposed frequently to alcohol and other addicting drugs
- Living in a family that tolerates drug use and/or excessive alcohol use
- Having a community that tolerates addiction and its consequences

On the other hand, even medical or religious exposure to potentially intoxicating substances does pose some risk of addiction for people who are biologically predisposed to addiction, especially for people who also have access to these substances for self-administration. Self-controlled exposure to alcohol and other drugs, especially by teenagers who are in peer groups without the presence of responsible adults, poses an especially high risk of addiction.

The human experience of getting high is more than the biology of the brain interacting with the drug. The setting in which the drug is taken influences the drug-taking experience. Similarly, the *set* of a drug user (a term used for the expectation that the drug user has when the drug use takes place) affects the drug experience as well.

The most high-risk picture for the development of addiction is not difficult to define. When a person with a high genetic vulnerability (e.g., parents or siblings who are addicted to alcohol and other drugs) and impulsive character traits is exposed to a highly addictive drug taken by a high-risk route of administration (smoking or injecting) in a setting that promotes drug intoxication with an expectation of getting good feelings (the setting and the set), the gun of addiction is loaded, it is aimed at the center of the brain, and the trigger is pulled. Sometimes addiction does not require all these high-risk factors to be present, but surprisingly often, especially in the most malignant cases of addiction, they are all lined up in just this way.

Blaming the Victim

As a physician, I am committed to the disease concept of addiction. How can a sick person be held responsible for the behavior that defines the disease? Is not this blaming the victim? We do not hold people with diabetes responsible for their disease, so how can a compassionate person hold alcoholics or other drug addicts responsible for their behaviors?

Although addicted people, like other sick people, are not responsible for their diseases, they are fully responsible for their behaviors during every stage of the disease. The addicted person's disease is a heightened vulnerability to drug-induced rewarding experiences, which has both biological and environmental elements. Addicts' behaviors, including their use of alcohol and other drugs, is entirely their responsibility, as is their use, or nonuse, of various recovery options, including the totally free and widely available 12-step programs, such as Alcoholics Anonymous and Narcotics Anonymous.

People with diabetes are not responsible for their disease, but they are responsible for their behaviors, including how they manage their illness. Adherence to proper diet and wise use of medicines are the personal responsibility of each diabetic person. The consequences of failure to care for the disease of diabetes mellitus are often added suffering and early death. The same is true for addiction. Denial and wishful thinking are deadly threats to people with all kinds of diseases. Addicted people, like people with diabetes, are responsible for the management of their diseases. As with addiction, genetics and behavior before the onset of the disease sometimes play important parts in the experience of the disease of diabetes.

Even in the absence of any therapeutic options, addicted people are responsible for all of their behaviors, including all of their use of alcohol and drugs. Addicted people are not likely to get well unless they are held responsible for their behaviors. Prevention efforts are inhibited by excusing alcoholics and drug addicts, because excusing removes socially imposed consequences for using alcohol and other drugs. Tough antidrug sanctions are a principal reason people choose not to use alcohol and other drugs or to stop using these substances. These sanctions are vital to successful prevention and treatment of addiction.

Think about how a family or a society could function if it excused alcoholics for their behaviors when drunk, behaviors that include inflicting injury on others and even committing murder, rape, and robbery. Is a drunk driver personally and legally responsible for killing an innocent pedestrian? In making the determination of personal responsibility for the drunk driving accident, does it matter whether the driver was an active alcoholic or merely a social drinker who had one too many drinks before taking the wheel? Think what a society would be like if it excused heroin addicts of their responsibility for robbing to get money to pay for their drugs, or cocaine addicts of their responsibility for selling drugs to others. It does not take deep thought to realize that excuses for addicts' behaviors make society unlivable and do immeasurable harm to addicts themselves.

This excusing is yet another well-meaning but misguided form of enabling. It is a principal environmental cause of addiction. Enabling is the ultimate form of both irresponsibility and uncaring. When it comes to addiction, enabling is love turned cruel, not by its intentions but by its inescapable consequences. Holding addicts responsible for all of their behaviors, for their personal

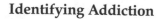

Identifying Addiction

- Addiction means powerlessness over use of alcohol and other drugs.
- Addiction both feeds on and causes self-centeredness, sensitivity to criticism, and dishonesty.
- Addicts are not responsible for their disease *but* they are responsible for what they do about their disease, at all stages of their disease.
- Abstinence is necessary for recovery from addiction, *but* abstinence is not sufficient for recovery.
- Getting well has a spiritual dimension that overcomes self-centeredness and dishonesty.
- Recovery most often comes from participation in the lifelong fellowship of a 12-step program, such as Alcoholics Anonymous and Narcotics Anonymous.
- Addiction is a family disease—family members commonly suffer from codependence, and they are part of the progression of the disease. They usually need to participate in the process of recovery, using Al-Anon, Co-Dependents Anonymous, Adult Children of Alcoholics, and other 12-step programs.

choices, is not blaming or controlling, it is simply being realistic. Recognition of the disease concept of addiction does not label addicts as "victims" who are not responsible for their actions; it offers both addicts and nonaddicted people a practical, understandable way to approach the otherwise bizarre and confusing behaviors of addicts and those around them.

Many well-meaning people today seek to soften the edges in dealing with addicted people by avoiding words such as *alcoholic, addict,* and *character defects.* They find such blunt, old words prejudicial and offensive. It is no accident that the 12-step programs and the best addiction treatment programs use these tough, clear words. By not using them, denial of the deadly disease of addiction is promoted. By using these words without apology or ambiguity, denial is stripped away and the real work of getting well from addiction can go forward. I use strong words in this book because I have learned to use them from my work with recovering people. Recovering people use these words to describe themselves and their behaviors when they were actively addicted to alcohol and other drugs. The addicted people in recovery with whom I have worked have characterized their lives when they were using alcohol and other drugs as filled with deceit and dishonesty when it came to the chemicals they loved to use. None has objected to my characterization of addiction, which focuses on two central features: 1) the loss of control over the use of alcohol and other drugs and 2) dishonesty.

Putting Limits on Personal Choice of Dangerous Behaviors

John Stuart Mill, the 19th-century English philosopher who helped to extend many of the modern values of individualism and the pursuit of pleasure that were embodied in the U.S. Constitution and the Bill of Rights, said that one person's right to swing his arm ends when it hits another person's nose. Drug users' arms frequently hit other people's noses. Most frequently, they hit the noses of people in their families and with whom they attend school or work.

A society does not have to wait until a nose is broken to define the limits of arm swinging. The highway is a dangerous common space in society, so, for all drivers, many limits on personal choice of specific behaviors are defined and legally enforced. Examples include wearing seat belts, obeying speed limits, and not driving after drinking. Being required to go through a metal detector before boarding an airplane or entering some public buildings is an example of a universal search that is growing more common in modern life in all parts of the world. The loss of privacy and personal choice of behaviors in each instance is balanced against urgent public benefits. This same balancing of privacy and social responsibilities underlies the limits society increasingly imposes on the use of alcohol and other drugs.

Although many people can drive without seat belts for their lifetimes without any harm to themselves or anyone else, most Americans are now required by law to wear seat belts whether they want to or not. A few complain about the infringement of their rights because of this legal requirement for all people who drive or who are passengers in automobiles. How can this government-ordered infringement on personal choice of some behaviors be justified when we do not hurt anyone but ourselves by our decision not to wear seat belts?

One answer is that the costs of my injury, if I do not wear a seat belt, are borne by you, and by everyone else, through lost productivity and increased health care costs. In this example, my choice of behavior—not wearing a seat belt—has harmful effects that extend beyond my own welfare to the welfare of others. Another more fundamental answer is that people in communities care about each others' welfare.

Therefore, in many situations, society reasonably defines the limits to which I swing my arm, whether I like it or not. I must wear a seat belt when driving or risk criminal punishments. Society arrived at this decision collectively and democratically. The seat belt laws are new. Thirty years ago, cars were not equipped with seat belts. Today it is not legal to drive a car without wearing a seat belt. This example makes clear that legal boundaries to arm swinging change over time. It also demonstrates an increasing use of laws to promote health-related behaviors and the lack of any political or constitutional barrier to these laws in many situations for all citizens. As more is known about the probable outcome of various behaviors, and as social attitudes toward particular behaviors change, the limits of arm swinging change.

Arm swinging is not only limited by laws. There are many other formal and informal social mechanisms to limit it. Laws and social customs reinforce each other. As the social tolerance for cigarette smoking diminishes, the laws against smoking get tougher. As the laws get tougher, the informal social customs about tobacco smoking become more intolerant. The limits on

cigarette smoking today are being redefined rapidly and profoundly in North America, not only by new laws about where
smoking is not permitted, but by informal and widely shared
social customs. A few years ago a smoker could ask, to be polite,
"Do you mind if I smoke?" The answer was invariably, "No, not
at all." Today that is so seldom the answer to this question in the
United States that few smokers even ask it. They either do not
smoke around nonsmokers, or they receive hostile social responses.

Like the laws regarding speed limits or seat belts, the laws
governing drug use are set politically, with the majority defining
the limits of tolerable arm swinging when it comes to drug use. In
the United States, the actions of the majority are limited by the
Constitution. Not only are the swinging arms of drug abusers limited by laws, but the highest law of the land also limits the ability
of the majority to restrict arm swinging generally, including the
arm swinging of drug abusers.

The balance of these conflicting values—the growing North
American intolerance of nonmedical drug use versus the limits
on the majority's power to legislate controls on personal behaviors—is now being hammered out. Those who want to swing
their arms farther by legalizing the currently illegal drugs, such
as marijuana and cocaine, must make their cases in the political
processes, to their fellow citizens, and ultimately to the legisla-
tive and executive branches of government at the local, state,
and national levels.

Those who want further restrictions on arm swinging, greater
restrictions on the use of alcohol and other drugs, must enter this
same political marketplace. Both are subject to review by courts.
This conflict of values is seen most clearly in the workplace and
other drug testing cases now coming to court. Over time, these
cases will define what employers, schools, and others can do legally to prevent drug use. The same legal struggle can be seen in
the question of roadblocks to identify drunk drivers. Can police
stop drivers randomly to check for alcohol intoxication, or must
they wait to see particular drivers weave or otherwise drive dangerously before pulling them over and giving them a sobriety
check?

Conservatives and Liberals on Drug Use

It is common, but wrong, to perceive conservatives as being hard-line on drugs and liberals as being soft on drugs. The same misleading attitude equates conservatives with a law enforcement approach to drug problems and liberals as favoring treatment. Consider the central political argument of legalization versus prohibition for drugs such as marijuana and cocaine. Some staunch conservatives are in favor of ever-tougher prohibition of such drugs as marijuana and cocaine, thus supporting the stereotype that conservatives take a hard line on drugs. However, many political liberals see drug abuse as slavery and take strong antidrug positions. Some committed conservatives favor legalization of currently illegal drugs on libertarian grounds, as they oppose virtually all government interference with people's personal lives. Some deeply liberal people also favor the legalization of drugs, also out of antiauthority and proindividual choice values.

What are the conservative and liberal views on drinking and driving or on the use of cigarettes? My point in bringing up politics is that many people mistakenly believe that the social response to drug use has been politicized in a partisan sense. This has not been true in North America, at least during the last three decades of the current drug abuse epidemic.

There are, however, fundamental political but essentially nonpartisan issues of values at the heart of the problem of addiction to alcohol and other drugs. No one, regardless of personal politics, can be comfortable with the conflicts that are created by addiction and by societal responses to it. Recognizing and intervening in someone else's use of alcohol and other drugs involve a loss of privacy, whether that process occurs in a family or in a community. Under what circumstances is the use of alcohol and other drugs safeguarded by legal and informal protections of privacy? These are legally unsettled and personally unsettling questions in all parts of the world today.

People who drive too fast, crash their cars, and die choose to drive fast. They do not choose to die. Most people who drive fast do not crash and die. Most people who do not wear seat belts never have an automobile injury (or die in a car crash). Yet to protect a minority of drivers who will crash or be killed or injured in an automobile, all drivers must obey the speed laws and use seat belts.

Drug users do not choose addiction, illness, or death. They simply choose to use alcohol and other drugs to get high. They believe they can do it safely. Some do; many do not. Is the use of currently illegal drugs a more protected privacy right than speeding or driving without a seat belt? Are drug-using behaviors less likely to harm others? Is it less intrusive to ask all air travelers to go through a metal detector than to ask all employees, or all school children, to take a drug test? I do not think so, but some people, equally well informed and sincere, disagree with me.

Drug Tests: Denial Busters

Drug tests use modern biotechnology to identify the recent use of alcohol and other drugs. Without drug tests, dishonesty hides addictive substance use and retards the forces in families and communities that would otherwise act to end illicit drug use. The modern drug test involves a comprehensive system designed to be safe and reliable. The first step is a screening test. If the screening test is negative, meaning that no controlled substance use is identified by the laboratory, that ends the testing on that sample. If the screening test is positive for the use of alcohol and/or other drugs, the second step is a confirming test on the same sample.

In the workplace, where concern is high over prescribed medicine use possibly being confused with nonmedical drug use, a third step is added. This safety check is the Medical Review Officer (MRO), a physician who is an expert in drug abuse. The MRO reviews the laboratory results and, if necessary, verifies the appropriate use of medicine before the test results are reported to the employer. Laboratory tests that are positive as a result of the appropriate use of prescribed medicines are reported to the employer as negative drug tests. The employer is not informed of the medicine use in such cases because the drug test result is returned to the employer as showing no drug use. The standard in the workplace today is to retain positive drug test samples for retest for at least a year if the employee disputes a positive drug test result.

This comprehensive drug test system does not produce false positives. This means that people can be drug tested with confidence that they will not be falsely accused of having taken a drug nonmedically. It also means that medical treatments will not be the basis for a positive drug test.

Urine drug tests generally are positive for 1 to 3 days after the most recent use of a drug. Hair tests for abused drugs identify drug use within 90 days before testing. Hair tests use the same reliable system as urine tests to detect drug use. Because of its longer window of detection, hair testing offers major advantages over urine tests, especially in preemployment testing and other scheduled drug tests. Hair testing is more resistant to cheating than is urine testing, and hair testing permits both collection of a second sample in disputed results and quantification of drug use intensity, permitting the distinction between a person who uses a drug only occasionally from one who uses it intensively.

Drugs are dream busters. Drugs rob individuals, families, and communities of their hopes, making life unmanageable for everyone. Drug tests are denial busters, exposing the nonmedical drug user to the healing forces of family and community life and giving good, immediate reasons to say "no" to illicit drug use. Because marijuana and cocaine are the most commonly used illicit drugs, they are also the drugs most often found on positive results of workplace drug tests. One of my patients called workplace drug tests "cocaine Antabuse" because drug tests give cocaine users a good reason not to use the drug, just as Antabuse, the medicine that makes people feel sick if they drink, gives alcoholics a good reason not to use alcohol.

The Social Contract for Drug Use

The "social contract for drug use," which forms the foundation of my thinking about drug policies, can be simply stated: *Self-controlled use, as well as sale, of addictive drugs is prohibited.* Examples of prohibited drugs are marijuana, cocaine, and heroin. However, when one of these drugs, or drugs similar to them, is judged by formal scientific standards to be useful in the treatment of an illness or disease other than addiction, then its use as part of medical treatment, controlled by an informed prescribing physician, is legal. Medical use of a potentially addicting medicine is not self-controlled. The use of medicines is not characterized by deceit and dishonesty.

Many dangerous and potentially abused drugs have legitimate medical uses. Morphine is a good example. Use of potentially addicting drugs within controlled medical practice is encouraged for medical purposes, as long as the illness being treated is not addiction itself and as long as the supply of the potentially addicting medicine is restricted to the patient and does not find its way into other hands. This social contract for drug use is relatively simple and easily understood. It is a solid foundation for successful personal, family, and community drug policy.

In North America, the nonmedical use of alcohol and tobacco is legally accepted for adults. In fact, until recently most people did not consider these substances to be drugs. Even today international treaties do not consider them to be drugs. On the other hand, the use of these two substances by youth is legally prohibited, unlike all other consumer products, underlining just how different alcohol and tobacco are from chocolate and blue jeans. Many formal and informal rules of conduct restrict the use of alcohol and tobacco by adults, making clear that these are not routine commercial products.

Proposals to Modify the Social Contract

Some people would like to change this basic social contract for drug use, for example, by making alcohol and tobacco use by adults illegal or by making marijuana and cocaine use legal for adults. Others would like to make some currently illegal drugs legal as medicines (e.g., marijuana and heroin). These modifications in the social contract deserve wide public debate. My view is that we should strengthen the prohibition of all currently illegal drugs and increase the social and legal restrictions on the use of alcohol and tobacco, especially for youth under the age of 21.

Whatever a person's views of these laws, unless the American drug laws are changed, every citizen has a duty to respect the contract on drug use as it is now in force.

Political disagreement with this social contract for drug use is inescapable and, to some extent, even desirable. Nevertheless, the use of illegal drugs outside the current contract is both unhealthy and criminal. The full force of informal and legal punishments needs to be imposed on people who violate this basic social contract. The contract is embodied today in the laws throughout North America at all levels of local, state, provincial, and national governments. It is internationally imposed on virtually all of the nations in the world through formal treaty obligations.

Some media coverage of conflicts of drug abuse obscures this fundamental, easily understood, and important social contract. This book attempts to explain and support the contract. I consider this contract to be a matter of prudent public health policy as well as a matter of civic duty. This social contract, in its original form, was the basis of the antidrug or clean-living social movement in the United States in the first two decades of this century.

Cigarette smoking, as described in Chapter 6, is a special case in the social contract because nicotine is not a controlled substance, and its use does not cause mental impairment as do all other addicting drugs. Nevertheless, the issue of cigarette smoking is relevant to the prevention and treatment of addictions to alcohol and other drugs.

Good Fun and Bad Fun

Pleasure or fun is inherently good. Some ways to have fun produce long-term good, and some ways do not. It is easy to think of addiction as a disease of pleasure and to conclude that pleasure itself is the problem. Active addicts, not wanting to stop use of alcohol and other drugs, often assume that my message is, "Just live an unhappy life and you can prevent addiction." This simple-sounding view is just plain wrong. Being against fun is a losing strategy for either the prevention or the treatment of addiction.

The goal of a good life is not to avoid pleasure; it is to maximize pleasure for yourself and others over time by fitting your fun into a full, productive life that reflects your highest values. Drugs and alcohol produce pleasure when taken, but the inevitable outcome of the pursuit of chemical pleasure is pain and suffering for the addict and for the people around the addict. Take a look at any addict and you will see a miserable person. Talk with the family of an addict and you will learn about the depths to which pain can penetrate the soul of an entire family.

There are two criteria for pleasure-producing behaviors to be good behaviors. First, fun must be able to persist over the long term. The excessive use of alcohol, as well as any use of an illicit drug, simply does not meet this requirement for healthy long-term pleasure. The selfish brain automatically seeks short-term reward. Culture and humane values insist that, socially and morally, acceptable pleasure be subjected to the long-term test. Where does today's pleasure lead? What is the likely outcome of a person's particular choices about addicting substances, not just for the person who uses the alcohol and/or other drugs but for the entire society? Active addicts do not think this way. They are dominated by the immediate reward of alcohol and other drug use, and they are blinded by denial to the negative long-term consequences of their substance use. Pleasure now, pain later—the pattern seen in addiction—is not a good deal for anyone.

The second, equally important requirement for healthy pleasure is that fun is good only if it can be openly and honestly shared with others who care about the person having the fun. One inescapable element of addiction is dishonesty. A person cannot be an addict without being a liar—to oneself, to those who care, and to the community at large. Behaviors that do not fit with the honesty principle simply are not good ways to have fun. The hardware of the selfish brain does not contain an honesty test. That test comes from cultural values. When it comes to pleasure-producing behaviors, including the possible use of alcohol and other drugs, consider the following question: "Can I tell those who care about me the truth, the whole truth, and nothing but the truth about what I do to have fun, whether it is basketball, sex, or my alcohol and/or drug use?"

Remember as you are reading this book that pleasure is generally good, not bad. These same two questions can be usefully asked about all feeling-driven behaviors, including feeding, sex, and aggression, as well as about the use of addictive chemicals: 1) Will the behavior produce pleasure over the long term?; and 2) Can the behavior be honestly and openly shared with those who care about you? In summary, there are two simple universal tests that can be applied to any pleasurable activity to separate good pleasure from bad pleasure: the long-term test and the honesty test.

Fun must have the capacity for persistence over time, and it must be socially acceptable. With those conditions, which are easily understood and not too hard for most people to follow, addiction generally can be avoided, and, if it occurs, it usually can be cured. Trying to skimp on those two requirements for fun enables addiction to grow.

Attendance at 12-Step Meetings

Before concluding this introduction to the story of addiction, I have a suggestion for every reader. As you will see in later sections of this book, I strongly support the 12-step programs based on, and including, Alcoholics Anonymous. These programs, the subject of Chapter 11, are called 12-step programs because they all use the same 12 steps to recovery that form the foundation of the program of Alcoholics Anonymous. At the meetings of any 12-step program, you can see for yourself the disease of addiction and the process of recovery. These meetings are easily accessible to virtually everyone in North America today. If you have a friend who goes to 12-step meetings, ask if you can go along for a few meetings. If you do not know anyone who goes to meetings, look in your directory for the telephone number for one of these three programs: Alcoholics Anonymous, Narcotics Anonymous, or Al-Anon. The first program deals with personal alcohol use, the second deals with personal use of other drugs, and the third deals with the experience of living in a family dominated by alcohol.

Ask for the time and location of an "open meeting" that is convenient for you. An open meeting is one that is open to people who either think they may have a problem with addiction or simply want to learn more about the subject. Plan to arrive at the meeting about 15 minutes early. Introduce yourself by your first name and say that you are new to the program and that you have come to learn. Ask if you can sit next to someone who can help you understand what is happening. At the meeting, soak up what is going on. If you are called on, although you are not likely to be, simply give your first name and say that you are not comfortable speaking or that you are there to learn. If, however, you want to enter right into the meeting, just say whatever you want.

Meetings usually last 1 hour. They are free, although a small donation may be accepted to help pay for space and coffee. One dollar is a common contribution at meetings, but a donation is not required. When the 12-step meeting is over, stick around and talk with the members of the fellowship. Ask them whatever you would like to ask about the nature of addiction and about what it takes to get well. The people at these meetings are the experts on addiction. They are writing the really big book on addiction, every day of their lives. If my book does nothing more than to let you know that these 12-step meetings are the place to find in-depth, real-life expertise about addiction, and if the book helps you find your way to meetings, I will be fully satisfied in my efforts.

Case Histories

These are the first of many case histories in this book. They give an idea of the range of experiences of people who are addicted.

Lonnie

Lonnie's parents first came to me for help when he was a senior in high school. Rebellious and willful, Lonnie was a more-or-less everyday pot smoker who did not do his homework and who had moved his girlfriend into his bedroom at home for his convenience. Neither his parents nor his successful, traditional older brother had ever had an alcohol or drug problem. Lonnie's parents were perplexed about what they could do about his outrageous behavior. When I suggested that they consider insisting that he stop using pot, with a regular urine test to enforce the standard, that they ask his girlfriend to leave, and that they require a modest level of school work if he was to use the family car, they were not surprised but neither were they interested in those ideas, which they considered conventional. His mother said, "We want to let him run his own life because that's the way we have raised our children. It's way too late for us to be prudish parents or narcotics cops."

I spoke with Lonnie, who told me that he liked smoking pot and having his girlfriend in his bedroom. He saw no reason to stop either practice. He had held a job as a salesman at a local waterbed store for over 2 years. His smooth-talking salesmanship and steady work performance got him a promotion to manager of the store. He told me he had big ideas for his future, including making a lot of money. He was never arrested or expelled from school.

When I had not seen any of Lonnie's family for several years, I called to find out what had become of him. His mother told me he had almost stopped using pot: "He still uses it every now and then to show that he has not knuckled under to the establishment." He had become a good, but uneven student in college, focusing on business. He had developed his own business selling rugs to incoming students for their dorm rooms, which proved quite lucrative. He was proud that he contributed significantly to his own college costs. Lonnie was looking forward to starting a business of his own when he graduated.

Lisa

Lisa's mother came to me when Lisa was a freshman in high school and had been expelled for the use of alcohol and marijuana. Lisa's mother, who became a single parent after her husband, an active alcoholic, had left her several years before, was worried about her daughter. I met with Lisa several times, but she had no interest in working with me because she wanted to do things her way, including continuing to use alcohol and drugs. Lisa was intelligent and attractive. When she liked her teachers and her courses, she got good grades. She wanted to be with her friends, not with her mother, with me, or with any other adult. She rejected my suggestion that she go to Narcotics

Anonymous meetings. She correctly saw that I was not friendly to her continued use of alcohol and drugs so, as she asked, "Why would I want to work with you?"

I lost track of this family until I got a call from Lisa's mother nearly 10 years later. She called to say that Lisa had been killed in a car accident the week before. She added that Lisa had dropped out of high school and had been in many addiction treatment programs in our area over the last few years, but each time she left she relapsed to drug use. Lisa had attended many Narcotics Anonymous meetings and would stop drug use for a while when she went to meetings. However, she repeatedly stopped going to 12-step meetings and quickly relapsed to drug use, progressing over the years from marijuana to cocaine and ultimately to intravenous heroin use. Over the telephone, her mother and I shared some sad moments and feelings of regret at our inability to help Lisa help herself.

These stories make several important points. Lonnie used a lot of drugs as a teenager and showed many other characteristics of a drug addict, but he did not have any relatives who were addicted, his family environment was unusually permissive to his drug use, and he had shown from an early age both a strong desire to succeed in life and the ability to stick over time with projects he cared about. He held one job for several years, and he had a good relationship with his parents. Lonnie was a *pseudoaddict* as described in Chapter 7.

By contrast, Lisa had a strong genetic history of addiction, and she lacked the positive outcome predictors that Lonnie had. Her experience, including using several addiction treatment programs without long-term success, is unfortunately common. Also common was the tragic ending of her disease with her death at a young age.

This concludes our overview of addiction. I hope it has whetted your appetite for what follows. In the next two chapters we explore the history of drug abuse and the current global drug scene.

Chapter 2

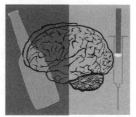

A World History of Drug Abuse

*In this chapter, I trace the history of drug use and abuse
from early traditional cultures to the modern "global
village" that the world has become.*

*I*n traditional or premodern cultures, drugs were not used
for pleasure in environments of high availability. There was not the
high tolerance for drug use and the low community control over
socially disapproved behaviors that exist today in North America.

Drug Use in Traditional Cultures

Premodern cultures, like wild animals, generally lacked the ability to supply drugs or to purify the few addicting drugs to which they had access. Even more important, traditional societies had high levels of social control over the behaviors of each and every community member. Everyone in the small village knew everyone else. If anyone's behavior, because of drug use or for any other reason, was a problem to the community, then direct, personal, and effective action was taken to stop the offending behavior. If the offending behavior did not stop, that individual was cast out of the community.

Traditional communities lacked not only today's diversity but also most of the opportunities for deceit and anonymity that characterize modern life. Lying was harder when everyone knew each other's every step throughout the day. In primitive cultures, being banished from the community meant certain death at the hands of hostile neighboring human communities or in the mouths of hungry carnivores. A solitary human being was utterly helpless.

Native Americans used tobacco without suffering from emphysema or lung cancer because their tobacco use prior to contact with Europeans was limited to ceremonial occasions. Native Americans did not have cigarettes or matches, which maximize the addicting properties of tobacco. Native Americans used tobacco in clay pipes smoked in community rituals. They did not use tobacco in manufactured cigarettes for personally controlled pleasure. The easily understood contrast between socially controlled traditional Native American ceremonial smoking of tobacco pipes and personally controlled modern cigarette smoking captures the distinction between premodern nonaddictive drug use and modern addictive drug use. Traditional societies treated the low-potency drugs to which they had access as medicines or limited their use to religious rituals. The drug use that did occur in these societies was low dose, infrequent, socially managed, and benign in terms of both physical health and behavior.

The use of opium and marijuana in Asia in premodern times was similar to Native Americans' use of tobacco. Opium and mari-

Drug Use in Traditional Societies

- Exposure was limited to single potentially addictive substances.
- Use of addicting drugs was restricted to low-potency materials.
- Routes of administration were relatively low risk.
- Use of addictive substances was controlled by religion and medicine.
- There was tight social control over all personal behavior.
- There were few drug-related problems.

juana use was limited to an oral route of administration, in teas, which were used infrequently as medicines. Traditional cultures limited the use of addicting drugs to low-potency materials by routes of administration that were relatively easy to control. The use of alcohol and other drugs generally was limited in village-based societies to one drug in each culture.

Early Alcohol Use

Alcohol use was a more complex story before the modern era because as soon as beer and wine could be produced, which in many cultures was thousands of years ago, drug-caused intoxication was possible. For traditional cultures, the relatively high cost of alcohol kept its use uncommon, as did formal and informal social controls over alcohol use. Even when premodern societies permitted sufficient use of alcohol or another drug to produce intoxication, that use was infrequent and managed in families and communities. An equilibrium was reached and maintained in traditional cultures over the use of alcohol and other drugs. Stable communities in premodern times were the

Golden Age for alcohol and drug use.

One of the sad paradoxes of the world experience with alcohol and drug abuse is that traditional cultures, which had achieved a safe equilibrium with the use of alcohol and other drugs as long as they remained isolated, have proven to be tragically vulnerable to modern alcohol and drug problems. To see Native Americans suffer from the use of alcohol, inhalants, and other modern drugs, and even cigarettes, or to see similar suffering among Australian aborigines, is to face the painful reality that traditional cultures are not prepared to withstand exposure to modern drugs and to tolerant values governing drug-taking behaviors.

Although some premodern societies lived comfortably with single reinforcing substances of low potency, they cannot cope as well as, let alone better than, modern cultures with the wide availability of many high-potency drugs. Today, the exposure of aboriginal cultures to tobacco, alcohol, and other drugs is producing a devastation comparable to the spread of infectious disease to which the previously isolated communities lacked immunity in the age of discovery. Traditional communities lack the limited but valuable cultural immunity that modern industrial societies are painfully and imperfectly developing to the use of alcohol and other drugs. Communities today that continue to function as they have for hundreds or even thousands of years are even harder hit by this modern biobehavioral plague than are economically developed communities.

Drug Use in the Era of a Shrinking Globe

The second phase of world drug history, the beginning of the world's first major drug problems, was linked to the first distillation of alcohol and the dissemination of drug habits as part of the age of discovery. These two events were accelerated by the move to cities and the breakdown of the village culture which took place in the preindustrial world between about 1400 and 1900. This was a period of transition from traditional cultures to the modern era.

When Europeans discovered the techniques for heating beer and wine so that the alcohol vaporized before the water did, and

Premodern Drug Use

- More than one drug, but low potency and lower-risk route of administration
- Use mostly limited to large port cities
- Use limited by cost and availability, except for alcohol in some areas
- Serious problems limited to alcohol and to a few nations
- Escalating but mostly low-level problems of addiction

then condensing the alcohol to separate it from the water, thereby raising the concentration of alcohol, the world experience with alcohol changed forever. Rum was made from sugar cane, vodka from potatoes, whiskey from grains, and brandy from wine, all using simple distillation. The social impact of cheap distilled alcohol on an increasingly urban Europe was sudden and devastating. The original European discovery of distillation was by the alchemists in the Middle Ages, who apparently learned these techniques from Muslim chemists. This discovery of alcohol distillation spread throughout Europe in the 1500s and 1600s. The "penny drunk" became the scourge of England and Holland and throughout much of Europe.

When distilled liquor was later exported into the growing global trade, the new threat of more potent distilled alcohol became global. Rum, for example, was part of the triangle trade of slaves from Africa to the Caribbean, molasses from the Caribbean to New England and Europe, and surplus rum from North America and Europe to Africa. Farmers from the American Midwest who grew grains in the early 1800s found that they could ship their crops more economically across the Appalachian Mountains or down the Mississippi River as whiskey than as corn or wheat. Taxes on whiskey were an important part of the new nation's political and economic history, reflecting the relative importance of alcohol in the cash economy.

Alcohol and the Emergence of Protestantism

It is no accident that in western Europe the Protestant Reformation was closely tied to antialcohol sentiments. The Reformation took place in the 15th and 16th centuries in northern Europe. When distillation of alcohol became widespread in these countries, the newly emerging urban communities in particular suffered intensely from an epidemic of drunkenness. Communities in northern and western Europe were the breeding ground for religious reformation partly because of the social disruption caused by the escalating use of distilled spirits.

It seems likely that Muhammad's prohibition against the use of alcohol, which has served to protect hundreds of millions of Muslims from alcoholism, was related to the early discoveries of distillation of alcohol, in that the discovery by the Muslim chemists did not lead to profound social harm. This harm was prevalent in Europe, however, where there was no similar religiously based prohibition against alcohol use to protect the population before the Reformation.

Tobacco, which had been used for ceremonial purposes by Native Americans, rapidly entered international trade as the habit of smoking became global within two decades of the initial European exploration of the Western Hemisphere. The properties of tobacco leading to physical dependence were observed quickly, leading to initial hostile societal reactions to tobacco use throughout the world.

Alcohol and Other Drug Use Since 1900

Although alcohol problems were severe in some cultures from about 1600 on, there were relatively few problems with other drugs until the last 100 years or so. Tobacco use spread rapidly after 1492, often despite strong legal and religious opposition. There also was a modest spread of the use of some traditional drugs outside old boundaries as a result of new travel and trade. Opium smoking came into wider use in Asia. Coca leaf chewing, which had been previously limited to traditional, religious uses in the Andes, was exploited by the Spanish conquerors in a cynical manipulation of native culture. The Spanish found that they could pay the tin miners in Bolivia with coca leaves, which was less costly than giving them food, housing, clothing, or money. Older medical and religious restrictions on drug use began to break down for marijuana, coca, and opium throughout the world after the 16th century, as colonialism disrupted traditional cultures.

Taking drugs by smoking was developed by Native Americans to use tobacco. This route of administration of drugs spread after 1492 to all parts of the world as a new and far more dangerous form of drug taking, especially for marijuana and opium. For the first time, opium was smoked widely only after the introduction of tobacco smoking. This change in the route of administration dramatically increased the addictive potential of opium. A similar change occurred for marijuana. When smoking replaced oral use of marijuana, the scene changed as cannabis intoxication and addiction became commonplace for the first time.

Modernization of Drug Abuse

Cannabis and opium use in the Middle East had a similar history as that in North America, with most traditional use of cannabis being restricted to oral, primarily medicinal use until about 200 years ago, when European imperialism introduced the smoking route of administration, thus disrupting the traditional social controls over the use of both cannabis and opium. Only then did the abuse of these two drugs become serious social and health problems in the Middle East. As the societies of the Middle East reasserted control over their own people at the end of the colonial era, the use of cannabis, opium, and other drugs, sometimes mistakenly called "traditional," was increasingly stigmatized and restricted to the lowest social classes.

No nationalist, anti-imperialist government anywhere in the world has ever promoted open use of opium, cannabis, or other so-called traditional drugs. In fact, the opposite has been the pattern with the breakup of colonial rule all over the world. China's hostility to the use of opiates is a good example of this universal experience. More recently Iran followed suit with a tough crackdown on drug use after the Islamic Revolution in 1979. These experiences also show that the extinction of drug habits is difficult as drug use evolves toward modern styles of addiction. Iran and China continue to have serious problems with increasingly modern and global patterns of addiction.

Coca leaf chewing did not spread worldwide at the start of the modern era, as did opium and marijuana smoking, because the coca leaves lost much of their psychoactive potential shortly after picking. When the early explorers brought coca leaves back home, the Europeans were unable to understand what the South American natives found so attractive about chewing the leaves of the coca bush. Because cocaine was available only when the leaves were fresh, coca chewing did not spread far from the Andes Mountains where the coca bushes grew.

Despite these disturbing changes as alcohol and drug use became global, especially in large port cities, the worldwide drug scene 150 years ago was, by contemporary standards, not menacing. It bore a striking resemblance to the earlier era of traditional cultures. The relatively high costs of the drugs, their difficult transportation, and their low potency led to a relatively low availability of drugs and low rates of drug-caused problems throughout the world. Most people in all parts of the world continued to have little access to alcohol and other addicting drugs until the 20th century.

During the 19th century, the industrial and scientific revolutions gave rise to modern drug problems as large, impersonal cities sprang up. The new urban environment that promoted more personal choice and less restriction, in contrast to earlier traditional behaviors and values, gave rise to the modern drug problem. The pursuit of personal happiness, often regardless of consequences from the community, increasingly became a goal for modern individuals. For millions of people, pleasure included the self-controlled use of alcohol and other drugs.

In the middle of the 19th century, cocaine was identified by chemists as the psychoactive component of coca leaves. It was purified so that users far from the slopes of the Andes Mountains had access to this powerful drug in a chemically pure form for the first time. Pure morphine and codeine were first extracted from the sap of the opium poppy at about the same time. Also, the hypodermic needle was invented in the middle of the 19th century, thereby allowing addicting drugs to be injected directly under the skin. As with the introduction of smoking, this was a new route of administration of drugs with threatening implications for the entire world. Old drugs became more addictive as a result of purification and of changes in their routes of administration. Smoking and injecting drugs of abuse posed serious new risks.

Drugs and Deviant Behavior: The Shift to Modern Values

In the 20th century, the ages-old short list of abused drugs was expanded to a virtually infinite number as modern chemists found molecule after molecule that produced reward in the brain's pleasure centers. Alcohol was joined by the barbiturates, cocaine by the amphetamines and methamphetamine, and cannabis by a whole new array of synthetic hallucinogenic drugs from LSD (lysergic acid diethylamide) to PCP (phencyclidine) and MDMA (methylenedioxymethamphetamine). The range of synthetic and semisynthetic narcotics was equally long, from methadone and hydromorphone (Dilaudid) to meperidine and heroin.

Modern travel and communication ensured that drugs were available in every part of the world. Drugs were, like spices 500 years earlier, the perfect product for the growing global trade because of their high value and light weight. The rise in the wealth of individuals in all parts of the world as a result of the Industrial Revolution meant that more people had the purchasing power to buy drugs in the rapidly expanding world market of alcohol and other drugs. The 20th-century trade in cigarettes, a global megabusiness, bears little resemblance to the tobacco trade of 100 or 200 years ago in terms of size and health consequences. Similar changes have taken place in the alcohol trade and, more recently and more dramatically,

Modern Drug Use

- Widespread exposure to multiple addictive substances
- Highly potent preparations and routes of administration
- Greater anonymity and behavioral diversity
- Impersonal communities tolerant of deviance
- Low social controls over individual behavior
- Reliance on the criminal justice system to reduce drug supply and drug use
- High rates of use and severe drug-related problems

in the illegal global drug trade of marijuana, cocaine, and heroin.

Of even greater menace than the explosive growth in the number, potency, and availability of drugs is the shift of values that has taken place in all parts of the world during the last 200 years. In earlier and simpler times, most people were born, lived, and died in close-knit, relatively stable, and isolated communities. They shared values and shunned outsiders who sought entrance to their communities. Modern police and criminal justice systems are far less effective in controlling deviant behavior than was the old-fashioned village social system. In the 20th century, the relatively inefficient and expensive modern social control systems became the major guardians of the public health when it came to nonmedical drug use.

Individuals and communities benefited in may ways from the changes from traditional to modern life. New creative forces and new ways of living and relating became possible. These changes, which continue to accelerate throughout the world, were both eagerly sought and widely practiced. Initially, the centers of greatest change were large port cities, the hubs of modern transportation and communication to which people flocked from nearby farms and distant lands. The newcomers in the rapidly growing ports brought their own values and behaviors, many of which were constructive. Along with these beneficial changes came drug-using patterns from all parts of the world.

In more recent years, universities have attracted people seeking changes in their lives, the way large ports did in the past. Universities are centers of communication and travel. They have also become the birthing grounds for new values, including new patterns of drug use in all parts of the world.

A Short History of Drug Abuse in the United States

The United States, a nation of immigrants from all parts of the globe, has had more than its share of addiction problems since its earliest years as a nation. The alcohol consumption per person in the country peaked in the early years of the 19th century and then slowly declined over the next 100 years with the progressive impact of antialcohol sentiment. These temperance values were widely incorporated into American religious sects, such as the Church of Jesus Christ of Latter-Day Saints (Mormons) and the Seventh-Day Adventists, as well as into many other American Protestant denominations. In 1849, Maine became the first state to establish the statewide prohibition of the sale and use of alcohol. Over the next 70 years, prohibition spread state by state until national prohibition was established in 1919.

At the end of 19th century, the United States experienced a massive patent medicine epidemic when cocaine was an ingredient of Coca-Cola (hence the name "Coke"), and heroin was sold to any willing buyer as a soothing syrup for babies and even as a treatment for alcoholism. In response to the terrifying effects of the widespread availability of addicting drugs, cocaine and heroin were restricted to use under a physician's prescription in the modern social contract for drug abuse discussed in Chapter 1. This response was embodied in the Pure Food and Drug Act of 1906 and the Harrison Narcotics Act of 1914. The widespread and destructive use of these drugs in the United States led to their prohibition. Prohibition did not lead to the widespread use of drugs, from alcohol and cocaine to heroin. Prohibition was a response to a serious problem, it was not the cause of the drug problem.

Prohibition of alcohol and other drugs led to dramatic reductions in the use of the prohibited substances and to reduced social costs and negative health effects. The cocaine and heroin problems that had been severe at the turn of the century all but disappeared in the United States by the mid-1920s. Alcohol problems fell sharply during the 14 years of national prohibition, which ended with the repeal of Prohibition in 1933. After the start of Prohibition, cirrhosis deaths, a good independent measure of excessive use of alcohol, declined from 29.5 per 100,000 people in 1911 to 10.7 per 100,000 people in 1929 (a fall of 64%). Admissions to state mental hospitals for alcoholic psychosis declined from 10.1 per 100,000 in 1919 to 4.7 per 100,000 in 1928 (a fall of 53%). Arrests for public drunkenness and disorderly conduct declined 50% between 1916 and 1922. Violent crime, often attributed to the prohibition of alcohol by opponents of Prohibition, did not rise in the United States during the years of Prohibition. Homicides did not rise during that period, despite the wide publicity given to gangs during this period, such as the Al Capone gang in Chicago.

There were negative consequences of the prohibition of alcohol and other drugs, however. Because the use of these substances was now criminal, Prohibition created the economic incentive for an illegal alcohol supply system, one that was rapidly taken over by organized crime. As health care costs fell under Prohibition, criminal justice costs rose, although the net effect of Prohibition was to lower the overall costs of the substances that were prohibited. (See Chapter 12 for a discussion of this issue today.)

With the repeal of Prohibition in 1933, the per person consumption of alcohol began to rise slowly but steadily in the United States from less than 1 gallon per person per year during Prohibition (when illegal alcohol or "moonshine" was used by some people) to about 2 gallons per person in 1945 at the end of World War II. Average annual alcohol consumption then rose further to a peak of slightly less than 3 gallons per person in 1981, a point still below the per person annual alcohol consumption in the United States 150 years earlier. After 1981 the long-term fall in per capita consumption, which had characterized the nation's experience with alcohol for the 100 years before Prohibition's repeal, was resumed, albeit at a slow rate of decline.

The American experience with illicit drugs was changed forever in the 1960s when the use of marijuana, cocaine, heroin, and other drugs became increasingly common. In 1962, before the modern drug epidemic, 4 million Americans had used an illicit drug at any time in their lives. Thirty years later that figure had risen nearly 20-fold to 77 million, or slightly more than one-third of all Americans over the age of 12. Those figures reflect the dramatic rise of the American drug epidemic, the world's first modern drug epidemic.

The most important development in the history of the American response to the problem of addiction to alcohol and other drugs occurred on June 10, 1935, when Alcoholics Anonymous (AA) was started in Akron, Ohio. In later years, the United States developed the largest national response in world history to the problems of addiction, including research, prevention, and treatment programs. Chapter 3 reviews the current status of this epidemic in the United States and in other parts of the world.

The United States: The First Modern Nation

From the 19th century to the present, the United States has stood at the forefront of worldwide changes in the use of alcohol and other drugs. This is not because America is inherently any more decadent or corrupt than any other nation. The United States was, quite simply, the world's first modern society, and it remains the world leader in new behaviors from fashion and music to drugs. North American society intensely values personal liberty, including relative freedom of individual choice from both legal and religious restriction. This was also the first society to experience widespread use of the products of modern science, including the new drugs that science has produced. David Musto, the distinguished historian of drug abuse, has called modern drug addiction "the American disease."

The Global Sweep of Addiction

Most of the drugs causing addiction today are not native to the United States. The brains of North Americans are not uniquely vulnerable to the effects of alcohol or other drugs. What has made North America the center of drug abuse in the world is that North America has been the breeding ground for the modern free-wheeling, consumer culture. The North American experience with drugs offers important lessons to the world. The problems that were once thought to be uniquely North American are increasingly understood to be global and, at root, human problems.

Although addiction is uniquely human and modern, the brain's vulnerability to alcohol and other drugs is nothing new. Problems have been caused by the use of alcohol and other drugs for thousands of years in all parts of the world. What is modern is not the interaction of the brain with specific addicting chemicals. What is new in the world is the exposure of large segments of communities to a wide range of addicting substances by high-risk routes of administration in environments that permit and even encourage the use of these chemicals.

People in all parts of the world share the drug problem today. Alcohol and other drug abuse will not disappear from any society or culture in the foreseeable future. Addiction is as inevitable as poverty and crime and as inescapable as sickness and death. Addiction is deeply rooted in biology and in human societies, especially modern consumer-oriented democracies.

Saying that the problems of drug abuse are inescapable does not mean that passivity is the best approach for individuals, families, or countries. As with other inescapable human problems, the rates at which drug problems occur are highly influenced by many factors over which individuals, families, and communities have substantial control. Because the personal anguish and social costs suffered as a result of drug problems are so great, it is vitally important that drug problems be understood clearly and that balanced, practical policies be found to minimize these life-and-death problems. Antiaddiction policies must be consistent with the resources and values of each family, each community, and each nation. There is also a major international dimension to policies that prevent addiction. Alcohol and other drug problems underline the increasingly interdependent relationships of all people on the planet. Today, both drug-using behaviors and drug supply are global, not national.

As travel and communication have shrunk the globe, it has become more common to speak of the world as a global village. That remarkable image offers hope of dealing more effectively with the universal human problems of addiction to alcohol and other drugs. It will not be easy to recapture the village ways of overseeing and managing individual behavior, especially given the new values that promote diversity and individuality. However, there is hope that addiction, like many other shared problems from terrorism to infectious diseases, will catalyze a new sense of community rooted in values that permit many of the positive features of modern life to flourish while eliminating the use of addictive drugs from the list of condoned personal choices. For this change to succeed it will be necessary for these values to go much deeper than laws and regulations. Feeling close to one another and linked by a shared vulnerability to addiction, it may become possible to have this sort of village experience even in the modern world. Such a change of values will require a new emphasis on the interests of maintaining healthy communities within which individuals can flourish.

Case Histories

Sandra and Peter are two sides of the coin of contemporary teenage drug use, one of which is a benign and even valuable personal exploration of biology and modern values, the other a malignant fall to the lower depths of human misery. Even Peter, however, eventually found a measure of redemption and stability, although at a terribly high and continuing price.

Sandra

Sandra was a scholarship student at a local private high school. She was sent to me by the school's guidance counselor because of her drug use and poor academic performance. The school was reluctant to suspend her because she was bright, and her educational alternatives in the public schools were not good. She was an activist who espoused the causes of life's downtrodden. She spent several sessions arguing with me about her use of marijuana and cocaine, which she felt were "no worse than alcohol," and which were, more importantly in her view, traditional drugs used for thousands of years in what are now called developing countries. Our work did not last long because she did not find my views attractive or helpful.

Several years later, Sandra called me to say she had stopped drug use. She had finished high school and was in college, majoring in anthropology. I asked her what her current views were on drugs. She said, "It took me a long time, but I now realize that the sort of drug use that went on in traditional cultures cannot be sustained in communities like mine. I now see that modern drug use is chemical slavery. To achieve my goals in life, and they are many and largely unchanged from when I saw you, I will need to have a clear mind as well as a strong body. Drugs robbed me of both." Sandra generously thanked me for helping her find her own road to these personal discoveries.

Peter

A few minutes before the start of an Alcoholics Anonymous meeting, Laura, the head of the meeting (called the secretary), asked Peter to lead the meeting and to pick out a topic for general discussion. Peter quickly took one last trip to the restroom, checked to see that his pack of cigarettes was full, and went to the front of the room of 30 people to sit in the big chair reserved for the leader of the meeting.

He opened with, "Hi, I'm Peter. I'm an alcoholic and a drug addict." He was greeted in unison with "Hi, Peter." He began his story, in the typical 12-step format. First he told about his life as an addict, then about his transformation to a new life, and finally about how he now copes with his new life. He said he did this to "authenticate" himself to the group.

Peter's father was a fireman and his mother was a secretary. He said, "I grew up a few miles from here, having a regular middle-class life, except that I was small for my age and I had real bad learning disabilities. When everyone else learned to read, I didn't, so everyone made fun of me. I just gave up on school.

I became a wise ass who made fun of the teachers and beat up on the other kids. I never went out for sports, and I never did my homework. My older brother turned me on to drugs when I was 10 and he was 14. He started me off on pills and alcohol, but by 14 I was into cocaine and acid. By the time I was 16, I was strung out on IV heroin. I have no idea how I got through junior high school or graduated from high school, but I learned nothing. I spent my time in the teachers' faces, giving them as hard a time as I could get away with. I hated myself and everyone else. Inside me I had a terrible anger that I did not understand and could not control.

"One night when I was 19 and living with some friends doing odd jobs and selling a little bit of dope to pay my bills, I came to our apartment and said to the guys, 'Let's go to the late movie and get high.' When we got to the theater at the local shopping center, it was nearly midnight. I was so bombed on booze and LSD that I couldn't sit in the theater, so I went out to the car to wait for my friends to drive me home. In the car next to mine was a beautiful new guitar lying on the seat. The car was locked, so I bashed in the window and took the guitar. I settled into the back seat of my car, playing the guitar and waiting for my friends to come out of the theater. Before they arrived, the guy who owned the guitar came back. He must have gone to the same movie. He was not pleased to see his window broken and his guitar in my hands. He asked me what I thought I was doing. I got real mad at him for interrupting me, so I got out of the car and attacked him, breaking his guitar over his head.

"When I drank, I felt that I grew a foot and put on 100 pounds of pure muscle. This had gotten me into a lot of trouble over a long period of time. I lost a lot of teeth and blood by treating my 'small man syndrome' with alcohol and drugs. This guy wouldn't quit fighting. He was upset that I broke into his car, and he was even more upset that I had ruined his favorite guitar. Pretty soon I saw two police cars heading across the parking lot toward us, along with a security guard from the mall. I took off for the darkness beyond the parking lot. The trouble was that I was too drunk to run and I had on cowboy boots. Don't ever try to run away from the cops in cowboy boots!

"The cops caught me and brought me back. I was so mad and so high that I called the cops 'fascist pigs.' I went at them with everything I had. I hit, scratched, and bit them. They let me know what they thought of me by handcuffing me and taking me out where no one could see us. There they beat me over and over with their night sticks and kicked me until I passed out. I woke up in jail with a broken nose and a broken left eye socket, so I could only see double. Don't think you have to be black to be beaten by the cops when they get mad!

"The judge sentenced me to 44 years on so many charges I cannot even remember them all. Theft, breaking and entering, fleeing from an officer, assaulting an officer, public drunkenness—you get the idea. They sent me to the toughest drug treatment program in the area, a 15-month residential program where I never got out for months at a time. Up in the morning before dawn, head shaved, work and meetings all day, and then I'd flop into bed late each night. We had to wear signs when we did things that were bad. I felt like a walking billboard, I had so many signs hung from me, front and back. They said things like, 'Smart ass,' 'Wise guy,' 'Lazy,' and 'Too dumb to study.' I was tossed out of that program after 18 months, and that was a 15-month drug treatment program. I went back to prison and then to a halfway house. I was on parole for a while. Each time I failed, as I had failed at everything I had ever done in my life.

"The judge called me back to court one last time and said, 'This is it, you damn dumb kid. We have tried everything we have in this state for you and you have messed it all up. One more slip and you are doing all of your back-up time. Let's see, how long is that? Just about 40 years left. I hate to spend that much of the taxpayers' money, but if I ever saw a hopeless case, you are it.'

"Somehow, although I had heard all that a hundred times before, this time I believed him. A light bulb in my head went on that day in court. I knew that I was a fathead and had no one to blame but myself for all of the trouble I was in and had been in for as long as I could remember.

"My brother had gotten into AA and straightened out. I had been to plenty of AA and NA meetings over the years, but I had not stopped using alcohol and drugs for more than few months at a time. But finally it was my sister, who never used drugs, who helped me the most. She gave me a place to live and helped me get a job. Mostly, though, I just went to AA and NA meetings, once or twice a day for over a year. I knew, without a doubt, that it was the only way I could stay off alcohol and drugs and out of prison. All I did was go to meetings, work, and sleep. When I had been to meetings before, I had always sat in the back and shared nothing. I just got my slips signed for my parole officers, and then I left as quickly as I could. I never did get a sponsor until after that day with the judge in court. This time I got a sponsor, and I started to sit in the front of the meetings. I said something at every single meeting. I worked the steps in the AA program for the first time in my stupid life.

"That was 4 years ago. I cannot tell you why I started then and why I didn't figure it out years before. I guess I just had not had enough alcohol and drugs. But there came a day when I had had enough, and I knew it. It happened in that judge's courtroom.

"Now I am a mechanic. My folks wanted me to do white-collar work like they do. They wanted me to be a college man. I like working with my hands. Sure, my fingernails have grease under them, but I do the job well and it is honest work. Will I ever get married? I am 28 now. I don't know. Maybe. Right now I don't have much time for women or for thinking about that.

"Last week my sister got mad at me. She wanted to know why I still went to so many AA and NA meetings when I had not used alcohol or drugs for so long. Why did I have so little time for her and for anyone else who is not in the program? I haven't been mad at her for a long time, but I got mad then. I asked her if she remembered what it had been like all those years that I was using alcohol and drugs. I told her that only by going to meetings every day can I avoid that. If I stopped going to meetings, I'd be right back there again. She said, 'I do not understand that answer, but I accept it. I just want you to know I miss being with you, and so do a lot of other people who are not in that program of yours.' I told her I was sorry she felt that way, and maybe someday I'd go to fewer meetings, but I doubted it.

"How do I feel now about being short and having a learning disability? I feel damn lucky to be alive. I like my body just the way it is. I can learn as much as I want to, if I work at it. My problems never were my size or my dyslexia. My problem was my rotten attitude. I cannot change my height, but I can change my attitude. I can stay clean and sober, one day at a time, by the grace of God and with the help of this program.

"So that's my story. As for our topic tonight, it would help me if we talked about 'working your program'—what each of us has found that works best for us. For me, the most important things are going to meetings every day, talking with my sponsor once a day, working the 12 steps, and praying. If I do those things, then my life works. If I don't do all of them every single day, then my life falls apart again.

"Oh, here is one more thing I learned over these 4 years of sobriety that may help someone else. After I had been straight for about 2 years, I found I didn't like my sponsor very much. He wasn't helping me. I was getting mad at him a lot. That scared me because getting mad was what used to get me to drink and use drugs. One day I thought, 'Hey, why not get a new sponsor instead of getting so worked up about this guy?' I did. It was the best thing I ever did. I started in a whole new direction in the program. I saw a lot of things I had overlooked before. Now I even feel good about my first sponsor. He was fine for me at the start, but we sort of outgrew each other. Being able to make that change without a slip to alcohol and drugs, and without a blow-up, was a big step forward for me."

Sandra's story is common today as large numbers of young people are caught up in the reckless use of alcohol and other drugs. Lacking a strong genetic predisposition to addiction and being strongly dedicated to her personal goals in life, Sandra was able, fairly easily, to walk away from drugs as she matured.

Peter's account, which focused on his life as an active addict, how he came to find the 12-step programs, and his new life once he was a member of the fellowship, is typical of the structure of speaker meetings, one of the common types of 12-step meetings described in Chapter 11. Speakers do not lecture or give advice; they tell their own unique stories, and they teach by example. At meetings people do not complain or blame others, they share their experience, strength, and hope the way Peter did. What works for the speakers often works for others at the meetings because these mutual-aid programs are not theoretical or led by professional experts. Instead, they are filled with one-at-a-time miracles of recovery.

Chapter 3

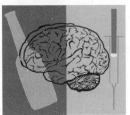

The Contemporary Scene for Alcohol and Other Drugs

In this chapter, I examine the contemporary drug scene in North America, profiling illicit users and projecting the costs, and also sketch the outlines of worldwide drug abuse.

After the initial peak of the illicit drug epidemic in the late 1970s, there was a decade-long but modest decline in the use of both alcohol and illicit drugs in the United States, as both became somewhat less tolerated, especially in more affluent and better educated segments of society and among middle-aged and older people. The problems caused by alcohol and other drug use over this period were increasingly concentrated among young people and in less-advantaged, less-educated segments of the population, in both rural and urban areas.

Despite these tentative signs of improvement, in the mid-1990s there was growing evidence of the intractable nature of the modern drug abuse epidemic, with large segments of the North American population caught in the grip of a generational drug problem and entire communities victimized by widespread addiction. Earlier hopes of returning to pre-epidemic levels of illegal drug use appeared unachievable. Public interest in curbing non-medical drug use, leading to public and private spending for law enforcement, treatment, and prevention, peaked first in 1972 and then again in 1987, but it was on the wane once more in the mid-1990s.

Worst of all, beginning with the 1992 survey and continuing into mid-decade, the national studies of teenage drug use showed the first significant increase in illicit drug use in more than two decades of study. A new generation of youth was deciding to use illicit drugs in ignorance of the painful consequences suffered by earlier generations. Marijuana and the hallucinogens were leading this new wave of drug use, and cigarette and alcohol use remained at high levels despite two decades of intense education programs designed to help North American youth grow up without using cigarettes, alcohol, and other drugs.

Drug Use Today in North America

The North American drug abuse epidemic, and the most serious costs associated with it, continue at historically high levels. As measured in surveys, the biggest decreases in drug use have been registered for the illegal drugs such as marijuana and cocaine, whereas the smallest decreases in drug use are with alcohol and cigarettes, drugs that are legal for adults. Drug use is falling far faster among casual users and more slowly, if at all, among hardcore drug users. Teenagers and high-risk populations, such as recently arrested individuals, have shown no fall in rates of drug use in recent years.

The first use of alcohol and other drugs is usually in the teenage years. Alcohol and other drug use peaks between ages 18 and 25 (see Figure 3–1). Males are slightly more likely than females to use most nonmedical drugs, except tobacco and stimulants, presumably because nicotine and the stimulants produce weight loss, a common concern of North American women.

The two major factors in the decision not to use or to stop the use of a nonmedical drug are the perception that the use is harmful to one's health and that drug use is socially disapproved. The declines in drug use in the last decade by North American youth were tied to the rising perceptions of health risks and to growing social intolerance over this time period. The recent rises in drug use among teenagers reflect the falling rates of belief that drug use

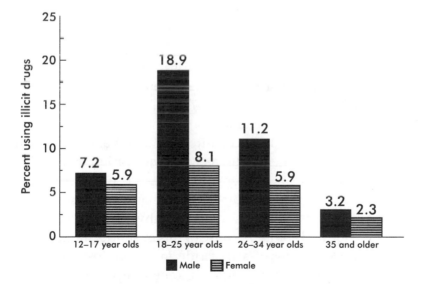

Figure 3–1.   Past month use of illicit drugs by age group, 1993.

Source.   U.S. Department of Health and Human Services, Public Health Service: *Preliminary Estimates from the 1993 National Household Survey on Drug Abuse.* Rockville, MD, Substance Abuse and Mental Health Services Administration, Office of Applied Studies, Advance Report Number 7, July 1994.

is dangerous and socially unacceptable.

A White House report estimated that in 1990 Americans spent a total of $40.4 billion for the major drugs of abuse: cocaine, $17.5 billion; heroin, $12.3 billion; marijuana, $8.8 billion; and all other nonmedical, illicit drugs, $1.8 billion. This entire sum was spent illegally, fueling organized crime throughout the world. That same year, Americans spent about $92 billion on alcohol and about $44 billion on tobacco products. In contrast, all prescribed medicines cost Americans $39.3 billion, and all over-the-counter medicines cost $1.3 billion in that year.

Drinking Your Share

American per capita consumption of alcohol for Americans ages 18 and older peaked in 1981 at about 2.75 gallons of pure alcohol per person per year and then fell slightly. In 1993, it was just over 2.3 gallons per person. The per capita consumption of distilled spirits, such as whiskey and vodka, has been falling slowly but steadily since the late 1970s. More recently, first wine consumption and then beer consumption also have begun to show modest declines on an annual per capita basis in the United States. (See Figure 3–2 for per capita alcohol consumption and cirrhosis of the liver rates throughout the world, which shows the United States to be in the middle of the rankings.)

In the 1990s, beer has accounted for about as much alcohol consumed in the United States as wine and spirits combined. Alcohol use in the form of beer continued to rise after the use of whiskey and wine fell, in part because many Americans do not recognize that beer contains the same ethyl alcohol that is contained in wine and spirits. Because of this misunderstanding, beer has gotten something of a free ride (as an almost soft drink), whereas distilled spirits have gotten something of a bum rap, as if distilled spirits were responsible for the majority of the nation's drinking problem. Most American alcohol-related problems are caused by the use of beer, the most common form of alcohol consumption.

Alcohol is alcohol regardless of how it is packaged. Slowly, more people are beginning to understand this simple but impor-

	Consumption of pure alcohol, quarts per capita			Cirrhosis deaths per 100,000 men in 1992, or most recent data
	1991	1992	1993	
Luxembourg	13.2	13.1	13.3	27.0
France	12.6	12.5	12.2	23.9*
Austria	11.2	10.6	11.1	41.6
Germany	11.5	11.5	11.0	33.1*
Portugal	12.3	11.3	11.0	40.6
Hungary	10.8	11.0	10.8	104.5
Denmark	10.5	10.9	10.6	18.8
Switzerland	11.3	10.7	10.6	13.7
Spain	11.6	11.5	10.6	28.9†
Greece	9.1	9.0	9.7	13.2*
Belgium	9.9	10.1	9.6	14.5¶
Czech Republic	9.2	9.3	9.4	27.0
Italy	9.6	9.4	9.1	34.8†
Slovakia	8.9	9.0	9.1	n.a.
Bulgaria	8.2	9.1	8.8	28.9
Ireland	8.1	8.2	8.8	3.2*
Romania	6.8	9.3	8.5	50.1

* = 1991; † = 1990; ¶ = 1989.

Figure 3–2.   The tipplers and the temperate: drinking around the world.

Note.   The wassail bowl and the champagne toast are synonymous with the end-of-the-year holidays, and beer frequently accompanies the end-of-the-season football game. But by and large, Americans are a more or less temperate bunch.

Citizens of Luxembourg are another story.

According to an international survey of alcohol consumption, Luxembourgers consumed 13.3 quarts of pure alcohol per person in 1993, almost three beers a day for every man, woman, and child.

The social pressures that have curbed drinking in the United States are not necessarily present elsewhere. Although drinking declined from 1991 through 1993 in half of the countries shown [in the figure], people drank more in other countries, especially those experiencing new freedom and wealth like China, South Africa, and the Czech Republic.

(continued)

	Consumption of pure alcohol, quarts per capita			Cirrhosis deaths per 100,000 men in 1992, or most recent data
	1991	1992	1993	
Netherlands	8.7	8.6	8.4	6.2*
Australia	8.1	8.0	7.9	8.8
Cyprus	8.5	8.5	7.9	n.a.
Argentina	8.1	8.0	7.8	15.0†
Britain	7.8	7.6	7.7	7.2
New Zealand	8.4	7.8	7.7	5.1*
Finland	7.9	7.6	7.2	16.7
United States	7.4	7.3	7.2	13.7†
Japan	7.0	7.0	7.0	19.1
Canada	7.3	7.0	6.9	11.1*
Chile	6.7	6.2	6.8	n.a.
Poland	7.5	6.7	6.7	15.6
Yugoslavia	7.0	6.6	6.6	n.a.
Uruguay	6.1	6.2	6.4	n.a.
Sweden	5.8	5.7	5.6	10.0†
Russian Fed.	6.0	5.3	5.2	n.a.
South Africa	5.0	5.1	5.2	n.a.

* = 1991; † = 1990; ¶ = 1989.

Figure 3–2.   The tipplers and the temperate: drinking around the world. *(continued)*

One of alcohol's side effects, liver disease like cirrhosis, strikes unevenly. It is not known, for example, why only 10 percent of alcoholics in the United States have the disease. But liver disease is generally higher in places where people drink daily, even in moderate amounts, than it is in those where most drinking is done on the weekend or special occasions.

The chart [above] compares beer, wine, and alcohol consumption by measuring the pure ethyl alcohol content of those drinks. The statistics were compiled by the Netherlands-based Commodity Board for the Spirits Industry. Only 51 countries listed supplied data. The cirrhosis death rates are from the World Health Organization, which did not have statistics for every country. *Note.*   Per capita consumption here is related to the total population, not to the population age 18 and older as was done on page 54.

(continued)

tant fact. Two and one-half gallons of pure alcohol consumed by an average U.S. adult during a year translates into slightly more than one drink per day for every person in the country ages 18 and older. A 12-ounce can of beer, a 5-ounce glass of wine, or a

	Consumption of pure alcohol, quarts per capita			Cirrhosis deaths per 100,000 men in 1992, or most recent data
	1991	1992	1993	
Venezuela	4.1	4.2	4.2	n.a.
Cuba	3.8	4.0	4.0	n.a.
Norway	4.3	4.0	3.9	5.6*
Brazil	3.8	3.6	3.6	n.a.
Iceland	4.1	3.8	3.6	1.5
Mexico	3.2	3.4	3.5	33.9*
China	2.9	3.0	3.4	n.a.
Colombia	3.5	2.6	3.1	n.a.
Paraguay	1.8	2.3	1.9	n.a.
Peru	1.5	1.7	1.2	n.a.
Israel	1.0	0.8	1.0	8.3[†]
Turkey	0.8	0.8	0.8	n.a.
Malaysia	0.5	0.5	0.5	n.a.
Tunisia	0.5	0.5	0.5	n.a.
Algeria	0.2	0.3	0.3	n.a.
Morocco	0.3	0.3	0.3	n.a.
Thailand	0.3	0.3	0.3	n.a.

* = 1991; † = 1990; ¶ = 1989.

Figure 3–2.   The tipplers and the temperate: drinking around the world. *(continued)*

Source.   Reprinted with permission from Cronin A: "The Tipplers and the Temperate: Drinking Around the World." *The New York Times,* January 1, 1995, p. 4E.

1.5-ounce jigger of distilled spirits each contain about 0.5 ounces of pure alcohol. One-third of Americans ages 18 and older do not drink alcohol at all, and about half of all the alcohol in the country is consumed by the top 10% of drinkers. Those heavy drinkers consume an average of six drinks a day, and the roughly 57% of Americans who drink more moderately consume an average of just over one drink a day, every single day of the year.

I found these data on American alcohol consumption to be so high that I doubted my calculations. To check my figures, I wrote to Enoch Gordis, M.D., the director of the National Institute on Alcohol Abuse and Alcoholism (NIAAA). He pointed out that the NIAAA survey numbers dealt with Americans ages 18 and older, whereas the survey data from the National Institute on Drug Abuse (NIDA) dealt with Americans ages 12 and older, but he confirmed that my math was correct. Dr. Gordis in his 1993 letter further noted,

> However, your text should emphasize that these estimates are based on sales figures, and that they greatly exceed self-reported levels of consumption. If we assume that the sales data correctly reflect true consumption levels, there are two possible sources of this discrepancy—the survey data underestimate the proportion of drinkers and/or they underestimate the level of consumption among those who do drink. If the proportion of adults who drink is really larger than our 63-percent estimate, then the average daily levels of consumption would be reduced.

Even if the 63% figure for the percentage of Americans who drink alcohol is low, meaning that fewer than 37% of Americans ages 18 and older do not drink any alcohol, and even if the 57% of moderate drinkers consume more alcohol than they report, these sales-based figures show that a relatively small proportion of American drinkers consume prodigious amounts of alcohol virtually on a daily basis. Although alcohol consumption in the United States remains high, it is nearly one-third less than it was in 1981, and it is 40% lower than the average consumption of alcohol in France.

Numbing Numbers: Drug Use Surveys

The U.S. Department of Health and Human Services has regularly conducted two national surveys of drug use for about 20 years. The responses give a good picture of the current trends in drug use in the United States. One study, called "Monitoring the Future," is a survey of American high school students conducted each year since 1975 by researchers from the Institute for Social Research of the University of Michigan. This series, popularly called the National High School Student Survey, gives the best look at the details of the changing drug patterns in the country because 18-year-olds are particularly responsive to current drug trends as well as relatively heavy users of drugs and alcohol. Lloyd Johnston, Ph.D., has headed this distinguished effort since it began. He has helped many other nations start their own school-based drug use surveys in recent years.

The second set of surveys tracks Americans ages 12 and older. The National Household Survey on Drug Abuse was first conducted in 1971. The two sets of surveys report alcohol and other nonmedical drug use at three levels: 1) use at any time in a lifetime (Lifetime Use), 2) use within the year before the survey (Annual Use), and 3) use within the 30 days before the survey (Current Use). The surveys sometimes report a fourth category, use more or less every day in the 30 days before the survey (Daily Use). The high school survey includes high school seniors, but it has recently captured drug use in grades 8 and 10 as well. Subsamples of high school seniors have been followed in later years, so the high school survey also reports use of alcohol and other drugs in college and in the years after high school for youth not in college.

Before looking at the results of these surveys, however, consider a few cautions. Both surveys are based on self-reports of the use of alcohol and other drugs. A staff member of the survey research team selects a classroom or a home carefully to reflect all high school students or all households in the nation in the same way that public opinion polls track voter sentiment. These are scientifically solid national studies conducted with great care.

Is the Drug Problem Getting Better or Worse?

- Drug use may have fallen in America for both legal and illegal drugs from the peaks of the 1970s and 1980s.
- Infrequent use of illegal drugs appears to be falling the most.
- Use of legal drugs (alcohol and cigarettes) and frequent use of illegal drugs is falling most slowly.
- Drug-caused problems, both health problems and crime, are falling slowly, if at all.
- Drug use in the most heavily affected communities is falling slowly, if at all.
- Drug use, especially use of marijuana and hallucinogens, is rising among teenagers.

There are two important limitations to these studies. First, there is considerable concern that a great deal of drug use is not reported in these studies. Data on American alcohol consumption, when compared with self-reported alcohol use, strongly support the view that self-reports understate actual use of alcohol. It is likely that illicit drug use is underreported to an even greater extent. Researchers have conducted studies to investigate the probability of such underreporting, but they have never conducted drug tests of study subjects to verify the survey results objectively. The studies that have been conducted appear to substantiate that many people are reliable in their self-report, even heavy illicit drug users.

The second concern with the national surveys is that some of the heaviest drug-using segments of the population are not counted fully in these surveys. For example, about 15% of 18-year-olds nationally have left school before May of their senior years, when the survey is administered each year. Many young people have left school because of their abuse of alcohol and other drugs. These high school dropouts, along with students absent from school the day of the survey, are not included in these studies. Similarly, some heavy drug users are not living in households. The only large groups of Americans not sampled in the household survey are those in prisons, hospitals, and colleges, as well as the homeless and those serving in the military. Some of these are populations with high rates of drug use, so not counting them leads to underestimates of the total number of nonmedical drug users in the country.

These limitations encourage caution in interpreting the national survey results, especially when these surveys are used to estimate the total number of users of specific drugs in the country. The two national self-report surveys each ask the same questions in the same way to similarly gathered samples over time. Although the surveys understate the total number of drug users in the country, they can be used to estimate changes, or trends, in the use of drugs and alcohol over time. The national surveys also give a lower boundary to the total drug use in the nation.

Because heroin use is relatively uncommon, with the total number of heroin addicts estimated at only about 500,000, about one-fourth of 1% of the population in America ages 12 and older, the survey data are not useful in assessing heroin trends. Estimates of the heroin addict population at its peak in 1972 were about 800,000. However, the surveys are useful for tracking the use of the other drugs on which we are primarily focusing: alcohol, marijuana, and cocaine. These are the "gateway" drugs because they are the most widely used drugs in the country and because they are widely considered, especially by drug users, to be relatively safe. These drugs are the gateway to less often used and more negatively viewed drugs, such as phencyclidine (PCP) and heroin.

Gates and Stepping-Stones

American youth for the last two decades have tended to use addicting substances in a stepping-stone fashion, beginning with cigarettes and alcohol, progressing to marijuana, and finally to cocaine. Not only do larger percentages use the first drugs in the sequence (except eventually more people drink alcohol than smoke cigarettes), but most of those who go to the next step in the sequence are those who used the preceding drugs more intensely and at younger ages. For example, youth who used alcohol earliest and most often were most likely to use marijuana, and youth who used marijuana earliest and most often were more likely to use cocaine. It is unusual for youth to skip steps in this drug sequence, so youth who did not drink alcohol or use cigarettes were unlikely to have smoked marijuana, and youth who did not use marijuana were even less likely to have used cocaine.

The other illicit drugs, most of which are used later and by fewer people than these four drugs, are almost always used after the gateway drugs. Heroin is the most infrequently used of the major drugs in American today. This is because it is widely perceived to be the most dangerous, not because it is less rewarding to the brain. The pattern of stepping-stones reflects the environment in which drugs are used, not their pharmacology.

Some people have suggested, usually in a sarcastic fashion, that the gateway drug theory means that if only alcohol or marijuana use would disappear, then all drug problems would disappear. This statement is based on the assumption that if youth did not use those particular gateway drugs, then they would not use any other drugs. This is an erroneous interpretation of the gateway drug concept. If, miraculously, alcohol and marijuana were to disappear from the face of the earth tomorrow, many people would continue to use drugs to get high. Which drugs are gateways to which other drugs is a matter of history and social attitude, not of solidly linked behaviors or of brain chemistry. For drug abuse to stop, the miracle would have to include all abused drugs, not just alcohol and marijuana.

Nevertheless, although alcohol, tobacco, and marijuana remain the principal gateway drugs in the world, young people who decide not to use those drugs are unlikely to use the stepping-stone drugs farther down the path into addiction. The gateway drug concept describes a pattern or a sequence, it does not describe causation. Alcohol use does not cause marijuana use. On the other hand, alcohol and tobacco use by youth does predict marijuana use, just as marijuana use predicts, but does not cause, cocaine use. The gateway concept is useful in focusing prevention policy goals on increasing the number of youth who choose not to use alcohol, tobacco, and marijuana. It is not appropriate to assume that the gateway drug concept means that alcohol, tobacco, and marijuana control the access to the brain's pleasure centers or that eliminating them would end the drug abuse problem.

The National Household Survey on Drug Abuse

The household survey showed that in 1993 the following percentages of 18- to 25-year-olds used these drugs within the prior 30 days (that is, they were current users): any illicit drug, 13.5%; alcohol, 59.3%; cigarettes, 29%; marijuana, 11.1%; and cocaine, 1.5%. Looking at that same 1993 survey, we find that the percentages of 12- to 17-year-olds using these drugs currently were any illicit drug, 6.6%; alcohol, 18%; cigarettes, 9.6%; marijuana, 4.9%; and cocaine, 0.4%. Among older Americans, and for drug use that means those ages 35 and older, the percentages of current users were any illicit drug 2.8%; alcohol, 48.8%; cigarettes, 23.8%; marijuana, 1.9%; and cocaine, 0.4%. For the highest-using age group, 18- to 25-year-olds, the lifetime use rates, not the current use rates, were any illicit drug, 50.9%; alcohol, 87.1%; cigarettes, 66.7%; marijuana, 47.4%; and cocaine, 12.5%.

The household survey also gave useful estimates for the total number of Americans who have used various drugs. In 1993, among the 207 million Americans ages 12 and older, a total of 173 million had used alcohol at some time in their lives, 148 million had ever smoked cigarettes, 70 million (or 34% of all Americans ages 12 and older) had used marijuana at least once, and 23 million had used cocaine. The current users of these four substances—that is, those who had used the substance at least once within the 30 days before the survey—were as follows: alcohol, 103 million; cigarettes, 50 million; marijuana, 8.9 million; and cocaine, 1.3 million.

Although those reporting current heroin use were too few to form the basis for an estimate, the household survey estimated that about 2.2 million Americans had used heroin at least once in their lives. Among all Americans 12 and older, 63% had never used an illicit drug, 25% had used at least once but not at all during the past year, and 12% had used an illicit drug at least once within the past year.

The household survey can also be used to track the total number of current users of illicit drugs in the United States from 1979 to 1993. The figures are as follows: 1979, 20.4 million; 1982, 21.9 million; 1985, 22.2 million; 1988, 14.5 million; 1991, 12.8 million; and 1993, 11.7 million. These figures, which show an overall decline of nearly 50% in the number of illicit drug users from 1985 to 1993, are useful in gauging the total level of illicit drug use in the country. They show a gratifying decline from the peak in 1985. The turnaround after years of steady rises was first recorded in 1988.

The surveys also show the likelihood of a person who has ever used a drug continuing to use it, in contrast to the likelihood that someone will use a drug and then quit. For 18- to 25-year-olds, the continuation rates were as follows: any illicit drug, 28%; alcohol, 71%; cigarettes, 45%; marijuana, 26%; and cocaine, 11%. These numbers mean that among American 18- to 25-year-olds in 1991, 71% of those who had drunk alcohol at any time in their lives were drinking alcohol within the 30 days before the 1991 survey. In sharp contrast, only 11% of those 18 to 25 years old who had ever used cocaine were still using cocaine in the 30 days before the survey. Heroin is similar to cocaine with a relatively low continuation rate of 12.5%. Only 28% of the 55% of American 18- to 25-year-olds who had ever used an illicit drug had used an illicit drug in the 30 days before the 1991 survey.

Continuation rates, like levels of use of the drugs within the society, reflect primarily the environment in which drug use occurs rather than any pharmacological property of the drug. Continuation rates are highest, as are overall use rates, for drugs that are more tolerated. The drugs we are looking at primarily in these surveys are scaled from the highest levels of use (and the highest continuation rates) to the lowest, as follows: alcohol, cigarettes, marijuana, and cocaine. The continuation rates for Americans age 12 and older in 1993 are shown in Table 3–1. This table also shows the number of Americans who used the major classes of drugs at various levels (lifetime, past year, and past month) and the changes from 1985 (at the peak of the epidemic) to 1993 (the most recent year for which information is available).

In the national surveys, cigarettes are included with the intoxicating drugs alcohol, marijuana, and cocaine. Cigarette smoking is clearly a different behavior from the use of these other drugs in that after a relatively brief period of occasional use at the start of smoking, usually early in the teenage years, cigarette smokers either use their substance from morning to night 365 days per year or stop use entirely. Few people smoke cigarettes only 1 or 2 days a week or less over many years, which is the most common pattern for use of alcohol, marijuana, and cocaine. Once more we see just how unusual cigarettes are when they are compared to the drugs of abuse.

The survey results demonstrate the high levels of use of these four substances and the impact of relative social tolerance of their use. The more tolerated a drug is in the society, the higher the rates of use and the more likely the use is to continue over long periods of time. Alcohol is more acceptable than is cocaine, so higher percentages of Americans use alcohol than use cocaine. Those people who use alcohol are more likely to continue to use alcohol than are those people who use cocaine likely to continue to use cocaine.

This information gives an interesting twist to the question of which of the four drugs is the most addicting. When the question is asked, "Which drug, once used, is most likely to be used 10 years later by the same person?" the clear winner is alcohol, with cigarettes a relatively close second. Cocaine and heroin trail badly. On the other hand, if the addiction question were rephrased as, "Which drug, once used more than a few times, is most likely to lead to a sustained period of compulsive, out-of-control use?" the answer is likely to be cocaine, with heroin a relatively close second. Here is another way to ask the question about which drug is the most addictive: "Once used, which drug is most likely to be used day and night, 365 days per year, for decades?" There is no contest on that one: Cigarettes have no peers. So, which of these five drugs do you think is the most addictive?

These survey data reinforce a mountain of other data to show

Table 3–1. Comparison of 1985 and 1993 National Household Survey on Drug Abuse (in millions of people 12 and older)

	1985 Past month	1993			Percent decrease from 1985–1993 past month	Percent continuation rate*
		Lifetime	Past year	Past month		
Illegal drugs for all ages						
Any illicit drug	22.3	77	24	12	46	16
Marijuana	17.8	70	18.6	9	49	13
Cocaine	5.2	23	5	1.3	75	6
Stimulants (amphetamines)	2.5	13	2.4	0.7	72	5
Heroin	0.16	2.3	0.2	0.08	50	4
Legal for adults						
Alcohol	112.3	173	138	103	8.3	60
Cigarettes	60.4	148	61	50	17.2	34

*The percentage of people who have ever used a drug who used it in the past month, 1993.
Source. U.S. Department of Health and Human Services, Public Health Service: *Preliminary Estimates From the 1993 National Household Survey on Drug Abuse.* Rockville, MD, Substance Abuse and Mental Health Services Administration, Office of Applied Studies, Advance Report Number 7, July 1994.

not only that addictiveness is related to pharmacology, the way the drug substance interacts with the brain, but that addiction risk is closely related to the social environment in which the use of addictive substances occurs. However, once a person has lost control of the use of any of these substances, or has fallen in love with the specific drug high, then the process of addiction has taken hold and the difficulty of quitting use of any of these drugs for prolonged periods of time is great.

Positive Trends

Let us shift our focus from the current levels of use to the trends in drug use between 1972 and 1993. Again, we focus on the current use of the four gateway drugs by the 18- to 25-year-olds. Current alcohol use peaked at 76% in 1979, cigarette use peaked at 49% in 1976, marijuana use peaked at 35% in 1979, and cocaine use peaked at 9% in 1979. Note that the alcohol rate fell from the peak of 76% to 59% in 1993, cigarettes from 49% to 29%, marijuana from 35% to 11%, and cocaine from 9% to 2%. Here again

Recent Positive Developments in the Drug Epidemic

- Growing recognition that the 12-step programs are the key to long-term recovery
- Greater use of driving-while-impaired programs to deal with drunk and drugged driving
- Drug testing at work, in the criminal justice system, and elsewhere
- Linking abstinence from nonmedical drug use to the "healthy living" agenda and to rejection of tobacco use

we see the pattern of environmental effects on the rates of drug use: bigger falls for the illegal drugs marijuana and cocaine, which are less socially accepted, than for the drugs that are legal for adults, alcohol and cigarettes, which are more socially tolerated.

The household survey also focused on the effect of race, education, and socioeconomic status on the rates of drug use. In general, whites were about as likely as blacks to drink alcohol heavily, more likely to smoke cigarettes, and less likely to use marijuana or cocaine (see Table 3–2). Higher income and higher education were associated with lower rates of use of illicit drugs and of both alcohol and cigarettes.

The effects of race, education, and income were more noticeable for heavy use of marijuana and cocaine use than for alcohol use, except at the highest levels of education and income where the rates of heavy use were also significantly lower for alcohol use.

The National High School Student Survey/ "Monitoring the Future" Study

In the 1994 National High School Student Survey, current use of alcohol was reported by 50% of high school seniors, cigarettes by

Table 3–2. Percent of people ages 18 or older who report heavy use of alcohol, cigarettes, and illicit drugs by race/ethnicity, United States, 1991

Substance	White	Black	Hispanic	Other
Alcohol	5.7	6.0	6.8	2.9
Cigarettes	18.3	11.9	8.4	12.5
Marijuana	2.2	5.1	2.3	1.6
Cocaine	0.6	2.3	1.6	1.0

Source.   Adapted from Flewelling RL, Ennett ST, Rachal JV, et al.: *National Household Survey on Drug Abuse: Race/Ethnicity, Socioeconomic Status, and Drug Abuse 1991* (DHHS Publ No SMA-93-2062). Washington, DC, U.S. Department of Health and Human Services, Substance Abuse and Mental Health Services Administration, Office of Applied Studies, U.S. Government Printing Office, Superintendent of Documents, 1993.

30%, marijuana by 19%, and cocaine by 1.5%. A total of 22% of U.S. high school seniors reported use of any illicit drug in the month before the study. Among American college students in 1991 the figures were as follows: any illicit drug, 15%; alcohol, 75%; cigarettes, 23%; marijuana, 14%; and cocaine, 1%. The percentage of 12th graders using any illicit drug and the percentage using any illicit drug other than marijuana are shown in Figure 3–3. This figure shows the alarming upturn in drug use recorded in 1993, after more than a decade of steady declines. The 1994 high school survey was a major wake-up call to everyone who had been lulled into the hope that illicit drug use was progressively declining in the United States and that someday soon it would fall to the pre-epidemic levels seen in the early 1960s.

The National High School Student Survey also reported racial and ethnic data for 1990. Drug use rates were higher for whites than for blacks or other ethnic groups. White high school seniors' rates were exceeded only by Native Americans, who had even higher rates for the use of marijuana, cocaine, and daily use of alcohol as well as for the use of cigarettes.

Focusing on marijuana use, the survey showed that for high school seniors between 1985 and 1989, 44% of Native American females and 42% of Native American males used marijuana at least once in the previous year, compared with 36% of white females and 40% of white males. For blacks the figures were 30% for males and 18% for females. The rates for male and female high school seniors who were Puerto Rican and other Latin Americans were 31% and 21% and for Mexican Americans 37% and 26%. For Asian American males and females the numbers were 20% and 17%, the lowest of any American ethnic group.

With respect to cocaine use, among white males the use within the past year was 12%, compared with 6% for black males. Whereas 30% of white males reported current cigarette use, only 16% of black males reported current cigarette use. For females the cigarette figures were 34% for whites and 13% for blacks. Native American and Hispanic males reported the highest levels of cocaine use in the past year, at approximately 15%. The University of Michigan researchers noted that there is now only a small difference in high school dropout rates between blacks and whites, so the different rates of dropping out cannot account for the substantially higher numbers for whites than blacks. The researchers concluded that "blacks are more likely than whites to perceive high risks for various forms of drug use,

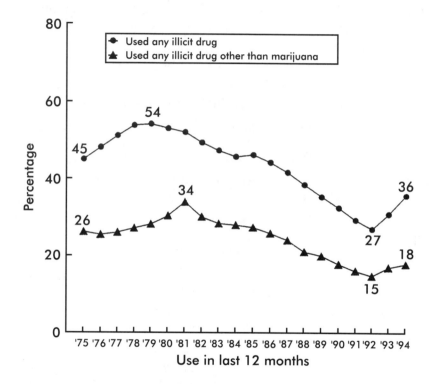

Figure 3–3. Trends in annual prevalence of an illicit drug use index for 12th-grade students.

Note. Use of "any illicit drug" includes use of marijuana, hallucinogens, cocaine, and heroin, or any use that is not under a doctor's orders of other opiates, stimulants, barbiturates, methaqualone (excluded since 1990), or tranquilizers. Beginning in 1982, the question about stimulant use (i.e., amhetamines) was revised to get respondents to exclude the inappropriate reporting of nonprescription stimulants. The prevalence rate dropped slightly as a result of this methodological change.
Source. Johnston LD, O'Malley PM, Bachman JG: "Drug use continues to climb among American teen-agers, as attitudes and beliefs about the dangers of drugs soften, U-M survey says," in *Monitoring the Future Study* (news release). Ann Arbor, MI, University of Michigan, Institute for Social Research, December 8, 1994.

and blacks also are more likely to disapprove of drug use."

It is not clear why the high school survey found lower rates of illicit drug use for blacks than for whites, whereas the household survey found little difference between the rates of use by blacks and whites ages 12 to 17, and, for Americans ages 18 and older, the rates of use by blacks were somewhat higher than by whites. It may be that black youth have learned from the devastating effects of drugs on older blacks and are now less likely to use illicit drugs.

The 1994 National High School Student Survey also showed the rise in cocaine use among high school seniors from 1975, with a sharp dropoff after 1986. This fall in the use of cocaine was mirrored by a truly remarkable rise between 1986 and 1987 in the percentage of high school seniors who saw great risk in even trying cocaine (33.5% to 47.9%). That was the sharpest change in perceived risk from one year to the next recorded in these studies. The change can be traced to the death of University of Maryland basketball player Len Bias, which occurred just 1 month after the 1986 high school data were collected.

The change in perceived risk translated into a fall in cocaine use by high school seniors and that this fall between 1986 and 1987 was not the result of a fall in perceived availability of cocaine at that time. In fact, high school seniors reported that cocaine was more available in 1987 than they had reported in 1986, even though they used cocaine less in 1987 than in 1986. The 1993 National High School Student Survey also showed the rates of selected drug use in the 8th, 10th, and 12th grades.

Social Problems Created by Drug Use

Having looked at the levels of illicit drug use (and the levels of use of alcohol and cigarettes, use of which is illegal for high school students) in the United States, we now turn to the recent trends in the major problems created by illicit drug use. One of the major social problems is serious crime, more than half of which is directly related to illicit drug use. The National Institute of Justice has studied booked arrestees in major cities starting in 1987 in its Drug Use Forecasting (DUF) program. Unlike the surveys that rely on self-report, DUF uses an objective drug urine test as well

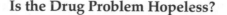

Is the Drug Problem Hopeless?

- Disadvantaged groups and youth are the most likely to see rises in the rates of use of alcohol and other drugs.
- Nonmedical drug use in most of the rest of the world will increase for the foreseeable future.
- Drug problems, such as crime, illnesses, accidents, and addicted infants, will persist at high levels despite a decline in the use of alcohol and other drugs for some segments of the population.
- Nonmedical drug use will not disappear from any community in the world and will persist at very high levels in many high-risk communities and population groups.
- New drug threats, like the crack cocaine epidemic in the United States in the late 1980s, can happen at any time with lightning speed, particularly affecting those already most heavily using illicit drugs. The most likely increases will be in the use of drugs that are widely perceived to be safe, as North American youth increasingly are seeing marijuana and hallucinogens to be.

as self-report at the time of arrest to identify recent drug use. In DUF sites reporting between 1989 and 1991, the average levels of illicit drug use immediately before arrest was steadily high during this time, perhaps with a slight fall from about 70% to about 60% over that 3-year period. Arrested females have somewhat higher rates of use than do arrested males for both 1990 and 1991.

For comparison, the hospital emergency room visits associated with drug use are compiled by the Drug Abuse Warning Network. The trends in drug-related emergencies between 1988 and

1993 were generally level, with the possibility of a slight decline over this period. This is in dramatic contrast to the household and high school surveys, which have shown strong declines in drug use over the last few years until the upturn in 1993.

Why did drug problems hold level even when self-reported drug use went down? One explanation is that many of the infrequent users of illicit drugs were discouraged from use by the lowering environmental tolerance for illicit drug use. In contrast, addicted users were much slower to quit their habits. Most of the social problems come from addicted, as opposed to casual, drug users, so the problem indicators did not fall in tandem with the use indicators. Another explanation for the diverging trends of use compared with problems is that the people who generate most of the social costs of drug use are in high-risk populations that have not responded significantly to the changing environmental forces resulting from declining social tolerance of both licit and illicit drug use.

A third and more disturbing explanation for the divergence between trends in drug-caused problems and self-reported drug use is that a growing percentage of users lie on surveys in response to the increasing social intolerance of drug use over the past decade. If increased lying were responsible for the declines in self-reported drug use, the survey trends showing declines in drug use could be giving a false sense of security about drug use in the United States. To answer this criticism of the survey research, it is essential that urine and hair tests be used objectively to assess drug use by survey respondents, as is now done in the DUF data from the criminal justice system.

Tolerance for nonmedical drug use has fallen further and faster in middle-class than in lower-class communities over the past decade. In any event, the persistently high drug abuse problem indicators and the 1994 high school survey results give pause to anyone who is tempted to become optimistic about the good news from the drug use surveys.

These data should not, however, be read to indicate that decreased social tolerance, the environmental approach to drug abuse, is ineffective in dealing with addicted drug users. Decreased social tolerance works for all drug users; it just works more slowly and requires tougher sanctions for addicted users. Recall that the powerful changes in the drug-using environment led to large reductions in the size of the American heroin-using population in the mid-1970s. Similarly, drug testing linked with tough sanctions for continued drug use, a classic environmental approach to drug abuse prevention, works well to curb drug use both in addiction treatment and in the criminal justice system, two of the toughest high-risk populations of addicted drug users. Drug tests linked to consequences also reduce drug use in workplace programs.

The Costs of Drugs

Drug users show as much variety of lifestyles and values as nonusers do. Nevertheless, there are common patterns of non-medical drug use in North America today. One important aspect of drug use is the cost to the user. How much do they pay for their drugs over the course of a typical year of use? In this book we focus on four drugs and one not-quite-a-drug: alcohol, marijuana, cocaine, heroin, and cigarettes. Although there are as many patterns of use for cocaine as there are for alcohol, here is a typical pattern for each of these five substances to give you a picture of the direct costs users pay for their drugs. We focus on the typical fairly heavy user, the kind of user I see in my clinical practice. Many addicts consume far more than this hypothetical average North American illicit drug user does, and many others consume less.

The most common intoxicant used by most North Americans is alcohol. People who are heavy drinkers commonly consume five or more drinks in a day, usually in an evening, at least twice a week. Assuming that each drink costs about $2, this comes to about $10 for an evening of drinking, or about $1,000 per year. (This estimate is calculated from $10 per drinking day times 100 drinking days per year.) Many heavy drinkers regularly consume twice that much most days of the year, in which case such heavy drinkers of alcohol might spend $20 a day for 300 days per year, or about $6,000. Of course, drinkers can pay a lot more than $2 a drink if they drink at expensive watering holes or if they drink expensive alcohol, say fancy brandy, fine wine, or champagne. Heavy drinkers on a tight budget can stay drunk for less than $5 a day. For purposes of comparison with other drug users, let us focus on typical fairly heavy drinkers who spend about $1,000 per year for their alcohol.

Marijuana costs users about $10 or $20 a day to use, once their use is fairly regular. Pot smokers often use their drugs about the way alcohol drinkers do, but pot smokers are more likely to use it during the day, and they are more likely than alcohol drinkers to be everyday users. For the sake of comparison with alcohol, assume that typical marijuana users smoke twice a week and that they pay $10 a day for pot use, which comes to $1,000 per year, or about the same as is paid by the typical alcohol consumer. Like alcohol users, heavy pot users may pay many times that amount. It is fairly common for marijuana users to spend $5,000 or more per year for their drug, especially if they give some away to friends, as often happens with all drug users, including alcohol users. Such sharing of drugs by friends is a major way that drug use spreads.

Cocaine is a less familiar pattern of drug use for most people. Coke users typically consume their drug in runs that often last for a few hours to a few days. On a single coke run, a user may spend $50 to $200. It is common for cocaine users to spend far more than that in a day or two of cocaine use. Some cocaine users take the drug in a regular, predictable pattern as commonly is seen for both alcohol and marijuana users. Cocaine users are more likely to have longer periods when they do not use cocaine at all, and then they are likely to use their drug in what would be called a "binge" if alcohol were the substance being used. To define a typical cocaine user, think about a person who spends $200 on a typical run and has about 40 of these runs of cocaine use during a year. That comes to $8,000 per year. However, it is not uncommon for cocaine users, once they become addicted to the drug, to use many times this amount, spending $20,000 or more in a year for the drug, a cost seldom, if ever, seen for either alcohol or marijuana use.

I listened as a famous musician described to a rapt audience his desperate struggle with alcohol and cocaine. His "bottom," the painful event that finally led him to get treatment and to stop all use of alcohol and other drugs, came when he decided to quit on his own, using his own willpower. He made it for 17 days until

> the voice of my disease spoke to me, saying, "You have been so very, very good for so long that now you need to reward yourself with just a little tiny bit of cocaine." I listened to that voice. Four days later, after I had spent over $5,000, I called a friend who I knew had beaten a cocaine problem of his own and pleaded with him to help me get into a treatment program right then. I had to admit that I could not do it on my own, in my own way.

There is no other drug that can cost users more than $1,000 a day the way cocaine all too commonly does.

Heroin is often used every single day, except when users are incarcerated or involuntarily separated from their drug. Heroin users often spend $80 to $200 a day, for a cost of $24,000 to $60,000 per year, assuming that the typical users find their drug for an average of 300 days per year.

Cigarette smokers often smoke one or two packages of 20 cigarettes a day, permitting them to use one or two cigarettes an hour while awake. At about $2 a package, and assuming that the typical physically dependent cigarette smoker uses cigarettes 365 days per year, this comes to about $750 to $1,500 each year.

None of these habits is cheap, to say nothing of the other costs paid by users, including lost work, lost potential growth in their lives, and severe negative health consequences as a direct result of their use of addicting substances. Alcohol, marijuana, and cigarettes are likely to cost moderately heavy users $1,000 to $2,000 per year, whereas cocaine is likely to cost $10,000 or more per year, and heroin is likely to cost $30,000 per year. Most heavy users of illicit drugs are also heavy users of alcohol and cigarettes, so many addicts routinely pay for more than one drug during a typical year of addiction.

Cocaine and heroin users spend more money on their drugs than do users of alcohol, marijuana, and cigarettes for two reasons. First, there is a higher level of physical tolerance to these drugs based on biology. That means that once users of cocaine and heroin have become familiar with their drug it takes much more of the drug to produce a high than it did when they first used it. Tolerance also develops to alcohol, marijuana, and cigarettes, but it is far less intense than for cocaine and heroin. For alcohol, marijuana, and cigarettes, experienced users consume two to five times as much as novice users. For cocaine and heroin, experienced users may take 20 times as much as they did as novice users.

The second reason cocaine and heroin users spend more for their drug is that those two drugs are more intensely prohibited than the other three. The price of these two drugs is inflated substantially by prohibition. If cocaine and heroin were sold like ordinary pharmaceutical medicines, a large habit would cost no more than an alcohol or a cigarette habit, about $1,000 per year. Because cocaine and heroin today are so expensive for users, they are especially highly correlated to income-generating crime, including both drug sales and theft. (For an interesting confirmation on these clinical estimates, see page 54. The cost issues related to proposals to legalize drugs such as cocaine and heroin are discussed on pages 426–428.)

Illegal drugs, unlike alcohol and cigarettes, offer users an apparently easy way to recoup some of their high costs. Many drug users sell illegal drugs to other users. As one drug abuser told me, most small-time sellers do not consider themselves to be drug dealers. Illegal drug users think that the people who sell drugs to them are drug dealers, and they think of their own customers as their friends. All of the illegal drug habits feed the criminal under world, which has devastating effects not only in the users' own communities but globally. Crimes, including political subversion and traffic in guns, as well as murder and drug sales, are the direct result of buying even small amounts of illegal drugs.

Earlier in this chapter we reviewed how many Americans are current users of these drugs and how much drugs cost users every year. We can put these two sets of numbers together to estimate about how many dollars each year the users of each drug spend on their "chemical lovers." This is how much money they devote to the stimulation of their brains' pleasure centers with each psychoactive chemical. Of course, these numbers are averages, meaning that many users of these substances use more, whereas many others use less than these estimates. We are considering only people who used each substance in the prior 30 days. Some of the users who did not use in the prior 30 days did spend money for each of the substances in the prior year. Both the estimates of the numbers of users and the amounts they have spent for their substances are far from precise. Nevertheless, these numbers give a useful snapshot of the typical drug user's costs each year.

For the substances that are legal for adults, in 1991 we find that 55 million cigarette smokers spent about $44 billion, or about $800 each per year, whereas 103 million alcohol drinkers spent $92 billion, or an average of about $900 each per year. Among the users of purely illegal drugs, the nation's 9.7 million pot smokers paid $8.8 billion, or an average of $900 each per year, and the 1.9 million cocaine users spent about $17.5 billion for an average cost of $9,200 each per year. The country's half-million current heroin users spent $12.3 billion, or an average of about $24,600 each per year (see Table 3–3).

These numbers help to show that the use of alcohol is relatively cheap. This reflects the large number of moderate drinkers and the relatively low cost of alcohol. Cocaine and heroin are truly expensive drug habits. Perhaps the most mind-boggling figure here is the average cost of $2,000 per month paid by users of heroin. When you realize that American heroin users as a group are mostly poor, relatively young men with little education, you realize the unique role heroin plays in criminal behavior in North America today. These survey-based estimates are similar to the clinically based estimates for typical users of the major drugs of abuse. These independent assessments tend to confirm each other and add confidence to the conclusions about the average costs of specific drug habits in the United States today.

Now that you have seen the most recent drug numbers, what do you think? Is the North American drug problem getting better or worse? Is there hope for the future, or are drugs a hopeless problem? Who is the typical North American illicit drug user today? These data show that illicit drug use appeared to be declining in the United States until 1993, when it rose again. Notice that

Table 3–3. Drug use in the United States: total users in 1991 and costs

Substance	Number of current users[a] (millions)	Cost per year (billions of dollars)	Cost per user per year (approximate dollars)
Alcohol	103	92	900
Cigarettes	55	44[b]	800
Marijuana	9.7	8.8[c]	900
Cocaine	1.9	17.5[c]	9,200
Heroin	0.5	12.3[c]	24,600

[a]*Source.*   U.S. Department of Health and Human Services, National Institute on Drug Abuse, Division of Epidemiology and Prevention Research: *National Household Survey on Drug Abuse: Population Estimates 1991* (DHHS Publ No ADM 92-1887). Rockville, MD, National Institute on Drug Abuse, 1991.
[b]*Source.*   Institute for Health Policy, Brandeis University: *Substance Abuse: The Nation's Number One Health Problem: Key Indicators for Policy.* Princeton, NJ, Robert Wood Johnson Foundation, October 1993.
[c]*Source.*   Office of National Drug Control Policy: "What America's Users Spend on Illegal Drugs" (technical paper). Washington, DC, Executive Office of the President, June 1991.

the problems created by illicit drug use, including crime and health problems, have remained persistently high, not showing the drop that the surveys of drug use showed. Some drug use problems, such as AIDS resulting from intravenous drug use, continue to rise. Declines in illicit drug use are uneven within the population so that, although there is hope in these numbers for many Americans, large numbers of people remain cruelly afflicted by illicit drug problems. The typical illicit drug user in the United States today is a person between the ages of 16 and 40, somewhat more likely to be male than female, with all racial, religious, economic, geographic, and ethnic groups well represented.

Drug Use in Canada and Mexico

This book focuses on the United States, which has the highest rates of multiple-drug use in the world. The United States also has the best information about the nature, extent, and trends in nonmedical drug use. Second place goes to Canada, which has generally similar rates of use and similarly sophisticated drug-use studies. In general, Canada's rates of use are most similar to the United States for alcohol and cigarettes. Marijuana use rates are somewhat lower in Canada than in the United States, and cocaine use rates are significantly lower. Canada has higher rates of illicit drug use on the West Coast, with somewhat lower rates in Ontario and even lower rates in the other Canadian provinces. As with the United States, the most recent Canadian research shows a worrisome upturn in the use of the illicit drugs, after a decade of declines.

A 1989 national study of alcohol and other drug use by Canadians ages 15 and older showed that among those ages 15 to 24, 81% were current drinkers of alcohol (that is, they drank at least once in the prior year), 30% smoked cigarettes, 16% smoked marijuana, and 5% reported cocaine use in the prior year. These figures are similar to those from the United States given earlier.

Among youth in Canada, alcohol and other drug use rose with age, so that 63% of 15- and 16-year-olds drank alcohol, whereas 80% of the 17- to 19-year-olds and 88% of the 20- to 24-year-olds drank alcohol. As in the United States, there was a recent modest downturn in the use of alcohol in Canada. For example, among 15- to 19-year-olds, the average drinks consumed during the prior 7 days fell from 3.3 in 1985 to 2.4 in 1989. This same Canadian survey looked into the percentage of various age groups that drank five or more drinks of alcohol on 15 or more occasions in the year prior to the survey. Five or more drinks of alcohol in a day is standard survey research criterion for heavy drinking, or alcohol abuse. In 1989, 20% of the 15- to 24-year-olds reported this level of drinking, whereas 13% of the 25- to 34-year-olds and 9% of the 35- to 44-year-olds reported this level of drinking. Of the Canadians ages 55 and older, only 4% reported drinking at this high level.

On the other hand, when the survey researchers asked subjects in each age group how many used alcohol twice a week or more often, the percentage among 15- to 24-year-olds was 21%. This figure rose with each successive age group until it peaked in the 45- to 54-year-old age group at 38%. Among Canadians ages

55 and older, the figure was down only slightly to 33%. The point here is that frequent, relatively modest drinking rises with age, whereas episodic heavy drinking is more concentrated in the 15- to 24-year-old age range.

The Canadian survey conducted in 1989 showed that 77% of Canadians ages 15 years and older were current drinkers, 16% were former drinkers, and only 7% had never drunk alcohol. A total of 6.5% of Canadians were current users of cannabis (marijuana), 23.2% had used it at one time but had stopped, and 70% had never used cannabis. With respect to the use of cocaine, 1.4% of Canadians were current users and 3.5% were former users. In Australia and New Zealand, rates of nonmedical drug use are most similar to those in the United States and Canada. These countries all have a relatively similar language and culture.

The drug use rates in Mexico are, as with those in Canada, more similar to those in the United States than to rates of drug use in many other parts of the world. However, Mexico has a long-established pattern of relatively heavy marijuana and inhalant use and a more recent and troubling pattern of heavy heroin and cocaine use. Drug use rates other than alcohol and tobacco began to climb in Mexico in the late 1960s when they also rose sharply in the United States and Canada. Cocaine use was uncommon in the early years of the drug problem in Mexico.

In Mexico, illicit drug use rates are the highest in the northwest region closest to California, and the next highest are in the central part of the country in and around Mexico City. The lowest rates of illicit drug use in Mexico are found in the south and in the northeast area near Texas. Alcohol use is lower in Mexico than in the United States or Canada, but it is rising. Mexico has particularly high rates of the use of inhalants.

In 1992, Dr. Guido Belsasso, the Anti-Drug Coordinator of Mexico, reported at an international conference on a survey of Mexico conducted by the Department of Education and the Mexican Institute of Psychiatry, which showed that 8.2% of the surveyed population had used an illicit drug at least once in the prior year. Inhalants, marijuana, amphetamines, and cocaine were the drugs of choice. Of these four drugs, levels of use remained stable between 1986 and 1989 for all but cocaine, the use of which increased significantly in those years.

The prevalence of illicit drug use is lower in Mexico than in the United States. For example, 4% of the male population in Mexico over age 12 had used an illicit drug compared with 37% in the United States. When drug use rates are studied among Hispanics living in the United States, the differences are smaller. For example, the lifetime prevalence of marijuana use in Mexico was 2.4% and among Hispanics in the United States it was 23.5% (compared with 33.5% for non-Hispanic whites). Cocaine showed a similar picture with 0.3% use in Mexico, 7.3% for Hispanics in the United States, and 12.4% for non-Hispanic whites in the United States. Mexican Americans born in Mexico have lower rates of illicit drug use than those born in the United States. Among Mexican Americans, higher levels of acculturation to the United States are associated with higher levels of illicit drug use.

Drug Use Outside North America

In other countries of the world, nonmedical drug use is growing, although it is often limited to one or two drugs. For example, heroin use is relatively high in Germany; in heroin-producing areas, such as the nations of Southeast Asia (including Thailand, Vietnam, and China); and in central Asian nations with well-established cultivation of opium poppies, such as Iran and Afghanistan. Cannabis use is high in the nations with long-standing cultivation of this drug crop, such as many Middle Eastern nations, Algeria, and Morocco, as well as in Jamaica and Mexico. Cocaine cultivation and local use of the drug, with its terrible effects, are increasing in Latin America, most intensely in the Andes Mountains nations of Peru, Bolivia, and Colombia. Drug use, especially of marijuana and cocaine, appears to be rising in Argentina and Brazil. Many parts of the world now are experiencing rising rates of both drug crop cultivation and nonmedical drug use as the illicit drug traffic spreads deeper into the economic life of most nations of the world and as urbanization and personal anonymity increase, along with tolerance for nonmedical drug use.

In June 1992, NIDA, the organization of which I was the first

director, published an important report on the global epidemiological trends in drug abuse, including the following summary by
Isidore S. Obot, Ph.D., M.P.H., from Jos, Nigeria. Nigeria is the
most influential nation in Africa. As a medical student, I spent
5 months there in 1960, shortly after the country became independent after 76 years of British colonial rule. Because of my continuing interest in Africa, I have been back to Nigeria three times
since my first visit.

Dr. Obot speaks eloquently, not only about what he sees occurring in Nigeria but also about what is now happening in virtually every developing nation in the world. His plea for more work
in demand reduction, including programs to help addicted people and public health programs to monitor accurately the levels of
drug abuse and drug-caused problems, should be an agenda for
immediate action in the world community today:

> Nigeria, the most populous nation in Africa, is experiencing a
> growing problem of drug abuse and drug trafficking. The prob-
> lem started with Indian hemp (cannabis) in the 1960s, but by the
> early 1980s, cocaine and heroin had entered the scene as the
> country became a transshipment route for drugs meant for
> Europe and North America. While cannabis and alcohol are still
> the most widely abused drugs today, and they contribute more
> to ill health than any other drug, the abuse of cocaine and heroin
> is on the rise. Lifetime use rates of cocaine and heroin/morphine
> are 1.6% and 2.3%, respectively, among university students, and
> 0.8% and 0.2% in the general population. About 50% of both
> students and adults drink alcohol regularly; 1.3% of students
> and 2.4% of the general population smoke Indian hemp. The
> abuse of a wide variety of other drugs, such as inhalants, central
> nervous system stimulants, hallucinogens, and prescription
> drugs, has also been reported. The health and social problems
> associated with drug abuse are increasing; drug abuse ac-
> counted for 9.1% of admissions into four psychiatric hospitals in
> 1984 and 15.1% in 1988. In response to the worsening drug situ-
> ation, a national drug control agency has been set up with pre-
> dominantly law enforcement functions. There is an urgent need
> for coordinated demand reduction activities, including a pro-
> gram of regular national epidemiologic surveys.

Here is part of the overview of the world drug abuse picture from the *Report of the United Nations International Narcotics Control Board for 1993:*

During the last two decades, the world has witnessed the "globalization" of the drug abuse problem and the situation has worsened drastically. The Commission on Narcotic Drugs no longer discusses individual situations such as the smuggling of heroin into China, the illicit traffic in opium from Turkey to Egypt or the supply of heroin to New York through the "French Connection." Some decades ago, the abuse problem was the concern of only a limited number of countries, but today countries that are not suffering from the harmful consequences of drug abuse are the exception rather than the rule.

The economic power and political influence of drug cartels are rising. While drug abuse has been "globalized," internationalization and cooperation among drug cartels have also increased. There is also clear evidence that trafficking organizations barter different types of drugs among themselves. Drug trafficking syndicates are increasingly becoming involved in other forms of organized and violent crime, making use of sophisticated technical aids and modern communication systems. Criminal organizations control drugs from the cultivation and production phases to the storage and distribution phases. Large amounts of drugs are stored at staging posts in certain countries to take advantage of weak or ineffective laws in those countries. There is evidence that drug trafficking organizations frequently make use of the territories of countries (a) that are not parties to the international drug control treaties; (b) that have formally ratified conventions without implementing their provisions; (c) that suffer from civil war, terrorist activities, political instability, ethnic conflict, economic depression or social tension; (d) that are not in a position to ensure governmental control over some parts of their territories; (e) and that are not able to maintain adequate law enforcement, customs and pharmaceutical control services.

More and more Governments are beginning to realize that international cooperation in drug control, which in the past was an expression of solidarity, has now become a matter of urgent self-defence. . . .

In the past, distinctions were made between supplier and consumer countries. It is now widely realized that such distinctions no longer have any meaning: consumer countries have become supplier countries and vice versa. The term "transit countries" has also lost its original meaning: they, too, are quickly becoming consumer countries and may also become supplier countries. The simplistic view that suppressing illicit drug production in some "supplier countries" and/or reducing illicit drug demand in "consumer countries" will automatically lead to the solution of the drug problem is no longer valid, if indeed it ever was.

It is necessary, however, to keep in mind that demand reduction efforts cannot lead to success without substantially reducing the illicit drug supply: if drugs are readily available and easily accessible, new drug abusers will soon replace former ones. At the same time, there is evidence that elimination of a given drug from the market does not mean the elimination of the drug problem but only a shift towards other drugs or substances of abuse. Consequently, without efforts to reduce illicit drug demand, actions aimed at reducing illicit drug supply will lead to only temporary successes. . . .

Without reducing availability and access to drugs of abuse in general, it is not realistic to expect lasting successes from demand reduction efforts. The legalization of any drug of abuse leads necessarily to increased availability of that drug. This is one of the reasons for the strong position of the Board against such experiments. The Board appreciates the overall support of Governments for its position on that matter at the 1993 session of the Economic and Social Council and at the thirty-sixth session of the Commission on Narcotic Drugs. It notes with satisfaction that the option of legalization was rejected by all who spoke on the subject at the forty-eighth session of the General Assembly. The Board hopes that the Government of Italy will remedy the situation in that country created by the issuance of a decree in June 1993 repealing the prohibition of the non-medical use of drugs, which is not in line with the spirit of the international drug control treaties. The Board appreciates that Portugal and Spain have recently enacted legislation that strengthens measures to prevent the non-medical use of drugs.

These two long and authoritative quotations are included to demonstrate the major points of this chapter: First, the abuse of alcohol and other drugs is not limited to North America, it is a worldwide problem. Second, the global addiction problem is worsening at an alarming rate.

Case Histories

Terry comes from where the American heroin epidemic began, in urban minority communities, and where the drug epidemic increasingly has settled in the early 1990s, largely now around the use of crack cocaine. I wondered how Terry's life would have been different if his mother had access to regular drug tests. She might not have used drug tests because of her denial. But if she had, she would have seen his drug use early. Knowing her as I did, I suspect she would have acted strongly to end the drug use of her much-loved son. I am not sure what Terry would have done under these circumstances at age 16, but knowing how important his family is to him, he might have stopped using drugs at that point. Because no one did drug tests on Terry, of course, we will never know what might have been. It is hard to imagine it could have been worse than it became for Terry, his family, and our community.

Terry

An attorney called to ask me to serve as an expert witness in a case involving a claim that Terry was making against a local Department of Corrections. While he was in prison, Terry was the victim of a stabbing injury that left him paralyzed from the waist down. I met Terry in prison, when he guided his wheelchair into the interview room. He told a sad but common story. He was serving a 10-year sentence for murder, the result of his shooting a fellow drug user whom he felt owed him money from a drug deal that went bad. Terry, who was only 19 when the shooting took place, told me, "I didn't like this guy anyway, so when we met and he said he wasn't going to pay up, I threatened him. He put his hand in his pocket, so I shot him before he could shoot me. Later I found out he was reaching for some money. He didn't have a gun, but by the time I figured that out, he was dead. I felt nothing at all at the time since I was so high on PCP."

This was Terry's second period of incarceration related to his drug use, which had begun when he was 13. He was a rebellious young inmate seeking a reputation for being "cool." Terry was a smart, attractive youth, the son of a solid middle-class minority family. About a year after he started to serve his second sentence, he was watching a movie on TV one Saturday night. The lights were out when he felt two or three thumps in his back. He called out and looked around, but he couldn't see who hit him. Terry tried to get up, but he couldn't move his legs. He called out, "Hey, I've been stabbed. I need help!" He was taken to a nearby hospital, but there was no treatment that could repair his severed spinal cord. Terry told me, "Now I have to figure out what to do with my life from a wheelchair."

I asked Terry's mother about his drug use in the community. She said, "I never knew Terry was using drugs. He was just a happy but wild kid." I said to her, "But he was first arrested and sent to prison for drug use at 15." She replied, "He told me it was just once that he had used drugs, and that the police had manufactured the charges that he was selling drugs. He was always nice to me, and I believed him." This mother was a well-respected community leader and a smart woman. She was also a sufferer from the denial that is part of both codependence and addiction.

Terry won his case against the Department of Corrections based on a jury's finding that the state had an obligation to protect him from harm while he was in prison. I talked to Terry several more times about what he would do now. We developed a plan that pleased us both. He wanted to become a high school teacher. He figured he could do a pretty good job helping kids avoid drugs and the many troubles he had from his own drug use: "They will have to pay attention to me because I will be in this wheelchair. The other ex-addicts they see look so good that many kids figure that they too can get away with drug use for a while. They think, 'Sure it can be bad but it's fun and exciting, and when it's all over, I'll be a cool guy like this teacher.' Well, when they look at me they will have a hard time saying that they can always put drug problems behind them. I sure can't."

Terry and I talked about how his long prison sentence gave him time to study to get his college degree, something he had not been able to do when he was on the street "ripping and running." We also talked about feeling grateful for what had happened to him, about the fact that he was alive (unlike the man he had killed) and that he had an opportunity to help kids (so some of them, at least, might avoid the fate that otherwise awaited them as drug addicts). His injury was a blessing of sorts because it led directly to his new goals in life. He had no goals at all before the stabbing made him stop, think, and plan for his future.

In the following case history, Scott is as typical of his community as Terry is of his. His addiction was as malignant and his environment was as permissive and as codependent as Terry's. Although Scott spent a lot of time in prisons, he had not killed anyone, and he was not seriously wounded despite his many reckless binges of addiction. This said more about his luck than about his good sense, a fact that he and his parents were quick to acknowledge.

Scott

Mike, a local dentist, called me for help with his 19-year-old son, Scott, who was "out of control." Mike wanted to get Scott into a local Job Corps program and needed a doctor to vouch for his son. Scott dutifuliy came in to meet me so that I could write a letter on his behalf. He told a story of having been "wild" since grade school, "always in trouble." Scott was smart and attractive. The teachers initially liked him, and he was popular with both boys and girls in school from an early age. He never did his homework, and he began to skip classes in the 7th grade. He started to use alcohol and marijuana at that time and continued using them, adding cocaine in the 10th grade, when he finally left school for good. He had been arrested for theft and drug sales and had spent a year in a state prison.

He wanted to develop a trade and hoped to make "a new life" for himself in the Job Corps. Mike had a friend who was a national director of the Job Corps, so he had no trouble getting his son a place in a program on the West Coast "so he can get away from the drug-using friends he has in this area."

Scott lasted 4 weeks in the Job Corps before he was tossed out for fighting, which he claimed was racially motivated. Over the next 5 years I saw Scott occasionally, usually when his father or grandmother wanted help to get Scott into some new therapeutic program. He went to the finest drug treatment programs in our area and in other parts of the country. He had therapy, including a stay in a psychiatric hospital, where he was put on a wide variety of medicines for psychiatric problems, which allegedly included bipolar disease, or manic-depressive illness. None of these efforts seemed to change the downward course of Scott's life, but over these 5 years he did learn more about his disease, and he came to recognize that Narcotics Anonymous had a lot to offer him. Nevertheless, he repeatedly relapsed to drug use and got into trouble. His parents continued to do their best to save him from himself. When he got jobs they were often in sales, where his attractive appearance was an asset.

I was impressed over the years by Scott's many friends, including girlfriends. Some seemed to be crooks, but many were quite lovely, successful young women. Each was attracted to Scott's outgoing personality and his limitless self-confidence: Here was a young man who appeared to have the answers to life's myriad problems! I suspect they were also attracted to the side of him that needed help and that offered to whoever would respond the siren song of "You can help me. You are the one who, with your love, can save me!"

Section II

The Brain and Addiction

Having explored in Section I the story of this book and the basic workings of addiction, we dig deeper in Section II. First, in Chapter 4 we look at the brain and how it works. Why is the brain so vulnerable to the effects of alcohol and other drugs? Next, in Chapter 5 we examine the three most commonly abused drugs: alcohol, marijuana, and cocaine. In Chapter 6 we explore heroin and other major drugs of abuse such as LSD and PCP, as well as nicotine, the dependence-producing chemical in cigarettes.

Chapter 4

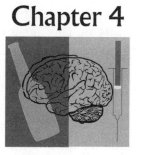

The Brain

Target Organ of Addiction

In this chapter, I explain how and why the brain can become addicted to feeling pleasure, even when that pleasure can be detrimental to the life of the addicted person.

ecause of the rapid progress in brain research during the

1980s, and in anticipation of accelerating progress to come, the

U.S. Senate and House of Representatives in the summer of 1989

passed a Joint Resolution declaring the period of 1990 to 2000 as the Decade of the Brain. Shortly thereafter, President George Bush signed a proclamation ratifying this designation.

One of the most promising aspects of the new brain research is the study of addiction. To understand how drugs work in the brain is to understand how the brain works. Drugs of abuse, as well as brain-altering medicines, produce their effects by traveling through the bloodstream to the brain, where they enter the brain cells. Each drug or medicine modifies the function of specific brain cells in unique ways. Nonmedical drug use distorts healthy brain functions, impairing the workings of the marvelous and fragile brain. A clear and sober brain thinks best. A brain high on alcohol and other drugs is a brain that is dysfunctional. Many of the ill effects of drug abuse on the brain persist, in some cases for a lifetime.

In the last two decades, the United States has invested billions of dollars in the fight against illegal drugs. Most of the money has gone to law enforcement and treatment, but hundreds of millions of dollars have been spent on research aimed at understanding how drugs work, from the physiology of the brain to the sociology of addiction. The study of abused drugs enhances the understanding of how useful medicines, such as antianxiety and antidepressant medicines, work. Painkillers, such as morphine, are a great blessing when used in medical treatment, but when used illicitly, they are a plague, showing that the way a drug is used is as important as its biology.

The human brain is a 3-pound gelatinous gray mass covered with deep wrinkles and connected to the rest of the body through the spinal cord and stringlike nerves that extend in an intricate web to every part of the body. Brain cells operate in a chemical bath maintained by the blood passing through and around them. Because the brain is exquisitely vulnerable to changes in this bath, the blood is separated from the brain by the blood-brain barrier, a filtering system that limits the movement of chemicals from the blood vessels into the brain.

The brain's principal fuels are oxygen, taken from the air by the lungs, and glucose, the sugar used by all of life as the most basic currency of energy, which comes from the food we eat. If the brain's supply of either oxygen or glucose is interrupted, even for a few seconds, consciousness is lost and in a few minutes the brain dies. Unlike other parts of the body, the brain does not regrow after injury. No other organ in the body is as sensitive to such brief interruptions in the supply of fuel. In addition to oxygen and glucose, some other chemicals pass from the blood to the brain through the blood-brain barrier, including abused drugs.

The brain produces neurotransmitters that affect adjacent nerve cells, and neurohormones that enter the blood supply and affect distant parts of the brain and other parts of the body. The brain is closely linked with the endocrine system, which produces hormones that control most bodily functions, and with the immune system, which protects the body against infection. The three integrated systems—the nervous, endocrine, and immune systems—are the principal guardians of the body's well-being and its ability to adapt to changing internal and external environments.

The Neuron—The Basic Cell of the Brain

The brain, the organ of the mind, is composed of billions of cells. Neuroscientists believe that in a single human brain there are between 100 billion and 1 trillion neurons, the fundamental cells in the brain, which were discovered just 100 years ago. The neuron is the fundamental building block of the network of nervous tissue in the brain and the nerves. It has three major parts: the *cell body,* the *axon,* and the *dendrites* (see Figure 4–1). The cell body contains genetic information in its nucleus as well as the metabolic engine for the neuron. The axon is the extension of the neuron that reaches out to make contact with other neurons to send messages. The dendrites are extensions of the neuron that receive messages from other nerve cells.

Chemical Messengers

Neurons send messages to each other across a minute space between the sending axon and the receiving dendrite. This tiny space is the *synapse.* When a message leaves a neuron, the swelling at the end of the axon releases chemicals into the synapse. These chemicals are stored in the axon in packets, called *synaptic vesicles*. For a signal to pass from one neuron to another in the brain, the sending axon must release chemicals into the synapse and the receiving dendrite must receive these specific neurotransmitters. The nerve impulse, received from another neuron, is sent along the dendrite through the cell body to the axon on to the next neuron in a continuous integrated electrochemical flow of messages. The neurons conserve energy by recycling the neurotransmitters released by their axons into the synapses. The neurotransmitters, having sent their messages, are taken back (*reuptake*) into the axon to be recycled again and again (see Figure 4–2).

Locks and Keys

A message can be sent only if the axon's neurotransmitter fits into the highly specific receptor site on the dendrite as a key fits into a lock. The neurotransmitters are keys. The locks, called *receptor sites*, are on the dendrites of the message-receiving nerve cells. The identification of this lock-and-key relationship, unique for each separate neurotransmitter in the brain, has been the central

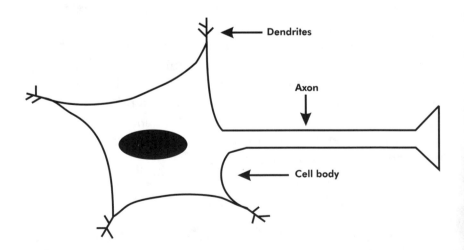

Figure 4–1.   The neuron.

discovery of neuroscience over the last two decades. The study of drug abuse has played an important role in this rapidly evolving science. Most drugs produce their effects by influencing specific lock-and-key complexes in the brain's synapses.

Each neurotransmitter in the brain is associated with specific brain areas or brain functions. Some neurotransmitters are relatively widespread in the brain, and others are more localized. Most synapses contain more than one neurotransmitter (key) and more than one type of receptor site (lock). The message is transmitted from the receiving dendrite through the nerve cell body to the sending axon as an electrochemical impulse that depends on the integrity of the entire nerve cell. Drugs that interfere with the cell membrane, as PCP, alcohol, and inhalants do, influence nerve cell transmission by a mechanism separate from drugs that affect the synapse.

Nerve cells have many, often subtle, influences on each other in complex networks, with some cells modifying the transmission from one neuron to another. Neurons primarily serve either excitatory or inhibitory roles in the brain. Drugs of abuse fit both categories. Some, called *stimulants,* such as amphetamines and cocaine, are primarily excitatory, whereas others, called *depres-*

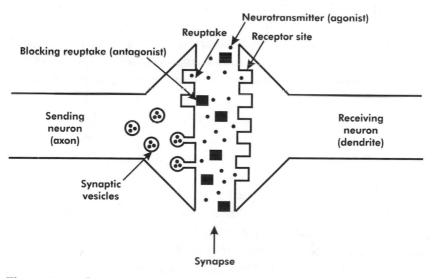

Figure 4–2.   Synaptic transmission.

sants, such as alcohol and the opiates, are primarily inhibitory. Reward, or pleasure, can be found by drug abusers from both stimulation and inhibition of particular groups of neurons in the brain.

The nervous system works as a balance of inhibitory and stimulant forces. Stimulating one side of the balance has a similar effect to inhibiting the other side. When it comes to drug abuse, the brain acts as if it seeks change, since many changes in feeling are experienced as desirable by drug abusers. Nonabusers of drugs do not like these changes of feeling. For example, the feeling of being drunk is attractive to alcohol abusers, but most people find it intensely unpleasant. Cigarette smoke makes nonsmokers sick, but smokers pay billions of dollars a year for the feelings nicotine produces.

Local and Long-Distance Messengers

Neurotransmitters work in the synapse in which they are produced. The brain also manufactures chemicals that carry messages to remote parts of the brain or to other parts of the body. Neurotransmitters are local messengers, moving across a single synapse to produce their effects. Hormones are long-distance messengers that are carried by the blood to act at distant sites in the body on organs other than the brain. The midbrain controls the functioning of the pituitary gland, the master gland located in the center of the head at the base of the brain. Hormones are sent out from the pituitary gland to manage vital body functions such as metabolism, sex, and reactions to stress through their effects on the thyroid, sex, and adrenal glands. This complex in the center of the brain is where pleasure and pain are handled, where hormones are managed by the pituitary gland, and where the brain controls all behavior. This is the final common pathway for all drugs of abuse.

Neurotransmitters are called *agonists* because they activate transmission across the synapse. The effects of specific neurotransmitters are blocked by equally specific *antagonists*, chemicals that block the receptor sites on the dendrites (see Figure 4–2). When the receptor site is occupied by an antagonist, the agonist (the external chemical stimulus or natural neurotransmitter activating that receptor site) cannot cause the nerve cell to transmit a message. Antagonists block the lock in the receiving dendrite, preventing the sending nerve cell's messenger, the neurotransmitter, from producing an effect. Scientists now use hundreds of agonists and antagonists, introduced into the blood or directly into specific parts of the brain, to study the brain in both health and disease.

Tolerance and Dependence

When a particular neurotransmitter system is excessively stimulated over a long period, the brain partially reestablishes an equilibrium by reducing the sensitivity of the particular neuroreceptors or by decreasing the number of these specific neuroreceptors. This is called down-regulation. There are limits to this process of adaptation, which is one mechanism of tolerance. This means that the more the brain is exposed to a chemical affecting a neurotransmitter over time, the less the brain responds to a particular dose of that chemical. Cigarette smokers do not commonly smoke more than 40 cigarettes (2 packs) a day, and alcoholics seldom drink more than about 10 ounces of pure alcohol (18 beers or a fifth of distilled liquor) a day, no matter how long they use these substances. The fact that people who are addicted to alcohol and other drugs do not use even more of these substances over time demonstrates the limits of drug tolerance.

Most nonusers are impressed by how much drug use tolerance permits. They cannot imagine liking the feelings produced by smoking 40 cigarettes a day or drinking 26 ounces of vodka a day. Tolerance is one of the most obvious effects of abused drugs. Addicted people use a lot more of a drug than do nondependent people, if nondependent people use it at all.

The other commonly observed effect of abused drugs is physical dependence. After everyday use of a drug for prolonged periods of time, when the drug use is abruptly stopped (sometimes called stopping "cold turkey" because "goose bumps" is a common symptom of withdrawal), there are withdrawal symptoms reflecting physical dependence. Both tolerance and physical dependence are caused by the brain becoming adapted to the regular presence of a chemical. Even though these two phenomena are apparent for many abused drugs, they are not the critical elements of the experience of addiction as is commonly thought. Both tolerance and physical dependence occur in response to most chemicals that affect the brain, whether they produce addiction or not. They reflect the brain's adaptation to a new chemical environment, one that includes the continuous presence, often at a high concentration, of a particular chemical. This traditional pharmacological definition of physical dependence is quite different from the use of the word *dependence* in the context of addiction. The narrower and older definition of dependence means that when the substance is removed, the user experiences withdrawal symptoms. The broader and newer definition of addiction reflects the fact that addicts depend on the use of self-destructive, pleasure-causing drugs to conduct their lives. Tolerance and withdrawal symptoms are not necessary for addiction to occur, although they sometimes occur in people who are addicted to alcohol and other drugs.

In this book, the distinction between physical dependence and addiction is made by using the term *physical dependence* for the narrower and older definition and *addiction* for the broader and newer definition. Physical dependence is the simple cellular adaptation of the body, especially the neurons in the brain, to the continued presence of a chemical that influences the function of the brain. In contrast, addiction is a complex, lifelong disease of the entire self.

This simplified explanation of how neurons work in the brain focuses on the synapse, the tiny but continuously active space between two neurons, one sending signals and the other receiving them. The activity in the synapse is affected by both abused drugs and psychoactive medicines. These chemicals enter the bloodstream, pass the blood-brain barrier, and become part of the chemical bath reaching all the synapses in the brain. Drugs influence a synapse in many ways. Psychoactive externally supplied chemicals facilitate or inhibit transmission between particular groups of axons and dendrites. Some chemicals act by blocking the reuptake or recycling of chemical messengers (neurotransmitters) from the synapse back to the sending axon. This is called *reuptake inhibition.* It facilitates transmission by prolonging the period the neurotransmitter stays in the synapse. Other drugs directly mimic neurotransmitters. They are agonists sending messages by themselves, fitting the lock on the dendrite in the synapse. Some drugs act as antagonists, blocking the effects of natural neurotransmitters or drug agonists. Many abused drugs produce their effects by more than one mechanism.

The Structure of the Brain

There are billions of neurons in the brain, which are interconnected in vast, continuously interactive networks. Although most neurons have only one axon, usually a relatively long extension of the cell, a single neuron may have as many as 10,000 dendrites. The dendrites of a single neuron can receive signals from the axons of thousands of different neurons. In the brain of a single person there are over 1 quadrillion synapses, more than the total number of humans who have lived since the brain evolved to its present form about 100,000 years ago. There are more different ways neurons can be linked through their synapses in a single human brain than there are atoms in the entire universe. Even in sleep the brain remains intensely active. Think for a moment about the complexity of this natural biological system, the human brain. It is not difficult to see why even today, with highly developed scientific techniques, the brain, especially the human brain, is the most challenging frontier of modern biology.

Glia—The Other Brain Cells

Neurons are not the only cells in the brain. The *glia* are even more numerous in the brain than the neurons. One kind of glia cell, the *oligodendrocytes,* are wrapped around the axon, providing a protective, insulating fatty sheath called *myelin.* When this protective sheath is lost, as in demyelinating diseases such as multiple sclerosis, nerve transmission is disrupted.

The *astrocytes* are the other major type of glia. These cells are essential to maintaining the blood-brain barrier that protects the neurons from disruption by many chemicals circulating in the blood. The glia also form the architecture or the structure of the brain. They are essential to the functioning of the neurons. Because the membranes that compose the blood-brain barrier are fatty substances, chemicals that dissolve easily in fat most easily pass through these membranes from the blood to the brain. Most substances eaten and taken into the blood are water soluble, and not fat soluble, so these chemicals do not reach the brain.

The kidney excretes water-soluble wastes from the blood. One key function of the liver is to modify fat-soluble chemicals to make them water soluble so that the kidney can excrete them more easily. This process of chemical breakdown is called *metabolism,* and the breakdown products are called *metabolites.* The delta-9-tetrahydrocannabinol (THC) in marijuana smoke is a good example of a fat-soluble abused drug. Alcohol is an unusual chemical because it is highly soluble in both water and fat.

Gray Matter, White Matter, and Dark Spots

Many neuron cell bodies, often dark gray, are located on the brain surface, making up the gray matter. The axons of these neurons, covered by white myelin, extend in pathways to connect with other groups of neurons throughout the central nervous system. These interlacing pathways are the white matter underlying the covering gray matter of the brain. The white pathways connect with other groups of gray cell bodies in various parts of the brain. Each of these separate collections of neuron cell bodies, dark spots in the white matter of the brain, fulfills a specific role.

The cerebellum at the back of the brain manages the body's movement and equilibrium, whereas the gray matter above the temples manages most voluntary muscle movement and speech. The central part of the brain has several areas with many cell bodies, or *nuclei,* managing the response to stress and pain and the experience of pleasure. These central gray areas are closely connected to the endocrine and immune systems.

Specific nuclei in the brain and their principal pathways are often served primarily by specific neurotransmitters. For example, the neurotransmitter dopamine is particularly important in the production of pleasure, including feeling high from nonmedical drug use. Central gray areas at the base of the brain that manage the experience of pleasure are the *nucleus accumbens* and the *ventral tegmental* area. They are connected by pathways responding to the neurotransmitter dopamine. The pleasure centers are closely connected to the pathways and the nuclei that manage pain, memory, and emotions as well as appetite, sex, fear, and anger. They are part of the brain's control center for behavior, so they are connected to the centers that manage movement and to the frontal cortex, the part of the brain that manages conscious thoughts (see Figure 4–3).

The brain areas that control pleasure, a major focus of this book, are the locations of the brain mechanisms of addiction. Ad-

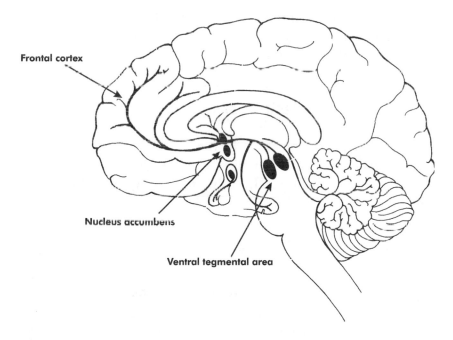

Frontal cortex

Nucleus accumbens

Ventral tegmental area

Figure 4–3.   A cross section of the human brain showing the projection from the ventral tegmental area (in the midbrain) to the nucleus accumbens and the frontal cortex. Addictive drugs produce their rewarding actions by increasing dopamine in the nucleus accumbens and ventral tegmental area.

diction, and other behaviors associated with appetites (such as feeding and sexual behavior), are primarily associated with the limbic system, the neuron network in the brain that manages feelings and emotions.

Neurochemistry

The first neurotransmitter was identified only 40 years ago. Today, scientists have identified over 60 neurotransmitters and speculate that there are 300 or more naturally occurring chemicals that are used by the neurons to send messages from one neuron to another. The first specific receptor identified was the opioid receptor discovered in 1972. Shortly thereafter the benzodiazepine receptor, the target of medicines such as Valium (diazepam) and Xanax (alprazolam), was identified. Brain cells are affected by everything that happens to the body: actions, thoughts, experiences, and the fabulous range of chemicals in the blood as well as the chemicals produced by the brain itself.

Three Neurotransmitters

This review focuses on three of the relatively well understood neurotransmitters, each of which has an important role in drug abuse: norepinephrine (NE), dopamine (DA), and the endorphins.

Three Major Neurotransmitters
- *Norepinephrine.*   Messenger for anger and fear, the flight-or-fight responses
- *Dopamine.*   Messenger for pleasure
- *Endorphins.*   Messenger for pain and stress

The catecholamines are a family of related chemicals based on the amino acid tyrosine, one of the fundamental building blocks of proteins. NE and DA, members of the catecholamine family, are major brain neurotransmitters. DA plays a role in the control of appetite and pleasure, including eating and sex. DA is the chemical that brings gusto to the brain. DA blockers are useful medicines in the treatment of schizophrenia, a major mental illness thought to be the result of excessive DA in certain brain areas. Parkinson's disease is associated with depletion of DA in the midbrain nucleus that controls fine movements and muscle tone. General DA depletion throughout the brain contributes to severe depression. Notice the range of brain activities associated with this single neurotransmitter, DA, from parkinsonism to schizophrenia and from depression to drug abuse.

Norepinephrine and Fear

NE is the neurotransmitter that governs the sympathetic nervous system, which is composed of the nerves that are not subject to voluntary control. These nerves manage the "flight-or-fight" response associated with the feelings of fear and anger. Fear stimulates the sympathetic nervous system as seen in increased heart rate, elevated blood pressure, and shutting down of the blood supply to the intestines so that blood flows to the muscles preparing for emergency action.

The NE neurotransmitter system that controls the sympathetic nervous system is found in all parts of the brain but in only 1% of the brain's synapses. More than half of the NE system is concentrated in two small areas associated with the alarm function of the brain, including the locus coeruleus, the central gray matter associated with panic attacks in agoraphobia. Some antidepressant medicines influence the NE system, with some of these medicines blocking the reuptake of NE in the synapse. These medicines also block the panic attacks associated with agoraphobia. Because depression is associated with NE deficiency, some chemicals that raise the level of NE in the synapse are effective antidepressants.

The Punch of Dopamine

Chemicals that influence the DA neurotransmitter system not surprisingly have many brain effects. Each chemical that affects the DA system does so in unique ways. For example, although cocaine and Thorazine (chlorpromazine), a medicine used to treat schizophrenia, both affect the brain's DA system, they do so in entirely different ways. Cocaine, which raises DA levels in the synapse, usually makes the symptoms of schizophrenia worse. Thorazine, which reduces DA, is not a substitute for cocaine in the lives of drug abusers, and they, like most other people, find the drug unpleasant. On the other hand, schizophrenic people, thought to suffer from DA excess, are seldom happy people. This observation highlights the important point that the DA system is not simple or uniform; it is made up of a wide range of subsystems of neurotransmitters and neuroreceptors. For this same reason, although most antianxiety medicines affect a single receptor complex, these medicines are not interchangeable, any more than painkillers or antidepressants are interchangeable, even though many of them affect the same basic receptor complexes in the brain.

Endorphins—Nature's Heroin

The third highlighted neurotransmitter is different from the closely related NE and DA, both of which are small chemicals called *amines*. In the 1970s, as scientists sought to understand how heroin, the model abused drug, affected the brain, they discovered the specific brain receptor for morphine, the core of the heroin molecule. Having found the opiate receptor lock in the brain, they searched for the natural neurotransmitter key that fits this lock in the synapses of the pleasure centers in the brain and elsewhere in the body. This neurotransmitter turned out to be not a simple chemical, like NE and DA, but a series of relatively long chains of protein building blocks, or peptides. This family of natural neurotransmitters is now known collectively as endogenous opioid peptides, or endorphins.

The three broad classes of endorphins are the brain's own

morphinelike substances, the natural neurotransmitters that fit the receptor lock that morphine fits. The endorphin brain system moderates pain, promotes pleasure, and manages reactions to stress. Today more than a dozen natural endorphins are known, and at least five different types of opioid receptors have been identified in the mammalian brain. Scientists have recently discovered additional neuropeptides that are also neurotransmitters, some of which do not involve the opioid receptors. Endorphins act not only as neurotransmitters but also as neurohormones (affecting nerve functioning at more distant brain sites to which they are carried by the blood) and as neuromodulators (natural chemicals modifying the workings of other neurotransmitters).

Endorphin receptors are found not only in the brain but in other parts of the body as well. This helps to explain why, although drugs of abuse are used by addicts for their effects on the pleasure centers of the brain, these drugs also affect many other parts of the body. Opioid receptors are prominent in the intestine, so that opiates not only cause addiction but also cause the gut to become quiet. For this reason, opioid drugs are used in the treatment of diarrhea as well as in the treatment of severe pain.

Drugs and the Brain

The effects of chemicals on the brain are determined by how much of the chemical reaches the brain. This is called the *dose response*. At very low levels of any drug there is no brain response. As the level of the chemical rises, the brain's responses not only increase but change, so that low levels of a drug produce one response and high levels produce different responses. The brain, continuously active and functioning as a single integrated unit, is influenced by all of the chemicals taken into the body that pass the blood-brain barrier. The rapidly changing concentrations of drug chemicals in the synapse are governed by the chemicals' concentration in the blood and by the body's ability to metabolize and eliminate them.

Roadways to the Brain

Drug users take drugs by one of several routes of administration. These routes include entry through the gastrointestinal tract for drugs taken by mouth and through the lungs for smoked drugs. Drugs can be injected with a hypodermic needle under the skin or directly into the bloodstream. A few drugs, such as cocaine, can be absorbed through the nasal membranes directly into the blood, a route of administration that is similar to injection under the skin but that does not require a needle and syringe. When drugs enter the body by smoking, they reach the brain within 8 seconds without first passing through the liver. This route of administration produces effects that are similar to injection of drugs into the vein (intravenous use), which produces initial brain effects in about 16 seconds.

The most intensely rewarding drug experience comes when the brain is hit by a high and rapidly rising level of drug chemicals. When chemicals are used for medical reasons—not to get high— they are usually taken orally to avoid the rapid rise and fall of blood levels that drug abusers avidly seek. A few medical psychoactive chemicals are taken by injection rather than by mouth, because these particular medicines are not absorbed efficiently from the gastrointestinal tract or are quickly metabolized by the liver. With few exceptions, psychoactive medicines, unlike abused drugs, are taken by mouth. When brain-affecting medicines are injected in medical treatments, they are injected into muscles or under the skin. When drug abusers inject drugs they inject into the vein.

Most psychoactive nonmedical drug use is by intravenous injection or smoking to get the most rapid rise to the highest level of the drug in the brain. This rapid rise is highly reinforcing because it is particularly effective in stimulating the brain's pleasure centers. This is why smoking and intravenous injection are the routes of administration chosen by addicted people and why these routes of administration are so much more addicting than is oral use of the same drug.

Alcohol: An Unusual Drug

Alcohol at first appears to be an exception to the general rule that addicted people take drugs by smoking or injection. A closer look

Medicines and Drugs

- *Medicines.* Medicines are usually taken orally to produce a slow rise and steady brain levels of the medicine, for example, taking 2 mg of Valium three times a day or taking 20 mg of Prozac once a day. The medicine-user's goal is to obtain relief from the distress of an illness and to function better in everyday life.

- *Drugs.* Drugs are usually taken by smoking, snorting, or injecting intravenously to produce a rapid rise and spiking brain levels of the substance, for example, snorting cocaine every 10 minutes for 3 hours or smoking marijuana for 2 hours in an evening. The drug user's goal is to get "high" or "to party" rather than to get relief from an illness. When addicts seek to excuse their behavior by calling it "self-medication," they mean that they seek to obliterate their negative feelings and to replace them with a euphoria in which they do not care about functioning in their everyday lives.

at drinking suggests this exception is more apparent than real. Nonalcoholic drinkers consume low doses of alcohol, often with food, which slows the absorption of the alcohol out of the intestines and into the bloodstream. This pattern of drinking produces a relatively slow rise to low brain levels of alcohol. Nonalcoholic drinkers purposefully consume alcohol in ways that avoid the "buzz" of rapid rises to high levels of alcohol in their blood. Alcoholics, in contrast, consume large amounts of alcohol on an empty stomach, drinking fast to achieve the rapidly rising, high brain levels typically sought by addicted people. The faster the rise of drugs in the blood, and the consequent rise of drugs in the brain, the more reinforcing is the drug use. Alcohol is unique because it is quickly and completely absorbed from the gastrointestinal tract, rapidly passing the blood-brain barrier. Even when taken by mouth, alcohol is relatively fast-acting, especially when taken on an empty stomach, compared with other orally consumed brain-affecting chemicals.

Searching for the Root of Addiction

Addiction to alcohol and other drugs involves the use of a drug nonmedically in such a way as to produce a high, leading to loss of control and denial. Alcoholics and drug addicts use "alcoholically" or "addictively," meaning that they use alcohol and other drugs in the ways that lovers behave: recklessly, irrationally, and impulsively. Often when people think about the roots of addiction they think of social or economic factors such as race or income, but the root of addiction lies far deeper than demographic characteristics. The root of addiction is in the human brain.

In the 1950s, Robert Heath, a brilliant researcher at Tulane University, sought to understand the brain mechanisms underlying the commonly observed lethargy of many people with chronic schizophrenia. He implanted electrodes into the brains of disturbed patients. To his surprise, he found that patients reported feelings of pleasure following stimulation of certain clusters of neurons at the base of the brain. This finding was particularly remarkable because the brain itself has no sensory nerve endings and cannot feel in the way other parts of the body do. Nonschizophrenic people reported the same experiences when stimulated in these specific brain areas, which led Heath to shift his study to brain-stimulated pleasure rather than schizophrenia.

Shortly thereafter, other researchers found that centers in the brain, located close to these pleasure centers, produced sensations of intense pain. When the pain centers, also deep in the midbrain, were stimulated by electrodes, experimental animals became disturbed. They would do almost anything to avoid stimulation of these particular areas of their brains. Both the pleasure and pain centers are collections of gray matter, clumps of neuron cell bodies, at the base of the brain in the center of the head.

Two researchers in Canada, James Olds and Peter Milner, found that rats with electrodes in their brains would work hard to get electrical stimulation of their pleasure centers. They worked just as hard to avoid electrical stimulation of their closely related pain centers. The rats hooked up to the electrical stimulation pressed the bars to get pleasurable shocks to the point of exhaustion, in preference to water, food, or even sex. When these experiments were extended to human subjects, they reported that electrical stimulation of the pleasure centers not only produced good feelings but changed their moods, producing a sense of well-being and euphoria. This experimental, direct stimulation of pleasure centers in their brains also reduced the sensitivity to pain and minimized the effects of abused drugs.

Brain Research

The line of research just described confirmed the observation made over half a century earlier by Sigmund Freud that "our entire psychical activity is bent upon producing pleasure and avoiding pain." Freud extended this observation by noting that human beings, who could think about probable consequences of their behaviors over a long period of time, did not simply act to seek immediate pleasure and avoid immediate pain but pursued long-term goals of maximizing pleasure and minimizing pain. He described this longer view as delayed gratification and attributed it to the mental mechanisms that manage human behavior, which he called the ego.

Addicts appear to be prominent exceptions to this rule. Addicted people act, with respect to their alcohol and other drug use, as if they were enslaved to immediate pleasure, despite the prospect of even catastrophic long-term negative consequences of their drug use. This finding led some Freudian psychoanalysts to describe addiction to alcohol and other drugs as an ego defect, a defect in self-care. Because addicts often lose their moral sense, psychoanalysts also described a deficit in addicts' consciences, labeled superego defects.

Scientists today use chemical probes of the brain, rather than electrical wires as were used by Heath and Olds, to stimulate or inhibit specific brain areas. There are pleasure and pain centers in the brains of all animals, including human beings. These centers are governed by the neurotransmitters that powerfully influence behavior. All the abused drugs, working in remarkably different ways, affect the midbrain pleasure centers.

This final common pathway explains why addicts use seemingly diverse drugs. By a wide variety of separate mechanisms, all abused drugs stimulate the pleasure centers of the brain and inhibit the brain's pain centers. It is this pleasure, and the reciprocal suppression of pain and distress, for which addicts strive. They are not too picky about the precise pharmacology of how they get this effect although, like all consumers, they are governed by habit, fashion, and price. When addicts change from one drug to another, such ordinary influences on consumer behaviors are usually the cause for the change, not pharmacology.

In the last decade, the work on the brain's reward mechanisms has become one of the most productive areas of neurophysiological study. There are three areas of the brain with DA-containing neurons. The first brain area includes both the ventral tegmental area and the nucleus accumbens, the principal pleasure centers. The second area is the *substantia nigra,* the largest cluster of DA-containing neurons in the brain. The substantia nigra manages movements. Depletion of the cells in the substantia nigra produces parkinsonism, a disease associated with muscular rigidity. The third DA-containing area of the brain, the *arcuate nucleus,* is a major pathway to the pituitary gland and the management of the body's hormonal balances and immune system.

The study of drugs of abuse has zeroed in on the first of these areas, the ventral tegmental area and the nucleus accumbens. These cells beat in unison, releasing DA in rhythmic pulses. Scientists have discovered that all drugs of abuse cause the neurons in this area of the brain to release relatively large amounts of DA into their synapses. Each drug of abuse does this by a different mechanism. Nicotine causes the same release of DA from the same cells of the ventral tegmental area and the nucleus accumbens as is caused by drugs as diverse as heroin, alcohol, and cocaine, although it does so by an entirely unique mechanism. More important, nicotine stimulates these cells without producing intoxication or impairment, as the drugs of abuse do.

Animal studies of brain mechanisms also have shown that if the axons connecting the ventral tegmental area with the nucleus accumbens are cut, an animal stops working to get drugs. If the animal is physically dependent on alcohol or another drug, the animal will show withdrawal symptoms, even with those particular nerve fibers cut. These experiments made clear that the animal's drug-using behavior is shaped primarily by reward, by the release of DA in the ventral tegmental area and the nucleus accumbens, not by withdrawal symptoms, because the animals stopped using drugs when the drugs did not produce reward even though stopping the use of the drugs still caused withdrawal symptoms.

Neurophysiologists wondered if these cells were stimulated by nondrug pleasures. Three dogs with probes in their nucleus accumbens were given meat bones, one of the most intense pleasure experiences for a dog. As expected, the dogs were excited and happy, but surprisingly researchers found no release of DA in the dogs' nucleus accumbens. Worried that they had failed to tap the correct spots in the dogs' brains, the researchers prepared three more dogs and repeated the experiment, using all six dogs.

The scientists were even more surprised to find that after giving juicy meat bones to all six dogs, the first three dogs now showed release of DA from the nucleus accumbens, but that none of the three dogs added to the experiment did. Repeated experiments showed that there was a learning in the brain following pleasure stimulation. Only after repeating the experience of intense pleasure did these particular brain cells release DA.

The brain pleasure centers had to learn to fire in response to particular stimuli. Even more remarkable, the scientists discovered that much of the DA release occurred before the dog actually began to chew on the meaty bone. As soon as the dog knew it was getting the bone, or even anticipated getting the bone based on prior rewarding experiences, the nucleus accumbens cells released pulses of DA. These experiments showed that reward centers required training by repeated experience. They were highly influenced by anticipation. These centers in the brain were appetite centers, producing strong feelings of pleasure based on past rewarding, stimulating experiences.

This line of research is profoundly important to understanding the working of the addicted brain. The specific part of the brain that responded to all addictive behaviors was turned on by a wide variety of drugs and by many nondrug rewards. The ventral tegmental area and the nucleus accumbens required repeated experience to trigger the pulsing release of DA. The anticipation of rewarding experiences, based on prior brain stimulation, was itself powerfully rewarding. Finally, these experiments showed that reward shaped addictive behavior, not withdrawal as had long been thought based on the experience of heroin addiction.

This research explains why drug abusers easily switch from one drug to another and why withdrawal is an inconstant feature of addiction rather than a crucial aspect of addiction. The different drugs use different mechanisms to produce the same basic brain reward. Behavior is shaped by the reward of drug use, not by the pain of withdrawal symptoms. These experiments also show why addictive behavior tends to be repetitive behavior and why anticipation of pleasure (the *set*, or the expectation of the drug user) is such an important part of the drug experience.

This important research into the brain's pleasure centers has not yet explained the differential risk of addiction of different people and the differential risk for particular individuals to addiction with different substances or behaviors. Some people are more likely to have food addictions; others are more likely to have alcohol or drug addictions. It is not as if a person had a single addictive risk, although some people do appear to be especially vulnerable to many addictive substances or behaviors.

Addiction reflects the DA-based pleasure/reward mechanisms of the brain as people (and other animals) repeat experiences that they find to be intensely pleasurable. There are many doors into the reward control room in the brain. Food and sex are natural doors, whereas alcohol and other drugs are chemical doors. For each person, I imagine that some particular doors to the control room are larger than are other doors. This is the reason that some people use alcohol and like it and others use alcohol and do not.

The first group has big alcohol doors to their pleasure centers, and the second group has small alcohol doors. The size of each hypothetical door, and the ease with which it is opened, is partly determined by genetic factors. Groups with large doors and groups with small doors both can be addicted to alcohol use and other addicting behaviors if they repeat the experience of reward often enough.

There are some ways to stimulate this part of the brain that are relatively safe and other ways that are inherently unsafe. The environment of the person experiencing pleasure and the values of that person have a major influence on the relative risk of addiction. The substance and the route of administration play major roles in determining relative risk for drugs of abuse. Addiction to alcohol and other drugs is rooted in biology, but addiction is a uniquely human experience that involves far more than brain chemistry.

In specific synapses of the brain, scientists at last discovered the behavior control room and began to explore how it works and what goes wrong in addiction. The new neurophysiology resonated with the new clinical understanding of the experience of addiction, offering important insights for both the prevention and the treatment of addiction. This book is titled *The Selfish Brain* because the biology of addiction is the central reality shaping the experience of addiction. The brain says "yes" to pleasure/reward. That experience of pleasure is rooted in the DA-containing neurons in the brain's ventral tegmental area and in the nucleus accumbens.

How important are the feelings produced by the brain's DA-containing pleasure centers when it comes to everyday behavior? Sex and feeding are the models for all pleasure-driven behaviors. What happens to sexual behavior when a person feels no reward from sex? It stops. I have seen this many times in my practice of psychiatry. When a person does not feel sexual pleasure, even with an intense effort of willpower, that person's sexual behavior stops. The same phenomenon takes place with eating. People who are profoundly depressed lose their capacity to experience pleasure. They often stop sexual behavior and eating. People who have exhausted their brain's pleasure system by abusing drugs also reduce both sex and eating. They commonly lose the normal ability to experience pleasure from anything at all, which is one reason that chronic addicts are so miserable.

Many behaviors are driven by this same process of seeking good feelings and avoiding bad feelings. Feelings of reward not only add depth and color to life but are absolutely necessary to life itself. It is no accident that the mechanisms of reward are universal and powerful in all animal species. That is why these mechanisms are hardwired into our brains and why they are so powerful.

Reinforcement and Punishment

Not only have chemists and anatomists been active in new brain research, but psychologists have been involved as well. Addiction is more than a chemical reaction in the brain. Psychologists describe three types of behavior-affecting stimuli: positive reinforcement, negative reinforcement, and punishment. A good feeling is positive reinforcement. When a hungry laboratory rat is given a food pellet after a specific behavior, this is positive reinforcement. Relief of a painful experience is a negative reinforcement. When a painful shock is stopped by a rat pressing a bar, the rat has received a negative reinforcement. Both positive and negative reinforcement are rewarding; they lead the animal (or the human) to repeat the experience. Both positive and negative reinforcement

Shaping Behavior
- *Positive reinforcement* produces pleasure.
- *Negative reinforcement* relieves pain.
- *Punishment* is painful stimulation.
- Both positive and negative reinforcement encourage behavior.
- Punishment discourages behavior.

need to be distinguished from aversive control or punishment. For example, when a rat receives a painful stimulus, such as an electrical shock after a particular behavior, this is punishment. It discourages the behavior with which it is associated.

All three behavior-shaping experiences are common for both animals and humans. They each have direct application to the experience of addiction. The pairing of pleasure and pain is mirrored in the brain's structure. Pleasure and pain centers in the brain are closely related and generally reciprocally linked in the brain. When heroin addicts take their drug, they not only feel pleasure or euphoria but also feel a waning of whatever negative sensations they were experiencing when they took the drug. Tension and depression, as well as pain and self doubt, are dissolved in the high of the heroin use. Many abused drugs also have important roles in medicine as painkillers. Medicines used to treat several painful mental illnesses, such as panic attacks, can also, at high doses, produce feelings of euphoria. This is no accident; it is the result of fundamental brain biology.

This linking of positive and negative reinforcement is also deeply connected to the common confusion, among physicians and the public, of the use of potentially abused medicines with drug abuse, as was seen earlier in the role of withdrawal in maintaining addiction. Withdrawal symptoms are distressing. Addicted animals, including humans, find relief from acute symptoms of withdrawal to be reinforcing or rewarding. Scientifically, but confusingly, this is called *negative reinforcement*, because it involves removal of a painful feeling.

One reason cigarette smokers find pleasure in their hourly lighting up of a cigarette is that the jolt of nicotine, which hits their brains within 8 seconds after the first puff, begins to relieve the withdrawal discomfort caused by the wearing off of the nicotine effect of the last cigarette as the nicotine levels in the smoker's brain fall below the level needed to sustain the effect they seek. That is also why the first cigarette in the morning is uniquely satisfying. Addicted smokers have gone for an unusually long time without a cigarette when they wake up in the morning, so nicotine withdrawal symptoms are relatively severe, and their relief after the start of the first cigarette of the day is particularly reinforcing. This is an example of negative reinforcement. It is seen universally in addiction to alcohol and other drugs.

Paths to the Pleasure Centers

Abused drugs directly affect the synapses in the pleasure centers. Many other activities and substances have an impact on the firing of the pleasure-producing neurons. These centers and the brain mechanisms involving pleasure and pain play a vital role in the everyday life of all animals. Food and sex are obvious stimuli for these centers in humans, but so are more mundane activities, from exercising and watching television to reading a good book or buying new clothes.

Understanding the biological basis of addiction requires putting the uncommon and often mysterious experiences of addiction to alcohol and other drugs into a more easily understandable perspective. Begin by thinking about nonchemical pleasures. Assuming that nonchemical pleasures are inherently safe is clearly wrong. Far too much human misery is caused by nondrug pleasurable experiences, such as eating and sex, to permit such a simple assumption.

Paths to the Brain's Pleasure Centers

- All substances and behaviors that produce pleasure stimulate the brain's pleasure centers, the ventral tegmental area and the nucleus accumbens.
- Each pathway to the brain's pleasure centers is unique, but all can produce addiction in people who are vulnerable.
- The major protections from addiction are lack of availability and cultural warnings about prohibited or dangerous activities.

Addiction involves principally two features: loss of control (unmanageability) and dishonesty (denial). Addicts have such strong and highly valued experiences with particular pleasurable activities that they put those sensations, those experiences, above everyday responsibilities and risk serious harm to themselves and others by pursuing their addictive pleasures. Addicts also lie about their behavior; they cover up and deceive others. Without these two features—loss of control and dishonesty—addiction cannot exist.

Making Excuses for Irrational Behavior

As a young resident in psychiatry, I attended a lecture on hypnotism that has stayed with me. I was fascinated when a professor hypnotized a patient in front of our class. He told the patient that 10 minutes after the patient came out of the hypnotic trance, he would go to the window and open it. The doctor gave the patient no reason to do this. It was a cold day, and the room in which the interview was taking place was cold.

The patient came out of the hypnotic trance and, after 10 minutes of general discussion with the professor, went to the window and opened it. The professor asked the patient why he had opened the window. The patient said, "I was hot and thought we would be more comfortable with the window open." The professor said, "But this is my office. Are you accustomed to opening other people's windows without asking them?" The patient politely replied, "No I'm not. I am sorry I didn't even think about asking your permission." Then the professor asked, "But it is cold in here now and it is even colder outside. Are you sure you want that window open?" The patient held his ground: "Yes, I am more comfortable with the window open right now, thank you."

As the professor explained that experiment to our group, he told us that the patient did not have any idea why he had opened the window. He was simply making up the most plausible excuses he could on the spot. Years later I thought of that experience as I saw hundreds of people addicted to alcohol and other drugs who sought to explain why they continued to use alcohol and other drugs despite the terrible things that often happened to them as a result of this use. Like the hypnotized patient, they did not know why they acted as they did. They simply made up excuses for what was irrational and self-destructive behavior.

The brain research on addiction has helped me to understand this mystery. People who are addicted act as if they were hypnotized, as if their pleasure centers, like the professor in the experiment, told them to do things in a voice that was not accessible to their conscious minds. So the addicts made up excuses that seemed to be as lame as that poor patient's excuses for opening the window on a cold day.

This is the process of denial. It is as if the disease of addiction whispered softly in the ear of the addict, "Do it again, right now. Go ahead. It's okay." Without consciously hearing the voice that gave the instructions, the addict acted as the voice directed. Even more mysteriously, denial can act to prevent the addict from seeing the addictive behavior at all. It is as if the hypnotic voice of the addictive disease said, "This is not happening at all. You are not doing it." It would be as if the patient in the experiment said, when challenged by the professor, "What window? I don't see a window. And if I did see a window, I can assure you that not only did I not open it, but I would positively refuse to open it. What do you take me for, a fool? Anyone can see that it is cold in here as well as cold outside today. Why did you even ask me such a ridiculous question?"

When you confront addicts about their addictive behavior, they deny it. Are they consciously lying, or are they deceived by their own disease? After many years of studying this fascinating process, I have concluded that the answer is "both." It is about as rewarding to ask addicts why they behave as they do as it was for that professor to ask that patient 30 years ago why he opened the window. To confirm once more the nature of the disease, I can ask the addicts I see in my practice why they continue to use alcohol and other drugs, but I no longer have hope of finding a useful answer to the question because I have learned that addicts have no idea why they are doing what they are doing when it comes to the use of alcohol and other drugs. Their reason, if they admit use at all, is usually "I do it because I like to do it." When asked why they lie about their use of addictive drugs, addicts give similarly direct answers that usually come down to, "Because if I told the truth, someone would try to stop me from using my drug."

Factors Influencing Addiction

Addicts act like people in love. They have lost control of their lives and become crazy in the pursuit of their particular addictive pleasures. The two most common traditional models for chemically produced addictions, heroin and alcohol, follow this pattern. Some people with eating disorders and some people with sexual addictions act in this same way. They live their lives with reckless disregard for social rules and for their own long-term self-interest, focusing only on immediate pleasure, despite the inescapable long-term pain that comes later.

Because loss of control over pleasure-driven behaviors is always a destructive pattern, and because it has been widely experienced in all societies at all times, every human culture has developed rules to govern all of the common pleasurable behaviors. These rules are seen in social conventions, in religions, in laws, and most especially in the family-based management of behaviors. Addicts not only have lost control of their lives, they not only deny their addiction-caused behaviors and the problems these behaviors cause, but they pursue their addictive behaviors in clear conflict with social norms, laws, and religious values. It is remarkable to see the ability of addiction to overcome even the most moral and sensible person. I have seen many physicians, teachers, ministers, and others of high intelligence and great moral strength turned into dishonest and irresponsible people by their addictions. Both they and those who know them well are amazed by this, because they underestimate the power of addiction to control human behavior, regardless of intelligence or character.

To produce an addictive behavior, the stimulus must be powerful. Relatively mild reinforcement will not produce this syndrome. Genetics plays an important role in vulnerability to addictions. Addictive behavior, often specific addictive behavior, to some extent runs in families. Age plays a powerful role. Most addictive behaviors are first evident in the teenage years and the early 20s. The risk of addiction is influenced by many other factors, from the availability of the particular pleasure-producing stimulus to the social tolerance for the addictive behavior. Pleasurable stimuli that are widely available and more tolerated are more likely to be problems than addictive stimuli that are less available and less tolerated in a society.

Protections Against Addiction

When we think of the role of brain biology in addiction, we need to keep in mind that the addicted brain exists in a social and historical context. The experience of addiction is part of a broad social reality. We can see addictive behavior in laboratory animals and observe that some stimuli are so seductive that almost all exposed animals lose control of their behaviors when they can self-administer a substance. Olds's rats were able to stimulate their pleasure centers, and monkeys used by other brain researchers were given access to cocaine intravenously. These animals all demonstrated addictive behavior in a simple, easily understood form based solely on brain biology. But in human populations, the experience of addiction to alcohol and other drugs is always more complex and far more interesting.

Sometimes people are protected from certain addictions by lack of exposure. Most North Americans today have never used or known anyone who has used heroin or cocaine, just as most people have never stuffed and vomited food (bulimia) or restricted the intake of food to a life-threatening degree (anorexia nervosa), syndromes that are serious, newly common eating disorders. Neither have most people gambled in a way that jeopardized their financial well-being. Sometimes people are protected from a particular addiction because they do not even consider such actions, and sometimes they are protected because they are not exposed to the behaviors or some aspect necessary for the behaviors (for example, hypodermic syringes containing heroin). Many people are protected by values and other cultural factors: "People like me don't do things like that." Most of us have been told not to engage in most addictive behaviors.

Often, our parents, teachers, and religious leaders tell us not to take risks with addiction. Some of us listen to that advice and others do not. Those who are not exposed or who have an inner values-based protection are relatively safe from addiction. Many of those who are exposed to particularly addictive behaviors, as most North Americans are these days to alcohol and tobacco, have a second level of defense. Some who try these behaviors are repelled or simply not interested in them. Some people do not like the taste of alcohol, or they find the experience of being drunk to be unpleasant. Many people are repelled by their first cigarette.

That initial repulsion, as well as the biologically based lack of reward from the initial experience with the addictive behavior, protects many people from addictions. People who are not protected by physical or psychological unavailability or by their lack of satisfaction with the addictive experience routinely progress to the first state of active addiction. This is where the mystery and the danger of this disease deepen.

Learning to Find Pleasure

Many of the most intensely pleasurable behaviors are not fun the first time even for people who become addicts. One must learn to get high or to have fun in addictive ways, the ways that the pleasure centers of the researchers' dogs learned to respond to meat bones. Typically, addicts learn by engaging in the addictive behavior with others who are doing it, usually those in their immediate friendship group. This sort of initiation is called "turning on" a friend. It involves teaching the person how to get high. This turning on is rarely, if ever, done out of meanness. It is done out of the enthusiasm the more experienced addicts feel for the pleasure that they have discovered and that they highly value. New drug users, who have yet to feel the full burden of their addictions, are the most likely to spread their addictive behavior because their enthusiasms are the most intense and their restraint is not limited by painful consequences of addiction.

Twenty-year heroin addicts over the age of 40 are not eager to turn on a 17-year-old neophyte. Neither are they attractive role models. Even with a good friend as a coach, people vary greatly, with some getting hooked quickly and others not getting hooked at all. Biology plays a major role in determining the level of reinforcement of a particular behavior. Some people have genetically large doors to their pleasure centers with particular potentially addictive stimuli. Others have small doors that are not easily opened to the same stimuli.

When I talk with addicts, I ask what their thoughts were the first time they used their favorite drug or first engaged in a particular addictive behavior. When the turning on occurred in early teenage years, and when the answer is, "It was like finding the most important thing in my life—something I had looked for but never found before," then I know the addiction is especially strong. When the answer is, "I did it for years and never had a problem, but then one day something happened and I lost control," I know the addiction is serious, but the chances of recovery are better, and the effort needed to get well is likely to be less.

Why Me?

Why do some people get addicted and others do not? Why do some people fall in love and others do not? Why does this person love that other one, whereas another person finds that one to be entirely uninteresting? There are no simple answers to these basic questions, but being in a receptive frame of mind, being in an encouraging environment, and being exposed to powerful brain-stimulating experiences go along with individual biological factors to shape the relative risk for particular addictive behaviors. Environmental and personal factors are both important in the addiction equation.

Another major factor in determining relative addiction risk is the behavior or the substance itself. Some substances and some behaviors are inherently more likely to produce intense pleasure than others. Prudent people, prudent families, and prudent communities limit these exposures, especially for youth under the age of about 25. They also erect clear boundaries so that those who have lost control can identify their affliction as early as possible. Trying heroin is a more risky behavior than is trying alcohol.

Smoking cocaine is more risky than snorting it. Frequent use of a drug is more risky than occasional use. For people with high addiction potentials, however, a single use of a particular drug can be addictive, and for people with low addiction potentials, even repeated intensive use of some drugs can fail to throw the addiction switch to "on."

The Myth of Self-Medication

The drug abuser's behavior has sometimes been explained as an attempt to self-medicate. Self-medication means the use of intoxicating drugs (such as alcohol, cocaine, and heroin) to treat unpleasant feelings (such as severe anxiety, depression, or pain) that result from an illness. Although distress from an illness may be a reason some addicts first came in contact with a particular non-medical drug, I am skeptical of the self-medication hypothesis as an explanation for persistent addictive behavior. Drug abusers do not abuse any medicine that does not produce reward or reinforcement. For example, people do not abuse arthritis medicines or antibiotics, two effective and commonly used classes of medicines that reduce distress. People with panic disorder do not abuse antidepressants even though they block panic attacks. Drug abusers do, however, abuse stimulants and narcotics. The reasons certain drugs are abused, but most medicines are not, has nothing to do with self-medication and everything to do with feelings produced in the brain's pleasure centers.

For people who have infections and arthritis, both of which can be terribly painful, the medicines used to treat their diseases are powerful. Once people with these diseases understand the importance of specific treatments, they are highly motivated to use the medicines. This is not self-medication, and these medicines have no appeal to drug abusers. Such medical patients, if they are denied access to their pain-relieving medicines, will exhibit "drug-seeking behavior" in the sense that they will take steps to ensure that they get the medicines they need. When drug addicts and alcoholics talk of self-medication, they refer only to their use of abused drugs such as alcohol and cocaine, never to routine, nonabused medicines such as antibiotics or antiarthritic medicines.

Because of my own professional involvement with both addiction and the anxiety disorders, I am drawn to the more complex aspects of the self-medication controversy in addiction, using anxiety as an example. Most clinically anxious people fear loss of control, so they do not drink alcohol or, if they do drink, they use alcohol exceedingly moderately. On the other hand, some people who suffer from anxiety disorders do use alcohol and find that it reduces their painful panic and anxiety, at least for an hour or so following alcohol use. A small percentage of all anxious patients get trapped in their use of alcohol, escalating their alcohol use over time in an alcoholic pattern.

Some anxious people become dependent on alcohol, using it in repeated doses throughout the day (*maintenance drinking*), and some anxious people use alcohol in a bingelike pattern (*binge drinking*). Most anxious patients who continue to demonstrate either of these patterns of alcoholic drinking when their drinking persists once the anxiety disorder has been treated have a family history of alcoholism. This makes it apparent that these people found not just brief symptomatic relief from their anxiety in the alcohol, but reward, or a high, with which they literally fell in love. It was the reward that produced the addiction, not the antianxiety effects of the alcohol.

Addicted anxious patients show the typical alcoholic pattern, which is easily distinguished from the common drinking behavior of the typical nonaddicted sufferer from an anxiety disorder. For these alcoholic people, their anxiety disorder does not explain their addiction to alcohol or other drugs, but occasionally it does explain how they became involved with alcohol in the first place.

The relationship of addiction to anxiety disorders is more complex than this initial picture suggests. Alcohol reduces anxiety only in the short run. Over hours, and even more over days and weeks, alcohol makes panic and anxiety worse. In fact, many alcoholics and addicts to other drugs, as part of their addiction, become clinically anxious, even sometimes suffering from panic attacks and other specific anxiety disorders. For most such addicted and anxious people, simply stopping drinking (which usually requires a program of lifelong recovery in Alcoholics

Anonymous) will terminate the symptoms of their anxiety disorder. In other words, for these alcoholic people, their anxiety disorder is secondary to their addiction in that their anxiety problem followed their addiction. Once the primary addiction to alcohol is under control, the secondary anxiety disorder diminishes or even disappears.

Anxiety disorders can also be used by addicts as an excuse for their addictions. Even worse, this connection of alcoholism and anxiety can be an excuse for physicians who prescribe addicting drugs to people who are addicted to alcohol and other drugs in the mistaken belief that such treatment will improve both their anxiety and their addiction. When anxiety coexists with addiction, I suggest considering the addiction to be the primary disease when it comes to treatment.

Addicts regularly speak of using drugs to "feel normal." This is the result of their having so disturbed the normal function of the pleasure centers in their brains that they feel lousy without their alcohol or other drugs. Nevertheless, the drugs that addicts seek for purposes of self-medication are the drugs that stimulate the brain's pleasure centers. Usually this drug-using behavior is simply addictive behavior hiding behind the rationalization of self-medication.

Whether the bad feeling being "treated" by the addicted person is anxiety, depression, anger, pain, or some other intensely unpleasant state, or whether the bad feelings are the result of prior drug use (as is commonly the case with hangover from drinking alcohol or withdrawal from heroin use), the reason the addicted person is using alcohol and other drugs over a prolonged period of time can be traced to the person's love affair with getting high, not to the discomfort of a preexisting disease. People who are not vulnerable biologically to addiction, and who experience anxiety, depression, pain, and other uncomfortable feelings, do not become addicted to alcohol and other abused drugs, even if they are exposed to them and find some temporary relief from their discomfort as a result of their use of these substances.

Although called pleasure, the drug high bears little relationship to the joys of stamp collecting, climbing a mountain, or talking with a friend. The drug user's high is far more intense and gripping—it is much closer to the experience of sexual orgasm or eating a large meal than it is to visiting an art museum. The drug high is a primitive profound brain stimulation, a sledgehammer blow to the brain's normally subtle pleasure system. Self-medication simply does not explain the experience of persistent use of addicting drugs despite the problems that this use typically causes addicted people.

Brain biology offers a useful way to think about the self-medication hypothesis of addictive drug use. Anxiety and panic are governed by the locus coeruleus in the brain stem. When the ventral tegmental area and the nucleus accumbens in the midbrain, the principal pleasure centers, are stimulated, they send signals to quiet the locus coeruleus. When an addicted person experiences physical withdrawal, the locus coeruleus sends out distressing alarm signals for days, making sleep difficult or impossible and producing profoundly uncomfortable anxiety and even panic attacks.

Drugs that stimulate the ventral tegmental area and the nucleus accumbens, as all addicting drugs do, calm the locus coeruleus. Once addiction has taken hold in the brain, when addicting drug use stops, the locus coeruleus is sent into action, helping to produce the painful withdrawal syndrome. With repeated alcohol and other drug use over time, the pleasure centers of the brain require more and more stimulation to produce pleasure, raising the risks of withdrawal when drug levels fall in the brain. What started as a self-controlled search for pleasure, and relief of discomfort from an anxiety or other mental or physical disorder, increasingly becomes a desperate out-of-control search for a feeling of normality, a way of escaping the brain's distressing alarm mechanism managed by the locus coeruleus.

For most people who do not have a preexisting vulnerability to addiction, the process of using addictive drugs to suppress uncomfortable feelings is short-lived as they learn that the stimulation of the brain's pleasure centers by the nonmedical use of drugs from alcohol to heroin is a fool's game. At best, they get short-term gains at the price of long-term disasters. For most nonalcoholic drinkers, one hangover or one episode of uncomfortable intoxication is enough to convince them that large doses of alcohol and other drugs are, in the end, no fun at all. In contrast, people who are biologically vulnerable to addiction are seduced in the process of repeated nonmedical drug use into persistent addictive behaviors despite the problems their alcohol and other drug use causes. For addiction-prone people, it is often difficult to sort out the positive rewards of addictive drug use (the pleasure from the stimulation of the pleasure centers of their brains) from the negative rewards (the relief of discomfort from the quieting of the locus coeruleus whether it is stimulated by withdrawal or an underlying mental disorder).

The All-Too-Human Disorder of Addiction

Addiction is a human disorder that can afflict anyone. No one is immune to addiction. Any pleasurable action can be addictive, meaning it can lead to loss of control and dishonesty. There are some simple, and old-fashioned, guidelines that protect people from addictions. The antidote to addiction is honesty with respect to alcohol and other drug use. That approach is fairly easy for most nonaddicted people to understand and even to practice. It is difficult for addicts to practice because the addiction has taken hold of their brains and has induced distortions in their thinking, including dishonesty. They rationalize their addictive behaviors to protect the forbidden fun of their addictive alcohol and other drugs use. When a person gets well from any addiction, the inner experience is similar to a person being released from slavery, the experience of a prisoner being freed from captivity. The slavery of addiction is especially painful, humiliating, and cruel because it appears to be self-imposed. Addiction is all the more mysterious because this awesome misery is a "pleasure disease" that makes addicts and those who love them miserable and because addicted people remain vulnerable to relapse throughout their lives.

Case Histories

Here are two stories about the use of prescription medicines that have abuse potentials, and about the boundaries of addictive behaviors.

Jeb

Jeb is a conscientious, 47-year-old, single scientist working for the federal government. He came to me for help with obsessive-compulsive disorder (OCD) because of his continuing morbid fear that when driving his car he had accidentally run over a pedestrian. He was a cautious driver with an unblemished driving record. Nevertheless, his unrealistic fear led to his driving around the block over and over again to check for "bodies." On many occasions when he came home from work, even after repeated checks to see if he had run over anyone, he could only get a bit of relief from these intrusive, unwanted, repugnant thoughts, which he knew were unreasonable, by watching the local news to see if there was a report of a hit-and-run victim being found on his commuting route. He did well in therapy with a combination of antianxiety and antiobsessional medicines.

As therapy progressed, he told me about his alcoholism. I was surprised by his labeling of himself as an alcoholic because his character was about as far from that of a typical addict as it is possible to be. He was not a risk taker. He was conscientious to a fault. He was introverted and barely social. He explained that he had started to drink in college, "when everyone was doing it," and that in his 30s his drinking had increased in a pattern he called "self-medication." He would often drink one or two beers when he got home from work late in the evening. He often experienced social insecurity on the infrequent occasions when he went out in the evenings with friends, saying he often drank "way too much," often five or six beers, for example. After each of these episodes, he felt sick the next morning with a hangover and swore to stop drinking in the future. He did not have a close relative who was addicted to alcohol or other drugs.

About 8 years ago a friend of Jeb's went into a local addiction treatment program and came out talking about what a big improvement this had produced in his life. Jeb thought more about his own drinking. He admitted himself to the addiction treatment program, which he found generally helpful, and stayed 7 weeks. He went to a lot of AA meetings and defined himself as a chronic alcoholic who self-medicated with alcohol for his anxiety symptoms. He stopped going to AA shortly after leaving the treatment program. He had never relapsed to alcohol use since then, although he guiltily told me he had sipped an aperitif with the family of his girlfriend one evening several years ago. He did not crave alcohol; he had no interest in ever drinking again and made no effort whatsoever to control or contain his desire to drink because he had no such desire.

I asked Jeb about how he used his antianxiety medicine. He said he often took a dose at 7 A.M. when he got up and then used one or two additional doses as the day progressed. His use of medicines was very moderate, in low doses, and it showed no tendency to escalate over many years of treatment. His use of medicines improved his life and did not lead to his relapsing to alcohol use. The medicine did not lose its effectiveness. He had never in his life used any other drug nonmedically (such as marijuana or cocaine). I asked Jeb if he ever self-medicated with alcohol the way he used his antianxiety medicine, starting in the morning and using it at low doses throughout the day. He said, "No. I never even thought of that. I didn't want to be impaired at work or when I drove." I asked if he ever self-medicated on the weekends, morning, noon, and night, when he was often quite anxious with his OCD. He said, "No. That's not how I ever drank or even thought of drinking." I asked him about the comparative effectiveness of alcohol and his antianxiety medicine in terms of his anxiety. He said the alcohol blotted out his feelings entirely, whereas the antianxiety medicine just made him worry less, but did not reduce his ability to drive, work, or think clearly.

Jeb's pattern of drinking was not normal. He clearly had a tendency to drink too much on the rare occasions when he drank at parties, but he never had an adverse result of his drinking (such as blackouts, accidents, arrests, loss of work, strained relationships), and he never drank in settings other than those commonly used for social drinking. If he was self-medicating with alcohol, it was a pattern that was easily distinguished from the pattern in which he used antianxiety medicine, as were the effects of alcohol use easily distinguished from those of his antianxiety medicine use. Jeb's use of the antianxiety medicine also was not the way active drug abusers treat these medicines. Addicts tend to use antianxiety medicines at high and unstable doses, and to mix them right in with their heavy use of other drugs nonmedically, most often alcohol, marijuana, and cocaine.

Was Jeb an alcoholic? I am not sure, but I would not label him an alcoholic despite the abnormality of his drinking. The fact that he did not go to AA meetings once he was out of treatment and did not seem to need meetings to stay abstinent reinforces this view. On the other hand, it was clearly helpful to Jeb to think of himself as an alcoholic. His public identification as an alcoholic was helpful to the many people he worked with and knew socially, since it encouraged them to look at their own drinking skeptically and to view treatment for addiction positively. It is also possible that I am wrong and that Jeb is an alcoholic whose repeated self-identification as an alcoholic is vital to his maintaining his sobriety. In the spirit of "if it ain't broke, don't fix it," I listened respectfully to Jeb's happy story of recovery and congratulated him on his success in overcoming this problem.

Timmy

Timmy was a 37-year-old chronic heroin addict whose mother paid for him to see me. When he missed an appointment one day, I called him at home. He said, "Oh, gosh Doc, I misplaced your appointment card and I thought I was to see you later in the week." He had pawned some family heirlooms, ancient dueling pistols, he had taken out of his mother's home. He needed to get them back before they were sold by the pawnshop. He wondered if his mother would pay for this debt, especially since he had already gotten money from her to buy the same items back from the same pawnshop 6 months before. He knew he was a liar, but he also knew his mother was codependent. He was sure that, when he told his mother how deeply he cared about these old dueling pistols and how mean the pawnbroker was, she would do what she had done thousands of times before. She would scold him, get him to say he was sorry and would never do it again, and then give him the money he asked for.

That did not surprise me, but what did surprise me in this conversation was Timmy's description of his own codependence. His girlfriend, Julie, was also a heroin addict, but she also liked to abuse antianxiety medicines such as Xanax and Valium. She wanted Timmy to give her $10 and drive her to a downtown public mental health clinic so that she could buy some pills that were sold on the street outside the clinic by patients who got them from their doctors inside the clinic. Julie would take large doses of the pills orally and then pass out in a drunken stupor for several hours. Timmy lamented his own weakness in repeatedly doing this for Julie, even though he knew it was a waste of their scarce money (neither worked) and it did her no good. Julie sometimes got her own pills to abuse, going to doctors and saying that she was anxious and had panic attacks and that these medicines helped her a lot. But when she got prescriptions herself, the medicines were relatively expensive to get at the pharmacies, and the doctors wanted to be paid in advance for visits to them. Julie found it was cheaper to buy the pills on the street, which were provided to welfare patients on Medicaid, than to get the drugs from private physicians, but both approaches worked well for her.

Julie's pattern of abuse of antianxiety medicines contrasts clearly with the pattern of medical use of these same substances by Jeb. Julie's experience also raises red flags for all doctors when it comes to the use of controlled substances in medical practice. For the social contract for drug use to work, physicians must know their patients and be able to distinguish addicted patients from physically dependent pseudoaddicts. Both the medical and nonmedical use of controlled substances reflect the workings of these chemicals in the human brain.

Chapter 5

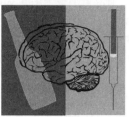

Gateway Drugs

Alcohol, Marijuana, and Cocaine

In this chapter, I review the drugs that usually initiate addiction—alcohol, marijuana, and cocaine—and focus on where they come from, how they have been used and abused, and how their use damages the body, mind, and spirit.

The introduction to the brain in Chapter 4 focused on the synapse, the tiny gap between nerve cells that is open to blood-supplied chemicals. Now we look at the most commonly used drugs of abuse to see how they affect the brain. This is called the drug's *mode of action*. It is the science of psychopharmacology. In this chapter we explore the three most widely used intoxicating drugs: alcohol, marijuana, and cocaine. These three drugs are called the *gateway drugs* because they commonly form the gateways into the use of other, less commonly used drugs of abuse. Most drug users begin with alcohol and then, if they are to progress further into addiction, proceed to use marijuana and, later, cocaine. In Chapter 6 we explore the use of heroin and several other dangerous drugs of abuse, including LSD, Ecstasy, and PCP. (See Drug Facts on page 491 for a short summary of the most commonly abused drugs.)

The most important drugs of abuse are alcohol, marijuana, cocaine, and heroin. The first three of these drugs are the focus of this chapter, and heroin is discussed in Chapter 6. During the 20th century, at an accelerating tempo, chemists have created an awesome number of molecules that are not found in nature but that have the capacity to produce brain reward and, therefore, addiction. Synthetic stimulants, including amphetamines and methamphetamines, and synthetic depressants, including the barbiturates, have been widely used in medicine for more than half a century. Synthetic stimulant drugs have much in common with cocaine. Synthetic depressants have much in common with alcohol.

Although thousands of chemicals can function in the brain as drugs, in the sense that they produce pleasure and intoxication, most drug problems throughout the world are caused by alcohol, marijuana, cocaine, and heroin, four relatively old and familiar drugs, and by a few other drugs that are closely related to them. Of these four drugs, only alcohol is swallowed and only alcohol use is legal anywhere in the world, and even alcohol use is not legal in the United States for people under the age of 21. All four of these drugs are easily produced with little chemical sophistication from natural agricultural products available throughout the world.

Alcohol and Other Depressants

Alcohol, a liquid, is swallowed. It is not smoked, snorted, or injected as many other drugs are taken into the body. Alcohol, although the simplest psychoactive chemical, produces highly complex effects on the brain and the body. Alcohol changes the neurons' membrane and opens the chloride and potassium channels at the synapse. Epinephrine concentrations in the blood rise after alcohol use, accounting for the raised heart rate and blood pressure following alcohol use. Alcohol affects the gamma-aminobutyric acid (GABA) system, producing quieting of the brain and temporarily reducing worry and tension. GABA is one of the brain's principal neurotransmitters, being particularly involved in the inhibition of stimulation. The GABA system suppresses the locus coeruleus, blocking intense anxiety and panic. That is why the benzodiazepines, which reinforce the GABA system, are effective in suppressing panic attacks. Alcohol does this much less well because it is short-acting, so that the initial quieting of the GABA neurotransmitter system and the locus coeruleus is rapidly replaced by overstimulation of these brain mechanisms as the blood alcohol level declines in the hours immediately after a drinking episode ends. Alcohol also affects the dopamine, norepinephrine, and serotonin neurotransmitter systems in the brain.

The effects of alcohol vary with dose levels. Some effects are even reversed with chronic alcohol use. Because alcohol is rapidly metabolized, withdrawal effects, which are opposite to the effects of intoxication, are seen a few hours after alcohol use stops. Although acute alcohol use has a quieting effect that reduces anxiety, the alcohol withdrawal effect is the opposite, with brain excitation and anxiety being prominent features. Alcohol withdrawal causes insomnia and sometimes epileptic seizures, expressions of pathological brain excitation following alcohol's initial brain quieting.

Because alcohol, like cocaine, heroin, and nicotine, is a short-acting substance, the heavy alcohol user is continually exposed to alternating intoxication and withdrawal effects that produce long-term disruption of brain functions. Alcohol can promote sleep shortly after use, but a few hours later, when the acute effects are replaced by withdrawal effects, the alcohol withdrawal actually creates anxiety and sleeplessness as well as nightmares. Following everyday drinking, especially drinking throughout the day (the way cigarette smokers consume nicotine), if drinking abruptly stops, the drinker can go into a severe withdrawal syndrome known as *delirium tremens* (DTs). This is a potentially fatal disease, including high fever, hallucinations (such as seeing pink elephants on the walls), and epileptic seizures. DTs are more commonly seen in maintenance drinking than in binge drinking.

Numbing the Brain

Alcohol is a depressant drug. Moderate use of alcohol leads to relaxation and lessening of inhibitions. Alcohol first affects the higher functions of the brain, including those managing self-observation and self-criticism. For this reason, drinkers feel relaxed and uninhibited, even as they sometimes say and do things that they later find embarrassing. Anger is often released after even relatively small doses of alcohol. It is common to find that routine evening alcohol drinkers, even when drinking fairly small amounts, become hard to live with as the evening wears on and they drink more and more. This is not normal drinking. Reasonable social drinking produces no negative effects at all. When evening drinking produces changed moods and behaviors, such as anger and irritability, it means that the line has been crossed into alcohol abuse. It signals the need for an intervention leading to treatment as described in Chapter 10.

In higher doses, alcohol can produce lack of coordination and digestive upsets, particularly vomiting, since alcohol irritates the lining of the stomach and triggers the brain's vomiting mechanism. Alcohol's role in body heat loss can be deceptively dangerous in situations in which hypothermia, or loss of normal body heat, may develop. Alcohol at first swallow gives a warm glow as blood flows to the skin, but the resulting heat loss, masked by alcohol's anesthetic effects, can have dire consequences that may prove fatal in cold environments. In even larger doses, alcohol can cause blackouts, periods when the alcohol user looks and acts more or less normal, although intoxicated. After blackouts, however, alcohol users have no memories of what happened to them during the blackout period. Blackouts are an early and relatively common symptom of excessive drinking.

Loss of consciousness after drinking large amounts of alcohol—"passing out"—can be extremely dangerous if vomiting occurs while the drinker is unconscious, because the vomited stomach contents can be inhaled into the lungs of the intoxicated person, producing asphyxiation or life-threatening pneumonia as stomach acid literally digests vulnerable lung tissues. Long-term use of alcohol leads to liver damage, internal bleeding, and, ultimately, brain damage. Alcohol use is highly correlated with the abuse of other drugs and with many types of cancer. Because many heavy drinkers also smoke cigarettes, the fact that heavy alcohol use multiplies the cancer risks of smoking is especially serious. The tetrahydrocannabinol in marijuana suppresses vomiting. Because many marijuana smokers also drink heavily, and because vomiting after heavy drinking can save the drinker's life by eliminating alcohol from the stomach, marijuana smoking can raise the risk of a fatal alcohol overdose.

The United States government's report, *Alcohol and Health*, from the Department of Health and Human Services summarizes the effects of alcohol on the body this way: "The range of medical

Alcohol

- The only drug containing calories
- The oldest and most commonly used intoxicant in the world
- Taken orally
- Rapidly absorbed and distributed to all cells in the body
- Metabolized to carbon dioxide and water in a few hours
- Produces few health effects in low doses, but produces severe health problems with high doses and after prolonged regular use
- Both the safest and the most harm-producing intoxicant

consequences of alcohol abuse is both immense and complex—virtually no part of the body is spared the effects of excessive alcohol consumption." The catalog of ill effects of drinking begins with the liver, the body's chemical factory, which is hit first by alcohol taken into the body through the stomach. The liver is the primary place where alcohol is metabolized (broken down) into carbon dioxide and water. Damage to the liver from drinking, which usually becomes severe after 10 or more years of heavy drinking, comes in three types: fatty liver, where yellow fat replaces normal red liver tissue; alcoholic hepatitis, when the liver is acutely inflamed and often seriously malfunctioning, with jaundice (the skin and the whites of the eyes turn yellow) as a common symptom; and finally, cirrhosis of the liver. Both fatty liver and alcoholic hepatitis may be reversible if the person stops drinking, but relapses to drinking can be disastrous to the liver.

With both fatty liver and alcoholic hepatitis, the liver is often enlarged, extending below the ribs on the right side of the body into the abdomen. The third sort of alcohol-caused damage is the chronic state following both fatty liver and alcoholic hepatitis, cirrhosis of the liver. In this end-stage disease, the fatty tissue and the normal liver tissue are both replaced by white scar tissue. This liver disease is not reversible, although when the person stops drinking, the cirrhosis (scarring) process may not progress further. The cirrhotic liver is small and does not work well to clean the blood, so jaundice, severe blood poisoning, and blockage of the blood supply from the intestines are common symptoms of this progressive and fatal disease. Chronic liver disease, including cirrhosis, is the ninth leading cause of death in the United States, reflecting a high level of alcohol abuse.

In the gastrointestinal tract, alcohol is a severe irritant, causing inflammation of the esophagus and stomach, often worsening peptic ulcer disease. Excessive drinking is a major cause of acute and chronic inflammation of the pancreas. Acute pancreatitis is one of the most painful of all diseases, producing an unrelenting knifelike pain in the middle abdomen between the rib cage and the belly button. This is an acute, recurrent disease that can be fatal. Heavy long-term drinking is often combined with nutritional diseases, leading to a variety of brain degenerations, including paralysis of nerves and memory deficits, many of which are not reversible once drinking stops.

Alcohol abuse also leads to anemia (loss of red blood cells) and a variety of cardiovascular diseases, including high blood pressure and stroke, as well as increased risk of heart attacks. Alcohol can also lead to degeneration of the heart muscle with the result that the heart no longer pumps efficiently. Chronic alcohol abuse is a significant contributor to cancer of the mouth, esophagus, stomach, larynx, liver, and lung. (See Chapter 9 for guidelines on how much alcohol is too much.)

The alcohol blocker Antabuse (disulfiram), introduced into medical practice in 1948, temporarily poisons the liver enzyme needed to metabolize alcohol to carbon dioxide and water. It allows the buildup of acetaldehyde, an intermediary metabolic product, in the drinker's body. Acetaldehyde is toxic and causes flushing of the skin, headaches, stomachaches, and elevated blood pressure. If a person drinks a lot of alcohol, Antabuse can even cause death. The alcoholic seeking motivation to avoid alcohol use needs to take Antabuse only once a day, usually in the morning when the determination not to drink is relatively high. Later in the day, when temptation to drink typically rises, the drinker is protected by Antabuse because of the fear of illness or death from drinking alcohol after using Antabuse. Because Antabuse poisons enzymes in the body for quite a while, the person must stop Antabuse use for 1 to 2 weeks before drinking alcohol; otherwise, disturbing and potentially dangerous symptoms are likely to result from drinking alcohol.

There are two serious problems with the use of Antabuse to treat alcoholism. The first is that it is specific for alcohol, which makes it possible for alcoholics to use other drugs and get high even when they take Antabuse. For example, they can use closely related medicines such as Xanax and Valium, or they can take quite different substances such as cocaine or marijuana and get high despite taking Antabuse. The second problem is that alcoholics can simply stop taking Antabuse. The people most familiar with alcoholism, those in Alcoholics Anonymous, generally take a dim view of treating alcoholism with Antabuse because it does not deal with the alcoholic as a whole person.

Antabuse treatment does not lead to long-term recovery. At best, Antabuse provides a relatively brief period when the alcoholic can get alcohol out of his or her brain and make some long-term decisions about getting well. I have found that Antabuse does not lead to recovery unless the alcoholic attends meetings of AA or NA. If Antabuse is used with psychotherapy, I have rarely seen it lead to prolonged, stable recovery from addiction. In fact, like psychotherapy for addicted people, it can become a "cover" for continued addiction as alcoholics delude those around them into a false sense that the problem of alcohol addiction is under control.

In 1995 the Food and Drug Administration (FDA) approved the use of naltrexone (ReVia) as a part of a comprehensive treatment of alcohol dependence. Naltrexone works by blocking the opioid receptor system that may play a role in the reinforcement of alcohol use. In two recent studies, the use of this medicine reduced craving for alcohol and relapse by about 50% during the 12 weeks of the studies. Although it is too early to know the ultimate place of this medicine, which had previously been used to treat heroin addicts (see page 198), in the treatment of alcohol dependence, naltrexone appears to offer new hope for at least some alcoholics. Equally importantly, the introduction of naltrexone underlines the importance of the new brain biology in the treatment of addictive disease.

Measuring Alcohol Intoxication

Acute intoxication after drinking results from alcohol traveling from the stomach and the intestines through the bloodstream past the liver and finally to the brain. The level of alcohol in the blood is called the blood alcohol concentration (BAC). To understand the relationship of drinking to the BAC, you need to know that all alcoholic beverages contain the same ethyl alcohol. The only important differences between one form of alcohol and any other for health are the concentration of alcohol in the drink. The other substances in the drink, mostly flavorings to disguise the generally unpleasant taste of alcohol, have little or no health effects. One 12-ounce can of beer contains about 0.5 ounce of pure ethyl alcohol. About 5 ounces of wine and about 1.5 ounces of distilled spirits (whiskey, rum, or vodka, for example) also contain about 0.5 ounce of pure alcohol. Each of these amounts of alcohol is considered equal to one drink. Thus, three beers is equal to about 15 ounces of wine, or about half a bottle of wine. This is also equal to three ordinary mixed drinks, assuming each drink contains about one 1.5-ounce sized jigger of distilled spirits.

When a person drinks alcohol, the alcohol is distributed more or less evenly throughout the person's body. Larger people (e.g., those who weigh more) have bigger bodies in which to dilute the alcohol they drink, and therefore their BAC is lower after each drink they take than is the BAC in people who weigh less. Many other factors influence BAC levels. For example, women generally metabolize alcohol less rapidly than men do, so their BACs tend to be higher even when they weigh the same. The biggest factors governing BAC, however, are not gender or weight, but how much a person drinks and how long after the drink is consumed the BAC is checked. This is because the liver is efficient at metabolizing alcohol. The liver can break down one drink of alcohol (0.5 ounce) into carbon dioxide and water in about an hour and a half.

A 160-pound man who drinks a great deal of alcohol in an hour has a BAC about as follows: after two drinks, 0.02%; three drinks, 0.05%; and four drinks, 0.07%. A 120-pound woman has a BAC after two drinks of 0.04%; three drinks, 0.06%, and four drinks, 0.09% (see Figure 5–1). The liver drops the BAC by about 0.015% per hour after drinking stops. It is unusual for normal social drinkers to get their BAC to over 0.05%. If a person were to drink one or two drinks over the course of a 2-hour period, a typical social drinking pattern, the BAC would never be greater than about 0.03%. Assuming that the person then had dinner with one glass of wine, by the end of the evening, approximately 4 hours from the start of the first drink, the BAC would be 0.03% or less. If that same person drank five drinks in 1 hour—not many nonalcoholics can do that, even if they try—the BAC would be about 0.07% 5 hours later if the person had no more to drink after that time.

Several years ago I worked with a group of judges who were away at a retreat, so no one was driving after dinner. We set up a

Breathalyzer and had them check their BACs at various times during the cocktail hour, during dinner, and then at the end of dinner. They were amazed at how low their BACs were even when they felt somewhat intoxicated immediately after drinking. None had even one reading of 0.08% or higher. They were surprised because the legal limit for driving in most of the United States today is 0.10%. When they had seen people in their courts with BACs in excess of this number, they assumed that they had had one or two drinks in the evening before being picked up by the police, be-

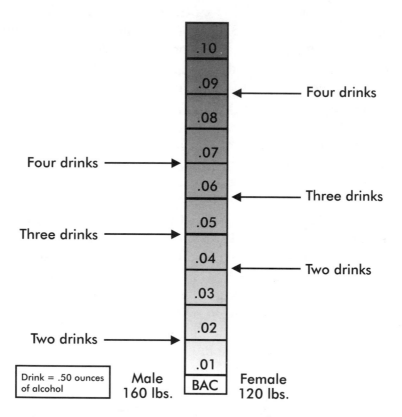

Figure 5–1.   Number of drinks and blood alcohol concentration (BAC) in 1 hour of drinking.

Source.   U.S. Department of Transportation, National Highway Traffic Safety Administration. *Improving Understanding of Alcohol Impairment and BAC Levels, and Their Relationship to Highway Accidents* (DOT HS-807-433). Washington, DC, U.S. Department of Transportation, 1989.

cause that is what the drunk drivers told them. The average number of drinks consumed by people picked up for drunk driving by the police is about 13 in the 5 hours before their arrest. Such drinking cannot be defined as "social" or "responsible" drinking.

In a recent study of new alcohol testing equipment, several of my colleagues gave alcohol to experienced alcohol-drinking college students who were at least 21 years old. We gave them as many drinks as they felt comfortable drinking in a safe setting, a hotel hospitality room. Over a 3-hour period these students drank three to five drinks each. None of them got a BAC of more than 0.05% at any time of the study. We asked the students how they would have felt if we had asked them to drink enough alcohol to get to a BAC of 0.10%. None felt they could have done that without feeling ill. As it was, one woman felt so drunk that she feared for how she would have driven a car right after drinking.

We did not let any of these students leave the test site until their BACs returned to below 0.02%, which took about 2 hours after they stopped drinking. This experiment was a confirmation that the current standard for impairment on the highway of 0.10% or even 0.08% is substantially too high. Normal social drinkers, even when they drink more than they feel comfortable drinking, do not get BACs into this range. When someone has a BAC of 0.08% or higher, that person is a heavy drinker who has drunk a large amount of alcohol immediately before the test.

Although the amount of alcohol consumed and the time over which it is consumed are the major determinants of the BAC, the presence or absence of food in the stomach is another important factor in determining BACs because food absorbs alcohol and slows absorption, thus giving the liver more time to break down the alcohol. Social drinkers often drink small amounts of alcohol usually with food to keep their BACs low because they do not like the intoxication caused by high BACs.

The effect produced by any level of BAC is different for different people. Inexperienced drinkers are often profoundly impaired with BACs of 0.05% or so, whereas experienced heavy drinkers can appear normal with BACs of 0.10% or higher. This is not because the livers of experienced drinkers are better at metabolizing the alcohol, but because their brains have learned to function reasonably with alcohol present. This is called *state-dependent learning*. It means the person has become accustomed to functioning with a drug in the brain. This is mostly a learning effect, not a metabolic effect. Young and inexperienced drinkers have severe behavioral effects far below the legal cutoff of 0.10% for drunkenness on the highway. Although heavy drinkers can appear normal in routine settings, they, like inexperienced drinkers, are not safe behind the wheels of cars if they have a BAC above about 0.04%.

The levels set for legal limits on the highways are averages and may not reflect the actual levels of impairment from alcohol seen in individuals, because there is so much variation in alcohol's effects. Even more variable is the effect of impairment from alcohol and other drugs in relation to specific tasks. When people are expected to do something routine they can often do it with a fairly high BAC, but when they are confronted with a divided attention task (e.g., adjusting their radio while still keeping track of what is happening on the highway in front of them) and when they are confronted by an unfamiliar experience (e.g., a biker unexpectedly entering the highway from a driveway), they are often profoundly impaired even with relatively low BACs.

One important paradox of chronic, heavy drinking is that alcoholics and other heavy drinkers can generally "hold their liquor," meaning that they show relatively minor effects from heavy drinking. But when their livers become adversely affected by their drinking, as often happens after years of heavy drinking, their livers do not metabolize the alcohol (or any other chemical) effectively. Then their alcohol sensitivity goes up, not only compared with their own previous prodigious abilities to drink but even compared with inexperienced drinkers. Alcoholics can be drunk and stay drunk for hours after one or two beers once their livers are damaged. This saves them a lot of money, but it is a terrible prognostic sign. Usually such increased sensitivity to alcohol means that death from irreversible liver failure is close at hand.

Any alcohol in the bloodstream is associated with impaired performance. For that reason, the U.S. Department of Transportation has set 0.02% as the maximum allowable level for commercial drivers. As recently as 10 years ago, some states had legal BAC levels as high as 0.15% for all drivers. Today, in states across the country, the permissible level of alcohol in the blood for driving is falling. The best social policy is to keep the nation's roads and highways drug and alcohol free. That means that, as a practical matter, the maximum permissible BAC should be 0.02% or less. In the United States we are now watching the social contract with respect to alcohol drinking change from the standard that one should not drive "drunk" to a better standard that a person should not drive within several hours after drinking alcohol.

My simple standard, outlined in more detail in Chapter 9, is that one should not drink more than two to three drinks in any 24-hour period and that one should not drive within 4 hours of the last drink. This will ensure that the BAC is well below 0.02% before driving. Heavy drinkers do not know how much they drink, so they often state, sometimes with complete innocence, that they only had "a few beers," when their BAC is 0.10% or higher.

I am reminded of a minister who was arrested for driving while impaired (DWI). Her BAC was 0.12%. She told me that she had had "no more than three drinks the entire evening." She was so upset with the arresting police officer that she argued with him and finally hit him, leading to an additional criminal charge of striking an officer. This was totally out of character for this generally calm and self-controlled woman. She was shocked when I reviewed with her the facts about BACs. She too suffered from denial, once more making the point that addiction distorts the thinking of all people.

In contrast to heavy drinkers who regularly understate their use of alcohol and its impairing effects on them, including their ability to drive a car, many inexperienced drinkers and most ordinary social drinkers not only feel impaired after one or two drinks, but they are afraid to drive for fear that they will be picked up by the police for drunk driving. This is a socially useful fear because it contributes to their drinking less, especially when they will be driving. However, in one sense, it is an unrealistic fear. Even if such people had an automobile accident and were taken by a police officer for a blood alcohol test, they would be passed as not impaired by alcohol because their BACs would be so low, far below the current minimum standard of 0.08% and even below the future standard of 0.04%. On the other hand, most of these inexperienced drinkers are impaired by low doses of alcohol, so their fears are well founded. No alcohol use before driving, which is the universal standard in Europe today, is the best policy.

The Alcohol Paradox: Safest and Most Destructive

Alcohol holds the apparently paradoxical position of being legal for adults in North America and throughout the non-Muslim world and at the same time being the world's most devastating drug. Alcohol is relatively safe, compared with most illegal drugs, but its wide use and relative social acceptance produce high social and medical costs. Why is alcohol so much more widely used than any other abused chemical, and why, despite its apparently safe use by many people, does alcohol cause more problems (in terms both of health and behavior) than all other intoxicating drugs combined?

The basic picture of addiction explains these apparent paradoxes. Alcohol is the most easily manufactured intoxicating drug, being made by simple fermentation of sugar. For this reason, alcohol production was discovered in virtually all early human societies (except the Eskimos, who lacked a supply of carbohydrates, including sugar). Alcohol is used orally, which somewhat limits its reinforcing properties. Until the discovery of distillation in the modern era, alcohol concentration was limited to that produced by wine (about 11%) or beer (about 5%) through natural fermentation.

Thus, almost all human populations have a long history of alcohol use and relatively well-developed cultural means of limiting alcohol's problems. Nevertheless, the introduction of distilled spirits had profoundly destructive effects in all societies when it first occurred, as described in Chapter 2.

Alcohol is the world's most abused drug because it is the world's most socially tolerated drug. Alcohol was used by 103 million Americans in 1991, whereas only 12 million used marijuana, the second most widely used intoxicating drug. Alcohol is more widely tolerated than any other drug, not because it is safe but because it is somewhat safer than most of the other drugs. Even more important, alcohol is more familiar than other drugs to most people in all parts of the world. Alcohol produces the most harm of any intoxicating drug because it is the most widely used drug.

When the social costs of alcohol use are related to the extent of use, it is the least problem-generating intoxicating drug on a per-use basis. But because alcohol use is so extensive, it produces the highest total social costs of any drug. Alcohol is generally the first drug that young people use. It is thus the ultimate gateway drug.

When any family, community, or nation attempts to deal with the problems of intoxicating drugs, alcohol must be a central focus of those efforts. The United States ranks midway between the high-consumption wine-drinking nations of southern Europe and such low-consumption nations as Algeria, Morocco, and Thailand.

When I speak to sophisticated North American high school and college students, some of whom oppose the restrictions of the 21-year-old legal drinking age for alcohol, I can count on one of the students to bring up the fact that there is no minimum legal drinking age in Europe. Anyone of any age can buy and use alcohol. According to these skeptical students, the youth of Europe have far fewer problems with alcohol than do their North American peers. This argument appears to go easily to the next step. It is the prohibition of youthful drinking in North America—and the "mistrust" that underlies it—that causes teenage drinking problems. How could the solution to this problem be simpler? Eliminate the drinking age and, presto, there will be fewer youthful drinking problems in North America! The logic here is as breathtaking as I have found it to be commonplace. Writ larger, this is a central argument used by advocates of fully legal drugs. In this misguided view, it is the prohibition of drugs that causes drug problems. Therefore, get rid of the prohibition and we can solve our alcohol and drug problems.

Before responding to this critique of current North American alcohol and drug policies, we need to have a few facts. Prohibition in North America came about because of the problems created by the use of addicting substances, not the other way around. The biggest cause of problems with alcohol and other drugs is not prohibition. It is the effects of the drugs themselves. In every situation, in every nation, prohibition reduces drug use and legalization raises drug use. It is both unbelievable and totally without foundation in experience anywhere in the world that legalizing drug use, or any other act of increasing acceptance of drug use, would have any effect other than increasing drug use and increasing the problems caused by that drug use. Reducing the drinking age or, even worse, eliminating it entirely would increase youthful use of alcohol, not reduce it.

Problems such as teenage drunk driving deaths would go up if alcohol use by youth were legalized in North America. The national experience with a decade in which the American drinking age for alcohol was reduced to 18 (roughly 1974 to 1984) was a clear lesson on this point. Drunk driving deaths for teenagers rose. When the legal drinking age was returned to 21, where it had been in the United States since 1933, teenage drunk driving deaths fell.

There is an important point buried in this common question: Why is it that Europe does not have legal drinking ages and yet has fewer adolescent drinking problems than now occur in the United States? The answer is that most European communities have fewer automobiles, and those they have are less likely to be driven by teenagers. Additionally, Europeans have had far tighter family and community controls over teenagers than do communities in the United States. European communities have not had the tradition of youthful peer group drunkenness and illegal drug use that has become commonplace in North America over the last three decades. Europe has a driving age of 18, in contrast to the usual North American age of 16 or, in some places, even 15.

The global cultural drift is toward the American model of teenage use of alcohol and other drugs. Today European youth are experiencing increasing levels of abuse of illicit drugs and alcohol. It is not difficult to predict that within a decade or less there will be far tighter legal and other formal controls on youthful drinking in Europe than exist today. Exchange students with whom I have talked make this point clearly. They see far more unsupervised peer drinking and drug use in the United States than in Europe, and they also see increasing evidence of the American pattern emerging in Europe. There are sound historical and biological reasons to restrict drinking of alcohol and smoking of cigarettes for teenagers.

When societies have tight controls over adolescent behavior, based on widely observed family and community values, it is less important to place legal controls over drinking and drug use by teenagers. To the extent that any community moves toward the modern high-risk approach to the teenage years—with looser adult supervision and greater socializing among adolescent peers—then there is a greater need for legal and other formal limitations on adolescent behaviors that are clearly destructive both to the youths themselves and to their communities.

As one 45-year-old woman patient of mine who grew up in the South American country of Colombia said,

> When I grew up, I was under my parents' watchful eyes every minute of the day. Now my teenage daughter, who is growing up in the United States, is free to go and come as she pleases, without the close, continuous oversight I had. She has risks that I never had. I do not begrudge her this freedom. I want her to have it, as I wanted it for myself. But I also see how hazardous it is for her and her friends.

It is not just alcohol; of course, drugs and sex also play big roles in the high-risk modern teenage lifestyle.

North American youth who want to adopt the European system for the alcohol drinking age might think twice about trading positions with their European peers who cannot drive until the age of 18, and who face during their entire lives a highway standard that calls for no alcohol in the blood of drivers of any age. Europeans are generally not as tough as North Americans on the drinking age issue, but they are a lot tougher when it comes to drinking behind the wheel of an automobile, for both youth and adults.

Alcohol as Medicine

In the heyday of patent medicines at the end of the 19th century, drugs of abuse were common ingredients in concoctions sold for virtually every imaginable ache or pain. This was no accident. Drugs of abuse produce powerful effects on the brain, including the effect of reward. They suppress pain. The brain is organized so that pleasure and pain are reciprocals. What produces pain reduces pleasure; what produces pleasure reduces pain. Many of the most powerful painkillers are abused drugs. In addition, some pleasure-producing drugs also cause physical dependence, which keeps the customer coming back, the way nicotine dependence sustains the sales of cigarettes.

Alcohol was a mainstay of patent medicines 100 years ago. In an era of growing hostility to nonmedical alcohol use, especially alcohol use by women, patent medicines were a relatively available source of the euphoric and analgesic effects of alcohol. Before the Pure Food and Drug Act of 1906 required labeling of all substances sold as medicines, the buyers of patent medicines had no way of knowing that alcohol was a major ingredient in the products they bought.

Today, alcohol is used commonly in over-the-counter medicines as a liquid in which to dissolve other substances. The amount of alcohol contained in these products is usually small, although it can cause problems, especially for alcoholics. Alcohol itself is not thought of as a medicine today. It is not prescribed by physicians, largely because alcohol lacks any specific medical benefit, and because it is likely to be abused. There were three primary indications for the past use of alcohol as a medicine: it was used as a painkiller, as a sleep-inducer, and as an antianxiety agent. Today there are safer medicines for all these indications. Nevertheless, recovering alcoholics, especially those taking the alcohol-blocking agent Antabuse, should read the labels of over-the-counter medicines carefully because some use alcohol as a solvent. The increasingly common label on over-the-counter preparations, "alcohol free," is a reminder of the history of alcohol's past role as a medicine.

Other Depressants

In the same way that stimulant drugs stimulate the central nervous system generally, so the depressant drugs depress the brain generally. These drugs work in a variety of ways to slow down brain processes. In medicine, depressants can calm someone who is pathologically stimulated (as in an anxiety disorder or epilepsy). These can be desirable effects, as can depressant use as part of anesthesia before surgery. Depressants also can reduce fear and cause amnesia as part of surgical anesthesia.

The depressants are used in medicine to treat anxiety and insomnia. The barbiturates were the most commonly used depressants until the 1960s, when the benzodiazepines replaced them in medical practice. Alcohol has many effects similar to those of the barbiturates and the benzodiazepines, but because it has no medical use and is by far the most widely used intoxicant in the world, it is treated separately in this chapter. Alcohol has a far shorter duration of action than either the barbiturates or the benzodiazepines, underscoring the role of pharmacology in determining abuse liability.

The whipsaw: intoxication and withdrawal. In overdose situations, depressants can suppress the brain so profoundly that consciousness is lost and breathing stops. During the first half of the 20th century, the barbiturates were widely used in outpatient medicine to treat insomnia and anxiety. They were a common cause of deaths from suicide throughout the industrial world. When depressants are abruptly discontinued after prolonged, everyday use, there is an overshooting of opposite effects associated with withdrawal—a pathological brain stimulation. When chronic nonmedical use of a stimulant is stopped abruptly, the drug abuser is exhausted and often sleeps for long periods of time. In contrast, when chronic nonmedical use of a depressant is abruptly stopped, the drug abuser often is pathologically stimulated. Anxiety, insomnia, and even epileptic seizures are common depressant withdrawal effects. Stimulant users after use of the drugs appear wired or uptight, whereas depressant users appear slowed down, drunk, or sleepy immediately after drug use.

For both stimulants and depressants, the effects of drug use are reversed during the hours or days after everyday use stops, during the withdrawal period. Therefore, depressants cause mental depression immediately after use but rebound or withdrawal stimulation after the depressant use stops. One of the most common signs of cocaine use in the workplace is sleepiness and lethargy, the withdrawal symptoms following acute overstimulation by cocaine.

Marijuana

Marijuana, or pot, is a plant product, like tobacco, and it is usually smoked, although it can also be swallowed. Marijuana is not injected or snorted as cocaine and heroin often are. Marijuana, unlike alcohol, cocaine, and heroin, is not a specific single chemical. Marijuana is a crude drug, a complex chemical slush. All four of the most commonly abused drugs in the world are simple agriculturally produced substances with long histories. Before the last half of the 19th century, these drugs were used by people in relatively simple and traditional ways. For example, cocaine was used by chewing the coca leaf, and opiates were consumed as opium, the dried sap of the opium poppy. Since the advent of modern chemistry, however, cocaine has been purified and has totally displaced coca leaf chewing, except for a few South Americans living in the Andes Mountains who continue to chew coca leaves. In the 20th century, heroin has replaced opium use throughout the world.

In contrast, marijuana is still widely used as a crude agricultural drug of abuse. The leaves and flowering tops of the plant *Cannabis sativa* typically are smoked. This plant comes in three forms: the drug plant, the hemp plant, and the intermediate plant. The common hemp plant contains little drug, but the drug plant contains large concentrations of psychoactive chemicals. Cannabis is available to drug users in three forms. Marijuana is the leaves and stems of the plant. It looks like common dried spice or herb leaves, much like dried parsley. Hashish is the resin of the cannabis plant. Hashish resin is dried and compressed into balls, cakes, or cookielike shapes. Hash oil is the concentrated chemicals in the hashish. It looks like motor oil.

The major cause of the high of marijuana is delta-9-tetrahydrocannabinol (THC), which is found in relatively high concentrations (roughly 1% to 6%) in the marijuana used by drug abusers. Hashish contains similar concentrations of THC, but hash oil can be 20% or more pure THC. Marijuana and hashish contain over 420 different chemicals, which fall into 18 different chemical families. Of these chemicals, THC is the major one that produces the high. THC is one of 61 chemicals in marijuana that are cannabinoids, or chemicals found only in the marijuana plant. Another common cannabinoid is cannabidiol, which, like all of the cannabinoids, is biologically active, meaning it affects the body of the marijuana user even though cannabidiol does not cause a high.

Once the marijuana is smoked, users inhale more than 2,000 different chemicals into their lungs to be taken in their bloodstreams to all the cells of their bodies. In terms of the complexity of the chemical exposure for the users, marijuana is unlike alcohol, cocaine, or heroin because it is a crude, not a pure, drug.

THC is highly soluble in fats, so it rapidly passes the blood-brain barrier. This property, combined with THC's insolubility in water, results in the unusually long retention of THC in the brain and other fat-containing tissues of the body. THC is trapped in the body's organs that use fatty building blocks, such as the brain and the reproductive glands. It is not quickly carried away by the water-based bloodstream as are water-soluble drugs. This means that THC persists in the brain and reproductive organs for days or even weeks after the drug was last used.

THC increases the heart rate and raises the blood pressure by stimulating the norepinephrine (NE) neurotransmitter system. THC can cause panic attacks and trigger agoraphobia among vulnerable people, presumably by this same mechanism. Other physical effects of marijuana use include increased hunger (called "the munchies" by marijuana users) and thirst, bloodshot eyes, and dilated pupils.

In high doses, THC can produce short-term or prolonged psychosis, supporting the view that the serotonin system of neurotransmitters also is affected by marijuana. It is possible that THC affects both the acetylcholine and GABA systems in the brain. The retained THC continues to affect the brain long after the marijuana high has passed. A study of young heavy marijuana smokers showed that their memory was still impaired 6 weeks after they stopped smoking the drug.

Marijuana smoke contains more tar and cancer-causing chemicals than even cigarette smoke. One marijuana cigarette has as much cancer-causing tar as 17 tobacco cigarettes. Marijuana smoke, like tobacco smoke, causes bronchitis, inflammation of the airways in the lungs, and chronic respiratory illnesses. THC also affects most other systems of the body. It reduces normal hormone function in both males and females, reducing fertility and causing miscarriages. Both alcohol use and marijuana use during pregnancy can produce the fetal alcohol syndrome, a specific congenital abnormality often associated with impulsive behavior and lifelong mental retardation.

The Dumb High

The most striking effects of marijuana are on the user's brain. With occasional use, marijuana produces sedation and slightly altered mental processes. Learning is slowed, and concentration and short-term memory are hampered. Reaction times are slower and perceptions of time and distance are distorted, making driving and other safety-related behaviors especially hazardous after marijuana use. Users are commonly unaware of their impairments after using small doses of marijuana. Larger doses can precipitate acute anxiety or panic, or schizophrenic episodes, particularly for novice marijuana users and for people subject to these mental health disorders. Long-term effects of marijuana use are still being researched, but there is growing evidence of permanent brain cell and chromosomal damage as well as the impairment of logical thinking. Some long-term users of marijuana show prolonged, perhaps lifelong, deficits in memory and motivation as well as irritability.

Although marijuana was not the first drug in the modern drug epidemic—a dubious distinction that belongs to the hallucinogens, especially naturally occurring mescaline and psilocybin as well as synthetic LSD—marijuana by 1970 became the central drug in the modern North American drug abuse epidemic. Because marijuana does not produce respiratory depression or other acute effects associated with overdose death (as heroin, barbiturates, and even alcohol do), and because withdrawal was not observed when chronic marijuana users refrained from use for a few days, marijuana had the aura of a safe high, the requirement for a new gateway drug. In the 1970s, marijuana mistakenly was the model for a "soft" drug as heroin was the model for a "hard" drug.

One of the more remarkable aspects of the marijuana story has been the difficulty scientists have had in understanding how marijuana works in the brain. Only in 1987 was the THC receptor in the brain identified, and not until 1992 was the naturally occurring neurotransmitter that fits this brain lock identified. The THC receptors, widely distributed throughout the brain, have been found in particular abundance in the cerebellum and the hippocampus, two primitive brain areas involved with motor functions, learning, and memory. These areas are connected to the pleasure centers of the brain, but it remains unknown what the natural brain function is for these receptors.

Experiments on rats have shown that THC causes impairments of short-term memory, which is similar to the effects pro-

Marijuana

- The crude drug that produces the dumb high
- Marijuana contains over 420 chemicals; marijuana smoke contains over 2,000 chemicals
- THC is long-retained in the body
- Causes many harmful physical effects, including harm to the brain, lungs, and reproductive and immune systems
- The most commonly observed brain effects are poor memory and reduced motivation, the "careless syndrome"
- The most devious drug of abuse with the most elusive bottom

duced when hippocampi in the rats' brains are damaged. Long-term marijuana use causes irreversible cell destruction in these same hippocampal brain regions. This may explain why people who have used a lot of marijuana for many years find that their memory is permanently impaired, just as heavy and prolonged alcohol use can permanently damage the users' livers as well as their brains and nerves.

Prolonged and even permanent changes after long-term marijuana use need to be kept in perspective. Whenever long-term drug users stop drug use, the damage to their bodies stops. The body often develops ways of compensating, partially or in some cases totally, for the harm done by the earlier drug use. The permanence of the damage done by any drug should never become an excuse not to quit drug use. Damage to the brain and other parts of the body should be a reason never to start and, if a person has started, an even more compelling reason to quit the drug use. This fact of life applies to marijuana as it does to all non-medical drug use.

One of the claims made for marijuana by enthusiastic supporters of this drug is that, unlike alcohol, marijuana does not cause a hangover after heavy use. The scientific basis for this common observation is not reassuring. Alcohol is quickly eliminated from the body, usually within a few hours after drinking stops. The withdrawal or hangover experience after alcohol use reflects the brain's attempt to get along without the presence of the chemical. This does not occur for marijuana because THC stays in the brain for days after use of the drug stops. The fact that marijuana does not cause a hangover the way alcohol commonly does after heavy use is not an advantage at all. Marijuana stays in the brain for a long time so that the brain is still experiencing the effects from pot smoking days after the drug use has stopped, in contrast to alcohol use.

The Careless Drug

Marijuana makes users stupid and lazy. It is the "careless drug," because pot users often lose the capacity to care. In the most extreme form, this is called the *amotivational syndrome*, meaning that chronic pot smokers become listless and apathetic, not just when using the drug but all of the time. This tragic state is called "burn-out" by drug abusers themselves. Unlike cocaine, which often quickly brings users to their knees, marijuana claims its victims in a slower and more cruel fashion. It robs many of them of their desire to grow and improve, often making heavy users settle for what is left over in life. For this reason, marijuana is the most insidious drug. Its effects are both profound and subtle.

Heroin use encourages criminality, as heroin addicts steal and rob to get money to keep getting high. Cocaine makes users unstable and aggressive, as their brains get stuck on "go." Marijuana makes its users lose their purpose and their will, as well as their memory and motivation. Marijuana smokers do not often come into treatment for their addiction simply because neither they nor those around them can differentiate their true selves from the effects of their drug use. They commonly just sink lower and lower in their performance and in their goals in life as their pot smoking continues. Their hopes and lives literally go up in marijuana smoke.

It is no coincidence that the terrible 1987 train crash at Chase, Maryland, which claimed 17 lives, was caused by an engineer high on pot. He looked fine to his co-workers that day, but he drove his train through four warning signals into the path of a high-speed Amtrak passenger train. He performed his important and potentially dangerous job with an attitude of carelessness that I have come to recognize as the common result of marijuana use. Based on my experience with marijuana users, when I learned that an employee in a paper mill reached in to grab a piece of wood through a fast-moving belt, in total violation of the basic safety rules of the company, I suspected that his carelessness was the result of marijuana use. A drug test conducted while the employee was in the hospital confirmed my fears. That man lost the use of his right arm as a result of his injury. That was a hard way to learn about the so-called safe high of marijuana.

Marijuana as Medicine

Marijuana, like opium, coca leaves, and alcohol, has a long history as a folk medicine used to treat an endless variety of human miseries. Prescientific cultures, lacking modern purified, potent medicines, relied on commonly available natural psychoactive substances to reduce human suffering. The abused drugs, because of their effects on the brain's pleasure/pain centers, were attractive in this role. In addition, incorporating these abusable substances into folk medicines rather than making them available for personally controlled pleasure ensured that their use within the community would be controlled not merely by the user but by culturally responsible therapists. Thus, the use of folk medicines was not for recreational purposes but for medical purposes with strict cultural controls.

Until the middle of the 19th century, there were few chemically pure medicines, so the use of complex natural substances, such as opium and cannabis, was common. In the last half of the 19th century, modern chemistry purified chemicals used as medicines so that morphine was extracted from opium and cocaine was extracted from the coca leaf. Only in the late 1960s was purified THC extracted from marijuana leaves and resin and identified as the chemical that causes the high and many of the other effects of marijuana use.

Modern medicine, beginning in the first two decades of the 20th century, for the first time brought chemical science to the ancient art of medical therapeutics. Physicians from then on did not use unpurified and unstable natural products as medicines. They used chemically purified and stable pharmaceuticals to treat specifically diagnosed medical illnesses. For severe pain, for example, physicians prescribed morphine or, in more recent years, synthetic opiate substitutes, rather than prescribing a mixture of alcohol and opium, called *laudanum*, as occurred in the 19th century and earlier. By using a chemical that was pure and stable, physicians knew precisely what their patients were taking and could give their patients these substances free of a hodgepodge of inactive and potentially harmful substances. Physicians could be sure that the specific therapeutic substance was present in a known, controllable dose.

Marijuana, with over 420 chemicals, let alone marijuana smoke, with over 2,000 different chemicals, many of which are known to be harmful to the user's health, is not an attractive modern medicine. Nevertheless, marijuana smoke does have powerful effects on the brain and other parts of the body. Modern biomedical research into the effects of smoked marijuana has identified many effects, some of which may be found to have therapeutic potentials to treat specific illnesses.

Several years ago, dronabinol (Marinol), a synthetic THC, was approved by the FDA as a medicine in both capsule and suppository forms to treat the severe nausea and vomiting sometimes caused by cancer chemotherapy. When patients are treated with powerful medicines to kill cancer cells in their bodies, the medicines also are toxic to other rapidly dividing cells in the body, including those in the gastrointestinal tract and those that make both red and white blood cells. Some of these anticancer medicines also stimulate the brain's vomiting center. Nausea and vomiting after cancer chemotherapy are both extremely unpleasant and potentially dangerous, especially for people who are already seriously ill.

Doctors discovered that THC reduces nausea and vomiting for such patients. This led to strong political pressure from the promarijuana lobby to approve marijuana for medical treatment as a compassionate response to the suffering of cancer patients. Marijuana, or even purified THC, was not and never has been proposed as a treatment for cancer. The only proposed use for marijuana or THC in the treatment of cancer patients is to treat the nausea and vomiting associated with the use of chemotherapy.

Oncologists, the medical specialists who treat cancer, studied THC and found that it was helpful for some patients but that it had many unwanted side effects, including making it unsafe to drive a car and sometimes causing psychosis. Most cancer patients who were not previously drug addicted found the effects of THC to be extremely unpleasant. Oncologists did not want to use smoked crude marijuana as a medicine because it contained so many chemicals, some of which actually caused cancer and suppressed the immune system, and because the dose of THC reaching the patient could not be controlled accurately with smoking. In recent years, new synthetic medicines, unrelated to THC or marijuana, have been developed that have made THC obsolete in the treatment of nausea and vomiting from chemotherapy. On-dansetron (Zofran) is one example of these new, more effective, far safer, and more powerful antinausea medicines.

Marijuana has been proposed as a treatment for the wasting (loss of appetite and loss of weight, which can be life threatening) in AIDS because of marijuana's well-known tendency to produce "the munchies," or the desire to eat high-calorie foods. Not only is there no solid scientific evidence that marijuana or THC helps AIDS patients, but marijuana's well-known ability to depress the immune system and to cause cancer makes it extremely unattractive as a medicine for AIDS sufferers, who are literally dying from damaged immune systems. The fact that marijuana can cause some AIDS sufferers to feel high and therefore less upset is no more a reason to use marijuana as medicine for these sick patients than it is to give them alcohol or cocaine.

Marijuana has been proposed as a treatment for asthma, but, although THC does dilate the bronchi (which are closed down by asthma attacks) in the short run, the irritants in marijuana smoke actually cause lung pathology, including long-term bronchial constriction, after prolonged use. Therefore, marijuana is not likely to gain favor as an asthma treatment.

It has been proposed that marijuana can be used to treat glaucoma. THC does reduce the pressure in the eye for a few hours, as do many other substances, including alcohol. However, glaucoma is a 24-hour-a-day disease, so a person who is treated for glaucoma with marijuana has to smoke pot or take THC pills around the clock. Worse still, marijuana and THC are weak in their effects on pressure in the eyeball, so the person with glaucoma has to use not only around-the-clock marijuana smoke or THC but also routine glaucoma medicines. No controlled scientific studies have shown that THC or marijuana add anything useful to the other medicines routinely used in the treatment of glaucoma, all of which last longer, produce fewer unwanted side effects, and are more powerful in their effects in reducing eye pressure than is marijuana, or THC.

Marijuana has been proposed as a treatment for the spasticity of multiple sclerosis. No controlled studies have been conducted to show that THC helps with this serious problem, although cannabidiol, a nonpsychotropic cannabinoid found in marijuana, may prove effective. These preliminary results showing benefit from the use of cannabidiol have not been confirmed in controlled studies.

The National Institutes of Health recently completed a review of all the proposed medical uses of marijuana and THC and concluded that there was no longer any basis for the government to have a compassionate program to supply marijuana to sufferers from any illness whatsoever. None of the medical uses for marijuana so far proposed met even the minimal standards of safety and efficacy required of a proposed medicine. Thus, although THC capsules and suppositories remain available to doctors treating cancer patients for nausea and vomiting, there is no other approved use for THC, and there is no approved use for smoked marijuana as a medicine to treat any illness. When THC and marijuana have been used in experimental settings to treat various illnesses, doctors have found that the psychoactive effects—the high and the mental clouding—are unpleasant to most patients, except those who were previously drug abusers. Marijuana and THC are poorly tolerated and exceedingly unattractive to most medical patients.

Meanwhile, the promarijuana lobby has not been satisfied with the approval of purified, synthetic THC because they want to focus on very sick patients using smoked marijuana, the crude drug, as medicine. They want the public to see smoked marijuana as medicine—as a way of rehabilitating the negative image of marijuana. Promarijuana apologists insist on the use of crude, smoked marijuana, not THC or other purified chemicals for medical treatments. The marijuana-as-medicine controversy has become a political issue in North America.

The FDA and the National Institutes of Health oppose such proposals, as do the National Institute on Drug Abuse and the Drug Enforcement Administration. Virtually all of the medical organizations that speak up for the welfare of the patients in each of the proposed areas where marijuana might be used are also opposed to marijuana as medicine. Most of the proponents of marijuana as medicine are the same people who want to normalize and/or legalize illicit drugs, especially marijuana.

It is useful to remember that all abused drugs have powerful effects on the body. It may someday be discovered that one or more of the individual chemicals in some of the commonly abused drugs will play a uniquely useful role in the medical treatments of some illnesses. The biomedical research now going on into the effects of abused drugs may identify important therapeutic effects of some of these specific chemicals.

Even the most antidrug activist needs to recall the nature of the modern social contract for drug use. It specifies that, under the careful supervision of a physician, abused drugs will be available in medical treatments of illnesses other than addiction. Thus, medical use is not an enemy of drug abuse prevention, as long as the medical use of potentially addictive medicines meets the standards set for other medicines and as long as the use is properly controlled to protect both the patient being treated and the community from the potential harm such medicines can cause when they leak out of the medical care system.

To this contract for medical treatments with abused drugs, I add one additional element. Substances that are of high abuse potential and substances that are currently widely used nonmedically in the society should be required to meet a higher standard than substances not widely abused. Not only should they be shown as safe and effective in specific medical applications, the standard that any medicine must meet, but they should also meet the standard that they provide a significant benefit not currently available from nonabused or less abused medicines.

Thus, before THC or heroin, two widely abused substances, are introduced as medicines, they should be shown to offer specific benefits not available with less socially risky substances. Although it is possible that in the future some of the chemicals in abused drugs will meet this higher standard, none does so today. Certainly, smoked marijuana will never be approved as a medicine, any more than smoked tobacco or, for that matter, alcohol, will be approved as an acceptable modern medicine.

The marijuana-as-medicine advocates have several advantages in the current political debates over medical use. The pro-drug lobby is large and powerful in North America, and it has now concentrated on this issue because it has proved powerless in its earlier, more frontal assault on the prohibition against marijuana. To sharpen their attacks on prohibition and to gain supporters, promarijuana advocates have focused on the most feared illnesses that induce the greatest sympathy for their sufferers, such as terminal cancer, AIDS, and multiple sclerosis. They have exploited the widespread conviction that the government agencies that control the approval of medicines are too slow and too tradition-bound to approve many medicines that can help suffering patients with these illnesses, especially potential medicines that are controversial because they are abused drugs.

Finally, this lobby has capitalized on the interest in traditional medicines and on alternatives to modern scientific medicines, both of which have enjoyed a new vogue in recent years. Folk medicines have an appeal to many North Americans who fear modern science. Thus, the fact that marijuana was used for centuries as a folk medicine is seen, in this highly romanticized view, as evidence that it should be available today as a prescribed or an over-the-counter remedy.

Recall the free-for-all days of the end of the 19th century when patent medicines did contain abused drugs. Although the promarijuana lobby can score some points today by talking about folk medicines in ancient China, the patent medicine debacle of a hundred years ago not only is closer to home but virtually impossible to romanticize. Americans tried the experiment of using cocaine, heroin, alcohol, and other abused drugs as folk medicines, as over-the-counter products, at the beginning of the 20th century. It was an unmitigated disaster. We do not need to repeat that experiment at the end of the 20th century.

The way medicines are approved in the United States today not only favors medicines that are developed and sponsored by large, sophisticated pharmaceutical companies, but the current path to approval by the FDA requires the issuing of a potentially lucrative patent that permits the recovery of the large costs of gaining approval. Because no one can patent ancient drug substances such as opium and marijuana, there is no money in such remedies for modern pharmaceutical companies.

Government agencies that often sponsor biomedical research, including research into the effects of abused drugs, seldom promote specific medicines, and when they do they have a hard time gaining FDA approval. Thus, if any of the chemicals in abused drugs were to show promise as more effective medicines than the medicines currently in use, it would not be easy to get approval within the current system. On the other hand, patents can be granted for specific chemicals in these crude, traditional drugs.

Today, more than 70 chemicals found in marijuana or related to chemicals found in marijuana smoke are under active investigation by pharmaceutical companies in all parts of the world. The normal profit motive will reinforce the desire of these companies to find more effective medicines for serious illnesses. It is possible that someday, perhaps soon, one or more of these chemicals will become widely useful in the modern treatment of a disease. If so, we can all be grateful for one more benefit from the modern scientific study of abused drugs, because that study will have been the basis of the new medicine.

A persistent fantasy of mine is that someday there will be a clear-cut positive medical use from one of the chemicals in abused drugs, and I will be able to join with my longtime foes in the drug prohibition battles and support approval for the medical use of the substance. This would please me greatly because it would add credibility to my claim all these years that I do not oppose the medical uses of these substances on a political, or even an emotional, basis, but simply because none of the chemicals in currently widely abused drugs has met the minimum standard of showing promise that it is better for the treatment of any illnesses than currently available medicines. When I see that evidence, I look forward to joining in the battle on the side of the medical use of these chemicals. So far I have waited 20 years without having that opportunity.

Cocaine and Other Stimulants

Substances that stimulate the brain come from many natural and synthetic sources. Naturally occurring brain stimulants include cocaine (from the leaves of the South American coca plant), cathine and cathinone (derived from the khat plant of north-eastern Africa and the Arabian peninsula), nicotine (from tobacco leaves), and caffeine (from coffee beans and tea leaves). Synthetic brain stimulants include amphetamine and its chemical cousins, such as methamphetamine, 3,4-methylenedioxyamphetamine (MDA), and 3,4-methylenedioxymethamphetamine (MDMA). This is a diverse catalog of substances with diverse histories and diverse effects in all parts of the world. The most powerful stimulant effects are produced by cocaine and the amphetamines, whereas MDA and MDMA are powerful hallucinogens that are closely related chemically.

Cocaine and the amphetamines are among the best understood drugs of abuse. Cocaine can be smoked ("crack" or "freebase"), snorted up the nose, or injected intravenously. It can also be taken by mouth and swallowed. Amphetamines, in contrast to cocaine, are commonly used by mouth, but they are also injected or smoked ("ice"). The related hallucinogens, MDA and MDMA, are taken by mouth. These drugs all stimulate the central nervous system, increasing the heart rate and blood pressure. Stimulant drugs mimic the alarm function of the sympathetic nervous system, the NE neurotransmitter system of the brain. In moderate doses, the stimulant drugs suppress appetite and increase alertness, effects that some drug users find extremely attractive. Other effects of stimulants are to reduce pain, to bolster feelings of confidence and competence, and to produce sustained high-energy levels that obliterate fatigue. Cocaine and amphetamines have profound effects on the heart and on the brain. Epileptic seizures and heart stoppage are possible following nonmedical stimulant use, and both can cause sudden death. Seizures and sudden heart stoppage are possible outcomes of cocaine use, especially when the drug is smoked or injected intravenously.

Crack cocaine, the smokable form of cocaine, is more fat soluble than the older cocaine hydrochloride, which is snorted. Because of this higher fat solubility, crack cocaine penetrates the blood-brain barrier more quickly and then leaves the brain more quickly than powdered cocaine. Thus, crack or freebase cocaine is especially addicting, both because it produces a more rapid high and because it produces a faster and more intense crash following use.

Cocaine users may experience "coke bugs," an uncomfortable sensation that bugs are burrowing under their skin. These feelings can be so intense that cocaine users become obsessed, developing the delusion that there are actually bugs under their skin. They seek to dig out the bugs with their fingernails, creating terrible, but characteristic, sores on their arms, legs, and other parts of their bodies.

As with all abused drugs, limiting use of cocaine or an amphetamine to occasional small amounts becomes increasingly difficult as the addict loses control of the drug use while addiction deepens. The stimulants are among the most reinforcing of all drugs, making them the most powerfully addicting drugs. When drug addicts abuse stimulants, especially when they inject or smoke stimulants, they quickly lose control of their drug use and of their lives.

Stimulant Addiction: The Quickest Bottom

No other drugs bring users to their knees, forcing them to seek help, as fast or as powerfully as do the stimulants. Many recovering addicts harbor dreams that they can learn in the future to drink alcohol socially or use marijuana or opiates with some moderation. Few stimulant users, once they have become addicted, believe they can ever again use these drugs under any semblance of control. When they do relapse, as they often do, to stimulant use after a period of abstinence, it is seldom with the hope that their stimulant use will be controlled. Addicts relapse knowing that the ending of the stimulant-using episode will be disastrous. The lure of the stimulant high is so powerful that they simply do not, at the time, count the costs to themselves and others. For most cocaine addicts, their "bottoms" rise up and hit them between the eyes within weeks or months of starting to smoke or shoot the drug.

Long-term effects, and effects of larger doses of stimulants, include heart palpitations, anxiety and panic attacks, extreme irritability, insomnia, seizures, paranoid psychosis, and death. The fact that this list of consequences, widely understood by stimulant abusers, does not discourage stimulant use for millions of people speaks eloquently to the grip that stimulants have on the lives of many drug addicts.

Cocaine

Cocaine is a simple chemical derived from the coca leaves grown in the Andes Mountains of South America. It is the only naturally occurring local anesthetic. Although cocaine promotes the release of dopamine (DA) into the synapse in the brain, its major action is to block the reuptake of DA from the synapse by the presynaptic axon, especially in the areas of the brain associated with sensations of pleasure. DA cannot be retrieved effectively by the axon of cocaine users, so it accumulates in the synapse. Because the cocaine-affected neurons govern pleasure and general brain stimulation, cocaine use produces euphoria, an exaggerated sense of well-being, and heightened feelings of energy. The cocaine user's appetite disappears, and sleep becomes impossible for several hours after use. Cocaine use locks the brain into the "go" mode.

An enzyme that is present in the brain's DA synapses metabolizes the DA abnormally caught in the synapse of the cocaine user. The axon is able to make new DA only very slowly. Because most DA normally is picked up and recycled by the axon, this slow, gradual metabolic process of making new DA is not a problem for the brain in the absence of cocaine use. The metabolism of DA by this enzyme and the production of new DA by the axon are normally in balance. However, with repeated cocaine use, DA is depleted from the axon and finally within the synapse itself as the normally occurring enzyme eats up the DA trapped in the synapse. This DA destruction occurs because of the increased exposure of DA to the enzyme caused by the cocaine-induced, abnormally prolonged presence of DA in the synapse.

The effects from a single use of cocaine last less than an hour, so cocaine users typically take the drug in "runs," meaning they take repeated doses of cocaine every few minutes over periods of hours or days. The longer a cocaine run lasts, the less pleasure the cocaine user experiences with each use of the drug, as DA is progressively more depleted in the axon and later in the synapse. DA

Cocaine
- The most addicting drug
- Snorted, smoked, and injected intravenously
- Intense compulsion to continue use
- Quick, hard bottoms
- Harm to heart and brain, and to lungs if smoked
- A difficult addiction to overcome

depletion leads to the crash that characteristically ends a cocaine run.

Cocaine does not produce either the physical dependence or the withdrawal that fits the model addiction based on heroin addiction. Cocaine users do not use the drug every single day, around the clock, the way heroin addicts (as well as cigarette smokers and maintenance drinkers) do. When people stop cocaine use, they do not have a clearly defined withdrawal syndrome, although they predictably are depleted and exhausted. This fact misled experts on addiction for many years into thinking that cocaine use was not addicting. Today it is clear that after cocaine users take their drug in runs, the typical user feels tired and depressed, often intensely so. When cocaine use stops, users have a hard time adjusting to their lives and finding pleasure from any activity at all.

The "white lady" turns deep blue.   Heroin is often called "boy," and cocaine is often called "girl." The events at the synapse explain why cocaine users feel depressed and exhausted at the end of a run of drug use, an experience called the "coke blues." Cocaine users not only feel terrible after a run of cocaine use, but they find they are unable to experience life's normal pleasures. Their brain's DA pleasure system has been overstimulated and exhausted by cocaine use. The brain requires weeks or even months to reestablish a normal equilibrium in the DA synapses. After years of work with chronic cocaine users, I am concerned that after prolonged heavy abuse, the DA system of some chronic users may never again function normally, producing a lifelong state of diminished ability to experience normal pleasures.

Cocaine is available to drug abusers in North America today in two forms. The white, snowlike powdered form of cocaine was the first to be used widely in the late 1970s by celebrities and the risk-taking upper class, especially those associated with the fields of sports and entertainment. Because of the association of cocaine use with people on the fast track and its initial high cost, powdered cocaine took on an aura of sophistication, becoming known as the champagne of illegal drugs. Sports figures and risk-taking business people found cocaine attractive for its energizing qualities and promotion of the feeling of omnipotence. Crack cocaine, which became widely available in the United States after 1985, is composed of small pellets, or "rocks," which are smoked by heating with a flame to produce vapors that are inhaled like tobacco or marijuana smoke.

Although cocaine was initially seductive, heavy cocaine users frequently became paranoid and developed severe psychosis after repeated use. Perceptions became distorted, judgment was altered, and careers and families were destroyed as cocaine addiction deepened. The high cost of cocaine meant that many of the worst effects of chronic use were financial, as people literally put their financial security, and that of their families, up their noses.

Cocaine compulsion.   Cocaine is the only drug that gives users good feelings when initially used but mostly uncomfortable feelings when subsequently used. With most drugs of abuse, including alcohol, marijuana, and heroin, people who begin using these drugs experience euphoria during their initial honeymoon stage of drug use. As their addiction deepens, they are more likely to report that they feel "normal" after they use the drug than to report that they feel euphoria. With cocaine, this dismal pattern is exaggerated as long-time cocaine users not only report that they no longer feel high after cocaine use, but they report that cocaine use makes them feel paranoid and frightened. Despite the bad feelings, the compulsion to use cocaine not only persists but grows stronger over time with repeated use of the drug.

One young man described to me using cocaine alone in his apartment and pulling down the shades and double locking his door. He then crawled around on the floor, alone and terrified, fearing that the police would look in his window or break in his door. Despite these dreadful feelings, he kept using cocaine, spending thousands of dollars for this experience. This amazed him and gave both of us a new understanding of the word *compulsion* when it comes to repeated cocaine use.

Many chronic stimulant abusers describe an irresistible compulsion to use their drugs again if they have access to stimulants. This compulsion is not based only on the desire to get high or to feel pleasure. They know from repeated experience that they will never again feel the intense pleasure they found with their initial doses of the stimulant. Nevertheless, they are compelled by a dark inner force from their selfish, addicted brains, a force that they have great difficulty describing, much less escaping. Their primitive brain systems have a hunger that they cannot resist. Watching this phenomenon in my patients who abuse stimulants has been my closest encounter with the full power of the addicted selfish brain. This dreadful experience can only be compared to the brain force experienced by obsessive-compulsive patients to repeat their rituals: It defies language, logic, and common human experience. This force to repeatedly use stimulants simply dominates and obliterates the otherwise sensible person's willpower.

Cocaine use rose rapidly in the United States in the late 1970s and early 1980s among affluent drug users, most of whom were previously heavy users of alcohol and marijuana. Cocaine had been used extensively in the earlier American drug epidemic at the end of the 19th century as an over-the-counter medicine. Cocaine has been popular with intravenous heroin users since the 1920s, when hard-core addicts often injected cocaine along with heroin, in what was called a "speedball." The mixture of a stimulant with a depressant is a common pattern among drug abusers who are disturbed by the negative effects of one class of drugs alone. Heroin users, for example, often feel uncomfortably sedated or lethargic, so they add cocaine or other stimulants to their drug menu. Cocaine users often feel wired or uptight, so they often lace their cocaine with depressants, such as heroin, or even medicines, such as barbiturates or benzodiazepines, to blunt the unpleasant effects of their stimulant abuse.

When cocaine use took off in North America in the early 1980s, these earlier negative experiences were forgotten as cocaine was seen to be the new marijuana, the safe step beyond marijuana for people willing to use illegal drugs nonmedically to get high.

A historical turning point in the American drug abuse epidemic. Len Bias, the University of Maryland basketball superstar, died on June 19, 1986, of a cocaine overdose following his signing of a multimillion-dollar professional contract with the Boston Celtics. This event ended the widespread feelings of euphoria about cocaine as the safe champagne of abused drugs. America's amnesia about cocaine's dangers ended overnight when Bias died. Although other celebrities had died of drug overdoses, no other event in America's drug abuse history had such impact as the death of this American prince at the height of his powers. The media played the death at top volume for months. Many Americans participated in the national outrage and mourning over the death of this attractive, talented young man. In this sense at least, his death was not in vain, as it galvanized a major national response not only to cocaine but to all illicit drug use.

This was the most public drug abuse death in history. Bias's death produced a massive reaction, whereas earlier deaths of such media figures as Elvis Presley, Jimmy Hendrix, and John Belushi did not, in part because all of them were seen as jaded by their celebrity, whereas Bias was a college student when he died. In addition, Bias's death occurred when crack cocaine had recently hit North America like a destructive hurricane. The United States was also entering an election season, which added a political dimension to the public reaction, as representatives of both parties tried to outdo each other in their responses to the drug abuse epidemic.

Bias's death not only changed the nation's thinking about cocaine, but it also dispelled many lingering myths about drug abuse. For two decades, so-called drug experts had told the public that people use drugs because they suffer from low self-esteem or from some mental disturbance. Other claimed that drug use reflected failures in family life or economic disadvantage. Bias died in a college dormitory a few hours after he left his loving father. He was not depressed. He was certainly not financially or educationally disadvantaged. The one aspect of his story that did reinforce a stereotypical—and wrong—view of addiction was that Bias was black. As noted in Chapter 3, 80% of the users of illicit drugs in the United States are white. With that one exception, this most public of all drug deaths is a useful standard against which to gauge any theory of why people use illegal drugs. The simple answer, repeated throughout this book, is that users like the feelings that drugs produce, and they believe they can get away with that use, that chemical high.

After Len Bias's death, many Americans reassessed cocaine, finding it to be much more addictive and dangerous than originally thought. In fact, cocaine's popular image shifted almost overnight from "soft," like marijuana, to "the most addictive" of all drugs, "worse than heroin." Most of the media coverage of cocaine, which had been accepting if not approving before 1986, turned unrelentingly hostile to cocaine use in subsequent years. Suddenly, gone from the mass media were the latter-day Timothy Learys, who touted the virtues of cocaine use to gullible Americans. Prevention and intervention efforts aimed at cocaine use began after 1986 to target an audience that previously had dismissed the incipient dangers of cocaine use, especially youth who were frequent users of alcohol and marijuana.

Len Bias's death also helped dispel the idea that drug addiction was a result of poverty, poor family life, or lack of education, or that it represented a self-destructive or even suicidal act. Bias died in a college dormitory on the brink of a fabulously lucrative career. He used cocaine that fateful night to celebrate, to party, with his friends.

Crack: the ultimate addiction.   Crack is a smokable form of cocaine that was first widely used in about 1985, beginning in East and West Coast urban areas. Cocaine hydrochloride was the standard form of cocaine from the end of the 19th century until the early 1980s. It could be snorted or injected, a pattern of use that was also seen with heroin use over the same period of time. In the 1980s, a new technique for using cocaine was developed that involved creating what was called freebase, a chemical form of cocaine that was more fat soluble than the hydrochloride and that had a lower vaporization temperature (98°C versus 195°C for cocaine hydrochloride). At first, freebase cocaine had to be made with ether extraction from the hydrochloride, a process that was dangerous because ether is explosive. The terrible fire that burned the comedian Richard Pryor reflected this older technique of freebase manufacture.

In the mid-1980s, a new technique was developed to manufacture freebase: baking soda and water were used to make gray "cracks" or "rocks" of cocaine freebase. This was an easier and safer technique to create a smokable form of cocaine. After smoking crack, the cocaine hits the user's brain at very high levels within 8 seconds, by far the fastest and most powerful way to get a drug high. Even intravenous use takes twice as long, or about 16 seconds, to reach the brain. Peak effects occur within 15 minutes of using cocaine by smoking or injecting and within 30 minutes by snorting the drug. The high of the cocaine is gone within an hour, although impairment of thinking can last for days or even weeks after high-dose use of cocaine.

The rapid acceptance of crack cocaine by novice and veteran drug abusers can be attributed to several factors. Cocaine is a highly addictive drug. The first rush after using cocaine produces such a strong sense of pleasure that many one-time users are strongly motivated to recapture those feelings. Smoking drugs—modeled on the experience of smoking tobacco cigarettes and marijuana—is an acceptable activity for many people today. Especially with the recent media attention to the dangers of intravenous drug use, even many dedicated drug abusers have become more wary of needles and injected drugs than they were before the appearance of AIDS. Thus, those seeking intense drug highs, caused by rapidly rising high brain levels of abused drugs, have been attracted to drug smoking.

Even as heavy drug abusers began to avoid intravenous drug use as being too dangerous and as marking depraved addiction, they mistakenly considered smoking a more normal or safe way to use drugs. Although drug smoking does not spread HIV infection, it is as addicting as injecting intravenously because it delivers rapidly rising and high doses of the drug to the brain. All drug abuse lowers inhibitions and promotes antisocial behavior. Therefore, even when drug abusers do not inject drugs, they are at increased risk of HIV infection because of other high-risk behaviors, especially promiscuous sexual activities.

Women are more inclined to smoke rather than inject drugs, making crack cocaine smoking more attractive than intravenous cocaine use to female drug abusers. Women have long been especially attracted to stimulant use compared with other classes of drugs. Crack use by pregnant women has resulted in the tragically common phenomenon of the crack baby, the infant born addicted to cocaine with congenital problems and developmental handicaps.

Marketing tactics of drug dealers have influenced the spread of crack cocaine use. Distributors package crack in relatively small units, making the purchase more attractive and affordable to adolescents and those with lower incomes. Buying powdered cocaine used to mean spending several hundred dollars at a time. Buying crack after 1985 meant coming up with only $5 to $10. The entry cost for the cocaine market fell dramatically in the late 1980s. Milton Hershey took an expensive luxury item, chocolate, and introduced the nickel chocolate bar in the early 1900s, making chocolate, for the first time, affordable for nearly everyone. The same market shift occurred for cocaine in the late 1980s, when cheap crack largely replaced expensive powdered cocaine as the dominant form of the drug.

The profits of cocaine dealers skyrocketed as a result of this change, recruiting new users and sellers with an explosive rate of growth. In America's cities, the problems of crack cocaine use and crime became thoroughly and disastrously intertwined in recent years, not only because crack users stole property and sold drugs to buy their crack but because cocaine use itself made people aggressive and paranoid. Crack cocaine in the late 1980s overcame individuals, families, and whole communities with a ferocity never seen before with any other drug habit. Crack cocaine effectively dashed any hope of drug proponents peddling their permissive ideas to the American public about illicit drugs. The question that drug legalizers could not answer became "What about crack? How would you handle that drug if illicit drugs were made legal?" They could not answer because this drug habit was so disastrous to virtually everyone using crack and to those around them.

Cocaine as Medicine

When cocaine was first available to physicians in the 1880s, it was used to treat many conditions, including depression and drug abuse. Sigmund Freud tried cocaine and found it miraculous, recommending it to a good friend and to his fiancée. Within a few years, cocaine was found to have two characteristics that made it useful in medicine. It was a local anesthetic agent, and it stopped blood flowing locally. Ultimately, cocaine found a limited medical use as a local anesthetic, which continues to this day, in minor surgery and in surgery involving bloody procedures, such as hemorrhoidectomies and tonsillectomies.

However, in the last 50 years, a wide variety of synthetic medicines have been developed, such as novocaine, which have fewer disturbing side effects on the brain and the heart than does cocaine. These new synthetics have virtually replaced cocaine in modern medical practice. Nevertheless, cocaine remains available in the American pharmacopeia for a few medical uses. Cocaine is not available to treat depression or drug abuse, however. The late 20th-century prodrug lobby, which has shown much enthusiasm for the medical uses of marijuana and heroin, has yet to show any interest in either alcohol or cocaine as medical treatments.

Stimulants

Amphetamines and methamphetamine. The synthetic stimulants mimic the effects of cocaine by inhibiting DA reuptake, but their major effect is to release DA into the synapse. In addition, amphetamines and methamphetamine are direct catecholamine agonists. They fit the DA and NE locks on the dendrites. The synthetic stimulants turn on the receiving dendrites in this DA neurotransmitter system just as cocaine does, especially in the brain's pleasure centers. The synthetic stimulants also inhibit enzymes that break down DA and NE in the neuron. The combination of direct action at the receptor site and inhibition of the enzymes that metabolize DA causes synthetic stimulants to produce effects over a longer time than does cocaine. Therefore, depletion effects, such as depression and lack of pleasure, after synthetic stimulant use are even more prolonged and intense than the depletion effects of cocaine use.

Life on a run.   A run of stimulant use, whether cocaine or methamphetamine, ends with a reversal of the user's initial experience—euphoria is followed by depression, energy by exhaustion, pleasure by malaise. The major difference between cocaine and synthetic stimulants is that the synthetic stimulants produce effects for many hours after a single use rather than for only a few minutes, as does cocaine. Synthetic stimulants are often used orally, especially early in an addict's career of drug abuse, whereas cocaine is usually snorted or smoked. Experienced synthetic stimulant users, like other serious drug abusers, usually move from oral use to smoking (a concentrated form of methamphetamine that can be smoked is called "ice") or to intravenous injection to produce more rapid and higher peaks of the drug in their brains. The eager pleasure centers of their brains, once turned on to the intensely rewarding stimulant drug high, demand these rapidly achieved high levels of the drug.

In the 1930s and 1940s, stimulants were widely used orally in everyday medical practice, especially to treat obesity and depression. They were even sold over the counter without a prescription to long-distance truck drivers and others subject to fatigue. Synthetic stimulants were met with widespread enthusiasm, as cocaine and heroin had been at the end of the 19th century when they were introduced. However, within a few years it was widely recognized that the benefits of stimulant use, which appeared to be quick and powerful, were not sustained over time and that stimulant users quickly developed a dependence on the medicines that was hard to break.

Dedicated and unrepentant users of illicit drugs often make fun of antidrug slogans designed to discourage nonmedical drug use. They love to mock *Reefer Madness*, the antimarijuana film made in the late 1930s, for example. But when it comes to the stimulants, the drug culture itself came up with one of the most powerful of all antidrug slogans, "Speed Kills." That slogan grew out of the devastating experience in the late 1960s with the use of intravenous amphetamine and methamphetamine. Intravenous stimulant use not only made its users paranoid and sick, but it literally killed them with the violence that their drug use unleashed. "Speed Kills" also refers to a deeper truth about drug use in general and stimulant use in particular. It is a dream killer, a killer of the soul and a killer of hope.

Today the synthetic stimulants have two approved medical uses: to treat hyperactivity or attention-deficit disorder, especially in children, and to treat the rare sleep disorder narcolepsy. In modern medical treatments of these disorders, stimulants are used orally at low and stable doses with few, if any, problems, as long as the patient was not an alcoholic or a drug addict before these medicines were prescribed. In the treatment of both hyperactivity and narcolepsy, the euphoria experienced by high-dose stimulant users for obesity and depression is not seen. Tolerance to the beneficial effects does not develop even after long-term use. Thus, these medicines have become generally accepted but only in the treatment of these two specific and relatively uncommon illnesses.

More recently in the United States, some sophisticated psychopharmacologists are finding new medical uses for the stimulants, including rediscovering their role in the treatment of obesity and depression. Stimulants are also now more widely used to treat adult attention-deficit disorder. These new stimulant uses may trigger conflicts with drug enforcement officials because of the high abuse potential of these drugs.

Khat. The khat (or qat) plant is a bush with fleshy brownish-green leaves with serrated edges and a glossy top. It has been cultivated and used as a stimulant for centuries in the northeast corner of Africa and the Arabian peninsula in ways that are similar to the use of coca leaves in the Andes or the use of coffee in much of the rest of the world. Khat is typically chewed for hours at a time in social settings, usually by men, often producing animated conversations such as those that might occur at a coffeehouse. Cathinone, the psychoactive ingredient of khat, is an alkaloid with a chemical structure similar to amphetamine. Some people from khat-using parts of the world who have emigrated to other places have gone to considerable trouble and expense to continue to obtain khat. Because the material is psychoactive only while the twigs are fresh and green, it rapidly loses its value, much as coca leaves do.

Although relatively few problems have been reported in Africa or Arabia with traditional khat chewing, cases of amphetamine-like paranoid psychoses have been seen in other countries where people have used large amounts of the drug. In the reported cases, the psychotic symptoms disappeared within 5 hours after the khat chewing stopped. Effects from persistent khat use include stained gums and teeth, constipation, elevated blood pressure, and impotence.

A diplomat who served in the Somalian capital of Mogadishu during the United Nations peacekeeping mission in 1992 reported that most of the local gunmen were khat chewers who did whatever they needed to do to get their drug during the day (very much, he said, like American cocaine or heroin users), only to spend their evenings and nights talking together and chewing khat leaves. He told me that it was much safer to walk around the streets of Mogadishu in the evenings, when the gunmen were relatively happily occupied, than it was in the daytime, when they were seeking money to get their drug.

Although khat use is in a legal limbo in much of the world, it is an illegal drug in the United States, with importers of the drug being subject to arrest and imprisonment. It is likely that other parts of the world, including Europe, will make khat illegal in the future.

Case Histories

The triggering of panic disorder in vulnerable people is just one of the many ways drug abuse interacts with mental disorders.

Drug abuse can trigger psychotic episodes in people with schizo-phrenia and bipolar disorder and, through the chronic intoxica-tion resulting from repeated nonmedical drug use, it can lead to poor compliance with needed medical treatments of many men-tal disorders. In addition, some people with mental disorders use alcohol and other nonmedical drugs in a misguided effort to re-duce their discomfort, in what has been called "self-medication," leading to the compounding of the original psychiatric problem by the addition of a new problem, addiction.

In the case history below, Carrie's disastrous and prolonged panic attack was triggered by stimulation of the NE neurotrans-mitter system in her brain. The psychosis caused by being high on marijuana and the delusional experiences with the clock and with her husband appearing to be the devil reinforced her panic reac-tion, leading to prolonged hospitalization and disability. All this resulted from one use of marijuana by a young woman who had never previously been mentally ill or seen a psychiatrist.

Carrie

Carrie was 51 when she rolled up her sleeve and showed me the scars on her left arm from the time when she put her arm through a window in a mad effort to get out of her home at the age of 26. She had then been married for 2 years. She had grown up in Iowa in a family of teetotalers, vowing that she would not repeat the mistake of her parents, who she felt had sacrificed their social life to their decision not to drink alcohol: "I heard from lots of people in our community that they would have liked to have known my parents better, but the fact that my par-ents did not drink made their friends uncomfortable, so they just did not pursue the friendship." As a teenager, she made her-self drink alcohol to be social. She noted that shortly after she left college in the late 1960s, "all of a sudden marijuana was every-where and I realized it was just like alcohol. If I did not use pot, I would lose many of my friends, just like my parents lost their friends." She persuaded her husband to buy some pot and to set aside an evening for them to use it so that she could learn about this exciting new social drug.

About a year before her first use of marijuana, Carrie had experienced her initial panic attack while she was spending an evening with her mother-in-law, a woman who made Carrie un-comfortable. She commented that "although that first panic at-tack was upsetting, it was not a big deal and it passed fairly quickly." On the evening, a year later, when Carrie first used marijuana, she took two or three puffs and sat back, waiting for the magical high. She felt a strange, growing discomfort along with a sense that time was distorted. She looked at the clock and saw the hands rapidly moving backward around and around the clock. Her husband looked to her suddenly like the devil. She had an overwhelming feeling that she had to get out of her own home. She panicked, smashing her arm through the front window in a bizarre effort to get out of the house. Her husband, frightened by her disturbed behavior, tried to hold her, which scared her more. He finally called the rescue squad, which took her to a hospital.

Carrie was admitted to a psychiatric hospital when her dis-tress did not diminish in a few hours. She described to me how she paced the halls of the hospital, wringing her hands and sob-bing uncontrollably about what had happened to her mind. She stayed in the hospital for 6 weeks and was reluctant to leave even then, fearing a return of the panic attacks after she was at home alone. She stayed on the medicine Stelazine for several years thereafter and had a hard time stopping it because she feared that the medicine was all that kept her from repeating the dreadful experience. Over the next 20 years, she continued to have anxiety and panic problems but in time came to recognize these as symptoms of agoraphobia with panic attacks that had been triggered by her one experience of marijuana use. She showed no signs of schizophrenia or other psychotic mental ill-ness over those years.

Carrie does not know, and neither do I, if she would have had a terrible, prolonged panic problem if she had never used marijuana, but we both were sure that the "breakdown" in her life was set in motion by her single use of marijuana. As Carrie said to me, "Isn't it ironic? Now I barely drink at all, and I cer-tainly do not use any illegal drugs, including marijuana. But at that time I was going to do whatever it took to avoid what I considered to be my parents' mistake in not using alcohol and drugs. What a high price I have paid, and my husband has paid, for that seemingly innocent decision."

Frank

I have seen Frank once or twice a month in psychotherapy for 6 years. He is a drug addict who has never hit bottom. I have told him that I doubt if he can get well until he does hit bottom. His reply is, "It's only been 25 years that I have escaped a bottom. Maybe the next 25 will be different." Frank was a phenomenally awkward kid. He could not catch a ball or run, and he felt he was ugly. He had acne as a teenager and still did from time to time at the age of 40. He worked on his weight, but mostly he weighed in at about 250 pounds carried on a 5-foot 10-inch frame.

Frank has one great gift, however. He is good at math, and when computers came along, he became a genius with the most complex computer programs. He went to college at Cal Tech and did well academically, although he never dated. His way of relating to other young people was with drugs. He loved marijuana, and later he developed a major infatuation with cocaine. Frank also became a nationally ranked bridge player. He got married at one point to a woman who did not care much for him but found him to be a steady meal ticket. They broke up when she inherited some money and no longer needed his financial support.

About 15 years ago, Frank discovered sleeping pills when he was at a bridge tournament and could not sleep. A friend gave him a sleeping pill, and Frank found that it helped him sleep despite the excitement of the tournament. He was never without them after that. He got sleeping pills from me, even though he was an active addict, and he has stayed in therapy with me even though we both doubted that I am helping him with his drug problem. He also has seen other doctors in consultation while seeing me because I was concerned about my treatment of him, including his use of sleeping pills. He has never used more than the prescribed amount of the sleeping pills, and he has been honest with me about his use of drugs, even when it upsets us both. He never drank, finding no pleasure in alcohol. In recent years he has used marijuana only in social settings, mostly once or twice a month. He has never used marijuana on weekdays, and never during or before work. He calculates that he has spent about $150 on marijuana in the last year. He has a large supply of marijuana in his freezer, but he feels no compulsion to use it except when friends are over. Then he shares his marijuana with them.

Frank's cocaine use is a different matter. When he was married, he became frightened by his cocaine use. His wife was a heavy cocaine user, and Frank found that his life was thoroughly out of control because he had so much of the drug around so often. Once he left his wife, he was able to moderate substantially his cocaine use. He uses cocaine for about 5 to 10 hours, approximately once every 6 to 12 weeks, mostly at national bridge tournaments, where he claims that many of the people under the age of about 40 use cocaine. "How else," he asked, "could we stay up those terrible hours?" After using cocaine, he feels awful and misses work for a day or two. He tells me that, unlike marijuana, he cannot keep cocaine around his house because he simply uses it all up whenever he has any. He also never got a steady supplier of cocaine, fearing that it would then be too easy to get cocaine in larger quantities. He estimated that he has spent about $1,500 on cocaine in the previous year. He claims that "If I had spent $10,000 or $20,000, I would call that a bottom. But I can afford this much for cocaine, even if I know it is dumb."

Frank is impressed by the antidrug television commercials that show a man with a straw up his nose to snort cocaine. The man in the commercial watches money pass by him, only to be sucked up his nose. Then he sees a $200 TV go by and then get vacuumed up his nose. An elegant $100 dinner and theater evening go up his nose, an entire automobile, and then even a home. He says that "These ads work for me; they make sense to me because I know I waste a lot of money on cocaine, while the TV ads that show addicts with fried brains don't seem realistic."

I have done my best to get Frank to go into addiction treatment, but he refuses. I tried to get him to go to AA and NA meetings. He went for a while and even tried Rational Recovery, an alternative nonspiritual mutual-aid program. He never went for more than a few meetings of Rational Recovery.

Frank became sexually involved with a woman who was addicted to alcohol. He is amazed by how hard it was for her to live a stable life without regular attendance at AA meetings and a strict adherence to the nonuse of alcohol and other drugs. He said, "If cocaine were as available to me as alcohol is to Judy, I would have to go to NA or Rational Recovery meetings every day, just the way she goes to AA meetings." Here we see the role of the environment in the process of addiction. Neither Frank nor his girlfriend, Judy, were stable in their relationships with their drugs of abuse, but their problems were different because of the difference in exposure to the drug. They had another difference. Judy had an alcoholic mother, but Frank had no addicted relatives.

Frank also suffers from depression and social phobia, a morbid fear of social encounters. He uses several antidepressants to help him cope with these problems. Frank and I talk a lot about his need to get on with his life right now, including improving his work-related skills. He does many things right in his life, including, for the first time in his life, buying a home of his own, "so I can pay a mortgage instead of rent." This step into adulthood scares him a lot. Frank now, without too much access to cocaine, has been relatively stable for several years without any addiction treatment. He and I both know that his stability is relative and fragile. Despite the absence of some risk factors experienced by his girlfriend, he has at least one foot on a banana peel, and we both know it.

I wondered out loud to him one day what would happen if the defense contractor for whom he worked as a computer whiz started random drug tests. Frank's reply was simple: "It would depend on how often they tested me. I don't use cocaine very often, so if they tested me once every year or two I would probably just keep on the way I am and take my chances. But if they tested more often, or if they tested when I came back from missing work (often caused by his cocaine use), then I would quit using it. I don't want to lose my job. I'm an addict; I'm not crazy. At that point I would have a reason to stop using cocaine, at least as long as I worked for a company that did drug tests."

Frank also likes to tease me about suing me for malpractice because I encouraged him to buy his home: "When the bank comes after me, I will be at my attorney's office." I asked him about his sleeping pill use. "Oh," replied Frank, "I won't sue you for that. That was my idea."

For all our joking, Frank and I both know that the issues that join us are serious. We are working to improve his life, which is seriously at risk. I feel sorry for him because I see him wasting an important life hanging onto the edge of addiction, not sick enough to have to go into treatment but not well enough to put drugs behind him for good. Frank lives like a person running a long-distance race pulling a large anchor behind him. I wonder what Frank's life would have been like if he had gotten well from his addiction to nonmedical drugs years ago. Today his biggest problem is not the dollars he has wasted up his nose; it is his lost opportunities for growth and achievement, the opportunities for happiness and for helping others. Frank continues to live with cocaine, his secret lover, to his own detriment. I am left to wonder if I am helping him or just adding to the problem by helping him stay back from the edge of his addiction, an edge that may lead to recovery once he falls over it.

Chapter 6

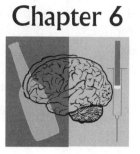

Heroin and Other Drugs of Abuse

In this chapter, I focus on heroin, the hallucinogens, and, a special case of addiction, nicotine, describing how these drugs work and the negative effects they have on the human body.

In Chapter 5, we looked at alcohol, marijuana, and cocaine, the three most widely used addicting drugs in the world and the drugs that are often the gateways into an addict's career. In this chapter we begin by looking at heroin, the most feared of all drugs and the one that literally opened the world's eyes to the desperate potential of modern high-potency drug addiction. Heroin and morphine addiction were common in the last decade of the 19th and the first decade of the 20th centuries as these opiates were widely identified with alcohol and cocaine as the three great scourges of humankind.

Heroin and Other Opiates

Heroin is a white powder which is most commonly injected intravenously, but it can also be taken by mouth or smoked (like crack cocaine). Heroin is much less widely used than alcohol, marijuana, or cocaine because it is feared by most potential drug users and because taking drugs by intravenous injection, as heroin is typically used, is seen by most people as a mark of depravity.

Opiates are the natural or chemically modified extracts of the opium poppy. Opioids are natural opiates plus purely synthetic substances that have similar effects, such as methadone. For practical purposes the entire class of opioids, natural and synthetic, can be considered to be opiates. Opiates modulate the sensation of pain by altering its emotional implications. They inhibit the transmission of impulses over pain-carrying brain neurons. Opiates have a wide range of other brain effects, including the effects on the feelings and behaviors associated with eating, anger, sex, and memory.

The opiates are powerful inhibitors of the body's reactions to stress, tending to reestablish normal physical and mental processes following acute stressful situations. They directly affect the opiate receptors in the brain. Heroin is a very short-acting opiate that rapidly penetrates the blood-brain barrier. The most potent ways to get high using heroin, or any drug, are to inject it into the veins or to smoke it. Because the addiction to opiates is so intense and the problems caused by opiate addiction are so severe, heroin addiction has been a model for all drug addiction throughout the world for nearly 100 years.

The Opiate Calm

The opiate effect is one of calming, tranquilization, and relaxation. Heroin acts directly on the brain's opiate receptors, triggering a warm glow, a sense of euphoria, and a self-centered loss of pain and distress. Opiates are effective in the medical treatment of pain, cough, agitation, and diarrhea. Opiates also affect most body systems. They cause loss of appetite and loss of interest in sex. The body quickly develops tolerance to most of the effects of the opiates. This means that after repeated opiate doses it takes more and more of the drug to produce the desired effect.

After repeated use many times each day, opiates produce virtually complete tolerance to their euphoric effects, as well as to sedation and respiratory depression. Opiates also cause the pupils to constrict, producing *pinpoint pupils* and also slow bowel function (which is why they are used to treat diarrhea). Even when opiate addicts use opiates at relatively steady doses, however, they continue to have pinpoint pupils and suffer from chronic constipation, because tolerance is incomplete to these common opiate effects no matter how long the opiate is used. Because of this differential tolerance to specific opiate effects, long-term opiate users have little risk of overdose unless they stop opiate use long enough to lose their tolerance to respiratory depression, and they are usually not sedated at steady doses. On the other hand, because of this differential tolerance effect, opiate addicts must raise their dose continuously to get high.

Opiates also produce physical dependence. This means that if the opiate drug is discontinued abruptly after prolonged everyday administration, there is a predictable withdrawal syndrome characterized by a reversal of the drug's major effects. In withdrawal, opiate users feel sick and have severe aches and pains, insomnia, and diarrhea. When heroin addicts take a dose, or a "fix," they eliminate any withdrawal symptoms they may have had since their last dose of the drug. Immediately after using heroin they feel calm and content. Unlike the other commonly abused drugs, such as cocaine, marijuana, and alcohol, it is possible for a person to take opiates on a long-term basis with relatively few visible effects on his or her behavior because of the phenomenon of tolerance.

Heroin is poorly suited for therapeutic drug maintenance because it is usually used intravenously or by smoking and because it has a very short duration of action. Heroin users typically take their drug intravenously six or more times a day to keep from going into withdrawal, more in the pattern of a cigarette smoker than of a one-a-day vitamin user or an evening drinker of alcohol. Active heroin addicts are battered all day, every day between a drowsy intoxication and uncomfortable withdrawal symptoms because of the short duration of the heroin's effects.

Nevertheless, heroin addicts do not eagerly switch to a long-acting substance that would let them avoid this discomfort because their primary goal is not to stabilize their lives or to avoid withdrawal but to get as high as possible as often as possible. If their goal was self-medication and not to get high, they would welcome the trade-off of avoiding withdrawal by using a less intensely rewarding, longer acting opiate such as methadone. Intravenous administration of a short-acting opiate—heroin—is the best way to get high from an opiate because it is the most powerful way to stimulate the brain's pleasure centers. For heroin addicts, all of the other effects of heroin use, including its high cost, are burdensome but acceptable side effects of the drug.

Methadone as Medicine

Methadone, being longer acting and orally effective, can be taken once a day and still prevent opiate withdrawal symptoms. Heroin addicts switch to methadone only when they hit bottom and are forced to quit heroin use by the negative effects of their use, usually by their families and the criminal justice system. Addicts seeking to get high do not use methadone because it is taken orally once a day, producing a relatively steady, unrewarding blood, and therefore brain, level of the opiate. On the other hand, if methadone is injected directly into the vein, it can produce a heroinlike intense and short-lived euphoria. When methadone is made available to addicts in dosage forms that permit intravenous administration, many addicts do inject it rather than taking it orally, once again making the point that opiate addicts typically seek the high, not the relief from withdrawal distress. For this reason, the methadone used in American methadone treatment programs is available only in dosage forms that are noninjectable. This ensures that the medicine is taken orally.

Methadone maintenance is the only form of chronic drug therapy not associated with intoxication or obvious impairment because of the virtually complete extent of tolerance to opiate effects on the brain (sedation and euphoria) of once-a-day oral methadone administration. It is not possible for people to function normally when taking continuous doses of alcohol, marijuana, or cocaine, but it is possible for users of methadone to act and to appear normal and nonintoxicated. Tolerance is far less complete to the brain effects of these other drugs than it is to opiates, which also makes these other drugs, such as marijuana and alcohol, unsuitable for therapeutic maintenance.

A heroin addict maintained on heroin, a marijuana addict maintained on marijuana, a cocaine addict maintained on cocaine, and an alcoholic maintained on alcohol are all chronically intoxicated and impaired. A methadone-maintained heroin addict, in dramatic contrast, is neither intoxicated nor impaired because of the complete tolerance to these opiate effects and because of the steady blood levels of the one-a-day oral drug dosage. Thus, methadone is useful as a treatment medicine, whereas the other drugs are not, not because of fashion or laws but because of basic pharmacology.

In recent years L-alpha-acetylmethadol (LAAM), a longer acting methadone-like medicine, has been approved for use in heroin addiction treatment clinics. It is taken only three times a week, rather than every day as methadone is used. This reduces the problems of take-home doses and diversion of the medicine into nonmedical uses, which has been a problem in methadone clinics. LAAM, taken orally, works the same way methadone does by reducing craving and preventing withdrawal while permitting patients to live normal lives.

Morphine is one of a large number of related chemicals called alkaloids found in the sap extracted from the opium poppy. Codeine is another closely related natural alkaloid found in opium. Heroin is produced in the laboratory by adding two small acetyl groups to the morphine molecule. The advantage to addicts that heroin has over morphine results from these two acetyl groups, which help the morphine molecule rapidly penetrate the blood-brain barrier. Once in the brain, the acetyl groups are taken off, and the effects of the drug at the synapses in the brain of addicts are the effects of morphine. Urine tests of heroin users find morphine, not heroin, because the two acetyl groups are removed from most heroin drug molecules before they are excreted as a water-soluble form of morphine by the kidneys.

Heroin: The Drug Nightmare

In 1898, heroin was introduced as an apparently safe treatment for a wide variety of common ailments, from cocaine abuse and alcoholism to infant colic and menstrual cramps. Within a few years, as heroin's medical and nonmedical use spread rapidly in the United States and throughout the world, heroin was universally understood to be a uniquely deadly drug. Medical scientists, humiliated by their failure to anticipate this disaster when heroin was first introduced, focused on learning how this particular chemical and related opiate drugs work. Heroin became the model for the study of drug addiction.

Physical effects of opiate use include lowered blood pressure

Heroin
- An early model for drug addiction
- Usually injected but can be smoked or snorted
- Produces intense physical dependence and overdose deaths
- The end-stage drug of abuse in North America
- Addiction to heroin can be treated with methadone, a synthetic, oral, long-acting opiate

and respiratory rates and constipation. New users often vomit after injecting heroin, but this effect is not seen in chronic, experienced heroin users once their brains become familiar with the drug.

High-dose heroin use, in the absence of tolerance, can lead to depressed respiration, coma, and death. This is the opiate overdose, or "OD." Overdose seldom occurs in opiate-addicted users, even if they take much larger than usual doses, unless they have lost opiate tolerance completely as a result of a period of a week or longer of not using any opiate at all. Heroin addicts die from overdose deaths with some regularity, underlining the important fact that heroin addicts frequently go through periods of involuntary withdrawal when they cannot get a supply of their expensive drug. When they resume heroin use, they lack tolerance. The large doses of heroin they had been taking previously with no problems can then be lethal.

The observation that opiate addicts frequently go through periods of abstinence only to resume heroin use as soon as their drug of choice is again available makes clear that mere detoxification is not a treatment of addiction to heroin or to any other drug. This may surprise many readers. It is also not widely understood by many physicians, even some who work in the field of addiction, because they continue to mistake addiction for physical dependence.

In medical practice, when morphine or other opiates are used to reduce pain, the desired effect of an opiate is not the rush but the steady brain level of the medicine. In medical treatment there is no advantage of heroin over morphine because there is no premium in medical care for super-rapid penetration of the blood-brain barrier. This fundamental pharmacological point has been missed by individuals who have argued in recent years, with much passion but little science, that the United States should make heroin available to treat severe pain such as that sometimes experienced with terminal cancer.

The study of heroin addiction has been fruitful for the scientific study of drug abuse. The discovery of the lock in the brain into which the morphine molecule fits led to the search for natural chemicals, neurotransmitters, that are the usual keys to this lock. One result of this search was the discovery of the endorphins, the brain's own natural morphinelike chemicals. This breakthrough opened the door to a range of previously unsuspected peptide neurotransmitters.

The discovery of the endorphin system led to a new understanding of the neurotransmitter systems in the management of pain and stress. One of medicine's longest searches has been for an effective, powerful painkilling drug that does not produce physical dependence or addiction. Despite intense, lavishly funded research efforts over more than half a century, no such drug has been found, suggesting just how tight the link is between pain relief and drug reward in the mammalian brain.

References to pleasure, drug-induced or natural, as resulting from the release of endorphins have become commonplace in the last few years. Many people now speak of going for a run, having sex, or eating a meal "to get an endorphin high." Although it is not clear whether these diverse activities actually lead to the production of endorphins, we do know that all of these pleasure-producing behaviors stimulate the midbrain's pleasure centers. The study of how heroin works has resulted in new understanding of the brain and the introduction of the language of neurochemistry into popular culture.

Heroin as Medicine

When heroin was introduced as a medicine, it was thought to be an excellent treatment for a wide variety of ailments, including coughs, alcoholism, morphine addiction, and infant colic. However, heroin was rapidly identified as a highly abused and dependence-producing substance. Heroin was removed from the American pharmacopeia in about 1930, meaning that it was no longer available to physicians after that time. Heroin was last used in government addiction treatment clinics in the early 1920s. Since then, heroin has not been available in the United States for any medical reason, although scientists studying heroin and its effects can obtain the drug for their studies. Heroin was removed from medical treatment around the world about the same time that it was taken out of American medical practice because of its unique abuse potential.

Heroin addiction was nearly as common and as widespread as alcoholism at the start of the 20th century. In the United States, heroin addiction became a model on which the understanding of all addiction was based. The use of heroin became far less common after the 1920s because it was so uniquely stigmatized as the most depraved form of addiction. Nevertheless, a new epidemic of heroin use occurred in the period of 1968–1973 in the United States when the number of heroin addicts rose from about 50,000 in the early 1960s to about 800,000 in 1975. In this era, once again, national antiaddiction efforts zeroed in on heroin. In the mid-1990s, heroin addiction is less a focus of national attention than are problems with cocaine, methamphetamine, and even marijuana, but the heroin problem remains large, with about 500,000 people being addicted. The potential for a new epidemic of heroin use remains both real and grave.

Over the years, heroin has had its backers for a variety of medical uses in the United States, primarily in the treatment of addiction or severe pain, especially the pain sometimes associated with terminal cancer. With respect to the treatment of addiction, heroin has one important advantage: Opiate addicts like heroin better than any other drug. It is therefore appealing to addicts and will attract them to enter programs that provide heroin.

In Britain, heroin could be prescribed to addicts by any physician until the late 1960s, when, for the first time in British history, they had a rapidly escalating heroin epidemic. After that, heroin could be given to addicts only in a few tightly controlled government clinics. In recent decades, the British clinics for addicts have all but abandoned use of heroin in favor of methadone, making these clinics more similar to the American methadone treatment centers. Nevertheless, British physicians continue to prescribe heroin routinely for pain and cough to nonaddicts, much as their American counterparts prescribe morphine and codeine. In contrast to the United States experience, the heroin addiction treatment programs in Britain permit addicts to inject methadone.

In the maintenance treatment of addicts, heroin has several serious disadvantages. It has a short duration of action, so the heroin addict has to inject the drug five or six times every day, 365 days a year. Heroin produces tolerance to its euphoric effect, so the heroin addict wants more and more of the drug. When a clinic attracts heroin addicts with the goal of stopping the purchase of the drug from the illicit drug trade, it is not easy for clinic doctors to settle on a heroin dose because addicts claim that they will buy heroin on the street if they do not get more heroin at their clinics.

When a person injects heroin several times a day, he or she is constantly swinging up and down between the drowsy euphoria after the injection and the withdrawal a few hours later. This roller coaster existence makes functioning in a family or on a job, or even driving a car, difficult. Opiate addicts choose heroin because it has a rapid onset and a short duration of action. The very characteristics that make heroin addicts unstable are what make intravenous heroin use so attractive to them. For these reasons, oral once-a-day methadone is much better than injected heroin in the treatment of heroin addicts. Heroin is a poor choice as a maintenance drug, as is injected methadone.

When it comes to the treatment of severe pain, heroin has no advantages over morphine and many synthetic opiates. Some well-meaning people concerned about severe pain, especially the pain of terminal cancer, a few years ago advocated the use of heroin as a compassionate way of improving on current treatments. The National Institute on Drug Abuse sponsored a controlled trial at the Memorial Sloan-Kettering Cancer Center in New York. The results confirmed years of clinical experience that heroin was an effective painkiller, but it was no better than other available analgesic treatments. Thus, heroin does not meet the standard required for highly abused drugs: that it offer significant advantages for some medical treatments compared with less-abused alternative medicines.

Agonists and Antagonists

Opiates, including heroin and methadone, are agonists, which are keys that exactly fit the receptor locks. This effect, unlike that of cocaine and many other abused drugs, works primarily by blocking the reuptake of naturally occurring neurotransmitters. Several synthetic chemicals are known to block the receptor sites for the opiates. They are called *narcotic antagonists.* When addicts take one of these opiate antagonists, they cannot get high from an opiate. After an addict takes a long-acting antagonist, such as naltrexone, injecting heroin produces no effects for a day or two after use of the antagonist. Morphine does not stop pain if blocked by a narcotic antagonist. People who overdose severely on opiates not only survive, but they rapidly wake from a deep coma when given a narcotic antagonist drug. The antagonists cover the receptor sites and block the effects of the opiate. Even if the opiates get to the receptors first, the antagonist knocks the opiate key out of the lock and closes the lock to the key as long as the antagonist stays in the synapse in the brain.

The effects of antagonists, like all medicines, last as long as they are present in the synapse at adequate levels. Two decades ago, when methadone was introduced as a treatment for heroin addiction, methadone overdoses were relatively common when a patient's methadone was taken accidentally, or for purposes of abuse, by people who lacked opiate tolerance. Methadone overdose victims, sometimes infants, were rushed to hospitals and treated with naloxone, the antagonist medicine used to treat heroin overdoses. Both heroin and naloxone, the first opiate antagonist to be widely used in medicine, have short durations of action, meaning they stay in the synapses at effective levels for a few hours. Methadone, by contrast, is slowly eliminated from the body, staying in the synapse at effective levels for 24 hours or longer.

When methadone overdose patients were treated with short-acting naloxone, which had worked well for heroin overdoses, comatose patients at death's door woke up just as heroin overdose victims did soon after receiving the naloxone. Because medical personnel assumed these patients were well, they were sometimes sent to their hospital rooms or put aside in busy emergency rooms. In a few hours they lapsed into a coma and, in some cases, died when the naloxone was eliminated from their synapses. Only later did physicians realize that methadone overdoses, in contrast to heroin overdoses, need to be treated with long-acting antagonists or with repeated doses of short-acting antagonists.

Antagonist therapy.   Naloxone is not effective orally, so it must be injected (like heroin). Naltrexone, a more recent addition to the therapeutic armory, is effective after oral administration (like methadone). An oral dose of naltrexone once a day, or even every other day, is sufficient to block the effects of opiates, including both heroin and methadone. The challenge today for drug abuse treatment is getting heroin addicts to take naltrexone. Because addicts want to get high, they are seldom motivated on their own to take the antagonist because the medicine makes it impossible to get high. Naltrexone has recently been approved to treat alcohol abuse (see page 142).

Naltrexone is used most by physician opiate addicts who are required to take naltrexone as a condition of maintaining their licenses to practice medicine. Although physicians are a tiny percentage of America's opiate addicts, they underscore the point that all forms of drug treatment, including the use of opiate antagonists, are highly dependent on the incentives established by nonusers to promote recovery by raising the cost of continued drug use. Physicians who have been identified as opiate addicts typically have strict supervision, including frequent urine tests, and strong incentives not to use drugs nonmedically. If physician addicts relapse to drug use, they lose their licenses to practice medicine. This is a major cost. Treating physicians with strict testing for drug use is a good example of the environmental approach to addiction treatment.

The discovery of opiate antagonists opened the possibility of finding antagonists for many other abused drugs, especially cocaine, which began producing severe problems in North America during the late 1980s. When scientists search for medicines to block the effects of abused drugs, they often use the model of the narcotic antagonists, such as naltrexone. One problem with this attractive approach to drug abuse treatment and prevention, however, is that drug users can get high on many different drugs, each acting on the pleasure centers of their brains through entirely different mechanisms. Antagonists that block one mechanism to get high do not block others. Addicts treated with opiate antagonists cannot get high on heroin (or any other opiates), and they cannot die from an opiate overdose, no matter how much heroin they take, as long as the antagonist stays in the synapses of their brains. But heroin addicts treated with opiate antagonists can—and all too frequently do—get high on alcohol, cocaine, and other drugs not blocked by the opiate antagonists.

The limits of antagonists. Although the search for an effective general drug abuse antagonist continues, this approach has not been promising. The research problem is reminiscent of finding a vaccination for the common cold. The cold virus changes too rapidly, and the illness is caused by too many related but unique viruses for this approach to work. As soon as a vaccine is developed for one cold virus, the virus changes and the vaccine becomes useless.

A similar problem exists with abused drugs: block one abused drug, and drug abusers and their suppliers, being at least as clever and far more motivated than the cold virus, turn to another drug that is not blocked by the antagonist. The pleasure functions of the brain are too basic and vital to permit only one door into this control room. Addicted people have discovered many doors over literally thousands of years. Block one door with a specific antagonist medicine and many others remain to be opened.

The challenge for both addiction treatment and prevention becomes finding ways to eliminate the desire to use any drugs to get high, by making all abused drugs psychologically unavailable. This involves changing the environment in which the decision is made to use or not to use any drug nonmedically. This helps change the heart and mind of the drug abuser. Such efforts lead to environmental prevention and recovery strategies that are largely nonpharmacological. These techniques attempt to change the "software," the values of people, not the "hardware," their relatively unchangeable brains.

Medicines may help in the war against drug abuse, but they are unlikely in the future to play more than the minor role that they play today. Methadone and naltrexone are helpful in the treatment of heroin addiction. Antabuse and, more recently, naltrexone are helpful in the treatment of some alcoholics. No other drug has been useful for the treatment of significant numbers of abusers of any other illicit drugs, and these three drugs themselves have proven to be a relatively minor part of the treatment of addiction.

Opiate Withdrawal

Withdrawal symptoms after prolonged heroin use resemble the symptoms of the flu: a general sick feeling, abdominal cramps, sweating, nausea, and diarrhea. These are, like all drug withdrawal symptoms, the opposite of the effects of the specific abused drugs. Although opiate withdrawal symptoms are extremely uncomfortable, they are rarely life threatening. Detoxification from opiate addiction does little to help a heroin addict over the long haul because the addict's primary problem is the desire to get high. Values, the inner environment, have to change for recovery to last.

The heroin addict's primary problems have nothing to do with withdrawal symptoms from discontinuing use. Nevertheless, detoxification remained the model for heroin addiction and, because heroin addiction was the basis for understanding of all drug addiction, the model for most drug treatment until the last decade. Unfortunately, it remains the model for understanding many medical and nonmedical drug-using patterns as people seek to explain drug taking based on the experience of withdrawal symptoms after discontinuation of drug use.

Other Commonly Abused Drugs

Hallucinogens

Hallucinogens are a complex, diverse, and remarkably controversial class of abused drugs, which are generally consumed orally. Hallucinogens are more widely used by high school seniors (3.1% used within the past 30 days in 1994) than is cocaine (1.5%). Hallucinogen use is increasing among American high school students as these drugs gain new users who are unaware of the problems caused by the hallucinogens a generation ago. Hospital admissions for lysergic acid diethylamide (LSD) use increased 100% between 1985 and 1992 in the United States.

The effects of the hallucinogens are highly variable from one person to another and from one episode of drug use to another. The most common physical effects, especially within the first hour of hallucinogen use, include dilated pupils, increased heart rate and blood pressure, dizziness, nausea, chills, and tingling, as well as loss of appetite and insomnia. These effects are similar to stimulant effects, reflecting the close relationship of hallucinogens to the stimulants, especially the amphetamines. These effects reflect the activation of the sympathetic nervous system involving the neurotransmitter norepinephrine. The hallucinogens produce changes in perception, feelings, and thoughts that are sometimes described as mystical or even religious. Feelings are exaggerated and moods are magnified. The ordinary often seems remarkable and even wonderful. Sometimes hallucinogen users experience panic, paranoid delusions of persecution, and other frightening and unpleasant feelings. Panic reflects the excessive stimulation of the locus coeruleus, the brain's norepinephrine-based detector of danger.

Hallucinogens are relatively easily separated from most of the traditional agricultural drugs, such as marijuana, cocaine, and heroin. They are not related to marijuana, although some of their effects are similar. When hallucinogens were first introduced in the 1950s, researchers called hallucinogens *psychomimetics* because they mimicked psychotic mental illnesses such as schizophrenia. Early advocates of their use rejected this name, claiming that it was used by people who were hostile to the use of these drugs. They preferred the term *psychedelic* from the Greek words for mind (*psyche*) and visible (*delos*). This term was invented by Humphry Osmond, an early researcher into the effects of mescaline and LSD, in correspondence with the novelist Aldous Huxley in 1956. Later Osmond himself adopted the term *hallucinogen* to describe this class of drugs, but his earlier name has stuck with many prodrug writers. The law enforcement community and the National Institute on Drug Abuse use the term *hallucinogen.*

Hallucinogens generally do not produce overdose death or physical dependence. The hallucinogens cause mild to profound alterations in mood, thought, and perceptions not otherwise experienced except in dreams and psychosis. Although the hallucinogenic experiences are generally dose-related, meaning that the larger the dose of the drug the greater the response, the effects of taking a hallucinogen are unpredictable.

The hallucinogenic drugs generally fall into two chemical classes: *indole derivatives* and phenylalkylamines. The indoles, which have more than one carbon ring, include LSD, psilocybin, and DMT (N,N-dimethyltryptamine). The phenylalkylamines, which have only one carbon ring, include mescaline, MDA (3,4-methylenedioxyamphetamine), MDMA (3,4-methylenedioxymethamphetamine, the N-methyl analog of MDA), and DOM (2,5-dimethoxy-4-methylamphetamine).

A dizzying alphabet soup of chemical variations on mescaline, LSD, and amphetamines has been synthesized and brought to the illegal drug market, including DOM, AMPH, PMA, DOET, and DOB. The initials by which these drugs are known are taken from their closely related but varying chemical structures. DOM, one of the more widely used hallucinogens, was synthesized in 1963 and introduced in San Francisco's Haight-Ashbury drug market in 1967. Drug dealers and drug users called it STP after the popular motor oil treatment. This name was based on the analogy that, just as STP helped car motors run better, this new synthetic drug helped the human brain run better. Later, the same initials were used to call the drug "Serenity, Tranquility, and Peace," a name in accord with the mood of the times.

The modern drug epidemic began when a few risk-taking, intellectual, antiestablishment leaders promoted what they called the consciousness expansion of hallucinogenic drugs, chemicals that disrupt thinking so profoundly that psychosis sometimes develops. Psilocybin and mescaline, naturally occurring chemicals found in certain mushrooms and cacti, respectively, were the initial hallucinogenic substances used. They often produce discomfort, nausea, and dizziness, which limits their appeal. The natural hallucinogens were quickly displaced by LSD, a powerful and purely synthetic hallucinogen free of these troublesome side effects.

A large number of synthetic and natural hallucinogenic compounds have similar effects. They each produce cross-tolerance to the effects of other hallucinogens, which means that when users do not respond to one hallucinogen because of excessive repeated use, they do not respond to any other hallucinogen. All hallucinogens are blocked by the same antagonist drugs. All hallucinogenic drugs inhibit the release of the neurotransmitter serotonin.

Although it is not known precisely how these drugs produce their profound effects on thinking, one hypothesis is that a part of the brain, the *pontine raphe,* which is richly supplied with serotonin receptors, acts as a filtering station for incoming sensory stimuli. This part of the brain screens sensations, sorting out the important from the unimportant. Drugs such as LSD disrupt the sorting process, flooding the brain of the hallucinogen user with jumbled sensory inputs that overload the brain's sensory processing circuits. When high on hallucinogens, users experience dehabituation—the familiar becomes new and the mundane appears remarkable because the brain's normal sorting processes for sensory inputs have been blocked. The brain, intoxicated by a hallucinogenic drug, is unable to assign relative importance to the many stimuli coming continuously to the brain, however routine and trivial they may be.

People high on hallucinogens can be utterly fascinated by the most ordinary experiences. They hear music in new ways, being profoundly moved by the simplest sounds or rhythms. They may look at the pattern in a carpet or a doorknob for hours on end. Ironically, such an effect, labeled by drug proponents as consciousness expansion, is more realistically seen as chemically induced brain immaturity or even stupidity. Like a 3-month-old infant fascinated by the sight of his hand moving across his field of vision, a person high on LSD or MDMA can become fascinated by a dripping faucet or a glowing light bulb. Similarly, simple loud music is popular with many stoned drug users. The stoned brain does not appreciate complexity or subtlety, and it finds the crudest and most banal stimuli to be amazing.

The hallucinogens are a unique group of abused drugs. They are most often used by youth, with most hallucinogenic drug use ending by about age 25. They are taken orally, which makes them unusual in the world of nonmedical drug use. Nonmedical use of prescription drugs such as sleeping pills, tranquilizers, and stimulants, as well as alcohol use, are the other common pattern of oral use of drugs nonmedically.

When hallucinogens were first widely used, scientists gave them to animals and drug addicts to see how rewarding these new drugs were. This is the standard test for the addictive potential of any drug. Hallucinogens were found in these experiments to be unique in another way. Experienced addicts and laboratory animals not only would not work to get hallucinogens, but they treated the hallucinogen high as if it were unpleasant.

The hallucinogen high is a mental experience that appeals mostly to risk-taking youth, not to experienced drug users. Hallucinogens are often an entry into the world of illegal drug use, but they are seldom drugs that illicit drug users stick with over long periods of time. Unfortunately, some youth never get out of this early phase of drug experimentation with hallucinogens because the psychotic reactions produced by the hallucinogens disorganize their lives and lead to suicides and accidents, as well as to long-term abuse of other drugs, most often marijuana, cocaine, and the synthetic stimulants.

Since they began playing concerts in San Francisco in the late 1960s, the Grateful Dead rock music group was intimately connected to the use of psychedelic drugs, especially LSD. Although they once actively encouraged LSD and other drug use, in later years the band took a more neutral stance on the use of drugs. The band toured the country, leading a ragtag following of "Deadheads," often dropouts from school who had adopted a drug-using lifestyle as they spend their lives "doing tour." They followed the rock group from city to city in a caravan of cars, campers, and trucks, wearing brightly colored T-shirts and selling pictures, T-shirts, tapes, memorabilia, and drugs to local youth who came to the concerts. The Grateful Dead concerts themselves were tightly organized and totally predictable musical events that began and ended precisely on time, which gave their often disorganized patrons a comforting sense of predictability.

In recent years, Grateful Dead concerts had featured Alcoholics Anonymous and Narcotics Anonymous meetings for followers who had given up, or who wanted to give up, the use of alcohol and other drugs. Deadheads who returned to home or school often thought nostalgically of their time doing the tour, feeling that the sense of free-living community they found there was not easily replaced in their everyday lives. A strong affiliation with the Grateful Dead is a visible marker of a commitment to nonmedical drug use (especially hallucinogen drug use) and to the "druggie" lifestyle. Today, many Deadheads are no longer young, as this remarkable phenomenon went on for nearly three decades, starting long before the birth of most of today's new followers. In 1995, Jerry Garcia, leader of the Grateful Dead, died in a drug rehabilitation program, apparently of a heart attack, which led to the breakup of the band. However, there are many second-generation Dead-style bands, most notably the bands Phish and Blues Traveler.

Although hallucinogens were the first drugs of abuse in the modern drug abuse epidemic, public attention rapidly left these drugs for heroin, marijuana, and, most recently, cocaine. This shift of public attention did not mean that hallucinogens were no longer used. Their use among youth has remained high for over two decades, continuing into the present. For example, in 1990, 6% of high school seniors and a similar percentage of college students used a hallucinogen at least once in the preceding year, down from the peak of 11% in 1975. Between 1990 and 1994, the hallucinogens have been more widely used by high school seniors, reversing the previous downward trend.

In 1992, a new status was accorded to the use of LSD and related hallucinogenic drugs such as Ecstasy. They were used in "raves"—large organized gatherings of youth (often held in warehouses or, in warmer weather, in open fields) in which synthesized music and laser light shows were featured. Raves began in England in the late 1980s and spread to Germany and other European and North American countries. These all-night happenings were promoted within the risk-taking youth culture for their accentuation of the emotional experiences of combining sound and light shows with the psychedelic experience of hallucinogenic drug use. Because Ecstasy and LSD produce disturbances in body heat regulation and because raves commonly involve extreme crowding, there have been a number of deaths from heat prostration at raves in both Europe and the United States. These experiences of mass intoxication are associated with loss of inhibitions, so the raves are also often associated with uncontrolled and un-protected sexual activity, leading to risks of sexually transmitted diseases, including AIDS.

Initially, raves were held without permits at undisclosed loca-tions. Teenagers had to call ever-changing 800 numbers or follow up on disguised clues distributed at teen hangouts and record stores to find the locations of raves. More recently, raves have been commercialized with broader appeal to affluent teens able to afford the $20 to $30 admission fees.

Raves are promoted as antialcohol, and many teenagers at raves do not think of LSD and Ecstasy as drugs because they are not smoked, snorted, or drunk the way marijuana, cocaine, and alcohol are taken. Teenagers are unaware that Ecstasy is an illegal controlled drug and that it can cause serious and sometimes pro-longed disruption of thinking and even brain damage. Ecstasy is an expensive drug, costing about $25 for a single dose. Many teen-agers who are introduced to nonmedical drug use by using Ecstasy later move to closely related stimulants such as metham-phetamine and to LSD, looking for lower-cost drug highs. Other youth drift into the use of marijuana, cocaine, and heroin after their initial fling with the hallucinogens.

As the hallucinogens have become more popular, treatment centers in Europe and the United States have seen increasing numbers of patients suffering from a combination of anxiety, panic, phobia, depression, and a range of persistent perceptual distortions. This has been labeled *posthallucinogen perceptual disor-der* (PHPD). The syndrome is not yet common, but the youth af-fected, often white male teenagers, experience severe disruptions in their lives during their crucial growing-up years. Some of these youth are so phobic they have trouble coming into treatment to get help. Many of them were not psychiatrically ill before their use of hallucinogenic drugs. PHPD interferes with the process of maturation, leaving sufferers less mature than their peers. As hal-lucinogenic drug use becomes more common, the adverse effects, including frighteningly distorted thinking and bad trips, also be-come more common.

There are three common types of chronic adverse reactions to hallucinogenic drug use: panic or anxiety reactions, depressive reactions, and psychotic mental disorders, including recurrences of distorted thinking called "flashbacks." A particularly frightening aspect of hallucinogenic drugs is the flashback phenomenon that occurs following use of a psychedelic drug such as LSD in about a quarter of users. A sight or sound may trigger an episode of panic in surroundings that remind the user of settings in which the hallucinogen was used. Flashbacks are often triggered by strong emotions and by marijuana or other drug use. Months, or even years, after the last use of a hallucinogenic drug, the user may experience an episode of panic or of perceptual distortion that lasts for minutes or even days. These unpredictable flashback experiences are not well understood, but they can have tragic consequences, including unpredictable behavior and accidents and even impulsive, panic-driven behaviors that can produce life-threatening suicidal actions.

Mescaline (peyote). The primary psychoactive chemical in the peyote cactus, mescaline, is found in the fleshy parts or buttons of the plant. Mescaline can also be produced synthetically. A dose of 300 to 500 mg of mescaline produces hallucinations and disturbed thinking, similar to the effects of LSD, from 4 to 12 hours. Drug abusers have been unable to distinguish LSD from mescaline in double-blind scientific studies.

Psilocybin mushrooms. Psilocybin and psilocin are psychoactive chemicals in more than 90 species of mushrooms, found in many parts of the world including the United States and Europe. Until recently, they have been eaten for their drug effects, mostly in Mexico and Central America. These psychoactive plants have been used for centuries in some Native American religious rituals. This use, like other psychoactive substance use in traditional cultures, was strictly limited to religious rites and had few harmful effects on the people who once used it because of this tight social control. These agriculturally produced psychoactive chemicals have effects that are similar to the effects of LSD except that they are said to be milder and to last for only 4 to 6 hours.

LSD. LSD was first synthesized in 1938. Its hallucinogenic effects were discovered in 1943 when a research chemist accidentally took some of the new substance. He became dizzy and noted that lights were intensified. He closed his eyes and saw fantastic images of amazing vividness in a frightening episode that lasted about 2 hours. This remarkable experience was called a "trip." Disturbing psychotic experiences with hallucinogens are called "bad trips."

LSD is usually bought in tablets, thin squares of gelatin called "window panes," or absorbed into paper called "blotter acid." The average dose of LSD today is from 30 to 50 micrograms, whereas in the 1960s the typical dose was 100 to 200 micrograms. This lower dose produces fewer adverse reactions, making LSD use more acceptable to novice users. LSD effects were achieved by pre-Colombian Aztecs, who chewed seeds of the morning glory family. LSD sold today is synthetic. To increase its hallucinatory effects, LSD is often spiked with PCP, strychnine, or methamphetamine. The effects of LSD last about 8 to 12 hours. LSD is a cheap high, with a dose costing as little as $2 in American high schools.

Hallucinogenic effects diminish rapidly within a few days of repeated use. LSD is the most potent of all commonly abused drugs, meaning that users take the smallest amount of LSD of any abused drug to produce a high. Intoxicating doses of alcohol are measured in hundreds of grams; intoxicating doses of marijuana, cocaine, and heroin are measured in tens of milligrams; and in-

LSD

- The most potent of commonly used drugs
- Easily concealed, cheap
- Not usually used by people over the age of 25
- Produces panic and psychotic reactions
- Causes flashbacks, weeks or months after last use

toxicating doses of LSD are measured in micrograms, or thousandths of a milligram. LSD is relatively difficult to detect in urine tests because there is so little of the chemical present in the urine. For this reason, LSD is easily transported and hidden.

The most common mental effects of LSD are perceptual distortions and visual hallucinations. Objects lose their boundaries and merge, the faces and bodies of people appear to be distorted, and senses and perceptions seem heightened and more vivid. There is an unusual attention to details, with exaggerated importance put on previously ignored objects and events. Concentration is disrupted, and recent memory and judgment are impaired. Personal identity is lost, which may promote mystical experiences of fearful paranoid delusions. The sense of time and normal relatedness is distorted or lost during the LSD intoxication. The overall effects of LSD use are unpredictable, ranging from euphoria to panic and depression.

LSD effects are sometimes described as similar to watching a theater in the mind. Like a person watching a motion picture and being absorbed in it, the LSD user may still be able to perceive the theater in which an event is taking place, meaning the user's everyday reality. The person intoxicated on LSD may be able to exist in these two mental worlds. LSD intoxication commonly produces novel perceptions such as, "My hand turned into a dog, grew wings, and flew out of sight." People high on LSD often feel that they are drifting in a void, between planets, or above the clouds, or they may think they are traveling magically within their own bodies. While high, they may "hear the color blue" or "smell a hot ginger sound." LSD specifically affects the locus coeruleus, the brain's novelty detector and the site of panic attacks in agoraphobia and other anxiety disorders. The locus coeruleus sounds the alarm when a person is confronted by a novel, exciting, and potentially dangerous setting or experience. People who experience panic attacks usually stay close to familiar people and experiences to avoid firing of the locus coeruleus. LSD intoxication makes the locus coeruleus more susceptible to panic attacks.

MDA and MDMA.   Many synthetic hallucinogens have been introduced over the past 30 years, including MDA and MDMA. This family of over 150 related synthetic compounds stands chemically between the hallucinogens and the stimulants. At higher doses these chemicals are hallucinogens, but at lower doses they produce stimulant effects, like amphetamines. Since the 1960s, one of these compounds has followed another as the psychedelic drug fad of the moment. They were synthesized and distributed by drug dealers to avoid prosecution as law enforcement officials scrambled to keep ahead of the illicit chemists' ingenuity. These compounds were typically introduced as not illegal and not harmful, often being picked up by risk-taking middle-class youth and the mass media as a new safe high, in the model of marijuana and LSD. They were called "designer drugs" because they were "designed" by illicit chemists to be "safe" and to evade drug abuse laws. The laws have now been changed so they are no longer designer drugs; they are simply synthetic, illegal drugs.

MDA, also called "the Love Drug," was in widespread use from 1960 to the early 1970s. Its popularity was replaced in the 1980s by MDMA, also called "Ecstasy," "DOM," "X," and "STP." These drugs typically produce drowsiness, a loss of inhibition, and a distortion in the sense of time and distance. Users claim that they can "control the high" and that the drugs are "nonaddictive." Users say that Ecstasy produces an intensification of mood (ranging from euphoria to anxiety and panic), an increase in sensory rather than verbal and abstract thinking, and a coming into consciousness of previously unconscious feelings and desires, often focused on the present moment rather than the past or the future. Ecstasy users describe a feeling of "connectedness" to other people, which led the originator of the drug's use to want to call it "Empathy." He changed the name to "Ecstasy" because he thought too few users would understand what "empathy" meant.

The chemical MDMA, an analog of amphetamine, was first synthesized in 1914 by the Merck Company in Germany. It was introduced into the nonmedical drug culture on the West Coast in 1978. Its use spread to the East Coast less than a year later. MDMA became popular in the early 1980s, when its legal status was uncertain, prompting its listing as a Schedule I drug (high abuse potentiation with no medical uses) in 1985. Since that time it has been an illegal drug. After oral administration of a dose of 100 to

150 mg, there is an amphetamine-like rush, often with nausea, after about 20 to 40 minutes, followed by a 3- to 4-hour period of feeling uniquely related to the rest of the world and an unusual muscular restlessness. Although Ecstasy users occasionally report feeling sexually stimulated, the drug regularly decreases the ability to have an orgasm in males and sexual arousal in females. It has therefore been called a sensual rather than a sexual drug.

Common acute effects of Ecstasy are jitteriness, jaw clenching, and anxiety. At higher doses, panic and paranoid reactions occur. Long-term effects include sleep disturbance and personality changes. Aftereffects can last up to 24 hours, including a hangover characterized by lethargy, fatigue, and the inability to feel pleasure, as well as loss of appetite and decreased motivation. Use of Ecstasy for a week or two may cause confusion, poor personal hygiene, memory impairment, and sleep disturbance, along with sweating, staggering gait, dizziness, and tremor. Residual effects that can last for weeks include exhaustion, depression, fatigue, nausea, and numbness. All of these symptoms reflect long-term serotonin deficiencies in the Ecstasy user's brain.

Ecstasy, like PCP, is a messy drug pharmacologically, affecting many brain neurotransmitter systems. It is a serotonin agonist that also affects dopamine and other neurotransmitters. Ecstasy's acute effects are attributed to a flooding of the overstimulated serotonin system of the brain. The acute effects of Ecstasy are to release serotonin and to prevent its reuptake. In addition, Ecstasy

---

Ecstasy or X

- The newest "safe high"
- Synthetic, closely related to amphetamine
- Can cause psychosis and long-lasting panic disorder
- Disrupts serotonin neurotransmitter system in the brain
- Expensive

is a serotonin agonist. The long-term effect of Ecstasy on the brain is to deplete serotonin. In laboratory animals, including in monkeys given doses similar to human doses, Ecstasy permanently destroys serotonin-containing neurons. Whether this effect occurs in humans remains to be demonstrated by future research, but the possibility is worrisome given the widespread use of this drug.

Because subsequent doses of Ecstasy deplete the serotonin system of the brain, they produce ever-lower positive responses and ever-higher levels of unpleasant side effects. For this reason, and because of its high cost, people tend to use Ecstasy less and less over time. This evolution of usage led to the common collegiate adage about Ecstasy: "Freshman love it, sophomores like it, juniors are skeptical, and seniors hate it." Because of the drug's demonstrated neurotoxicity and reports of lasting neurological disturbances in some Ecstasy users, this drug should be considered as dangerous despite its reputation in the youth culture as safe.

PCP.   PCP was studied in the 1950s as a human anesthetic agent. It was withdrawn from the market in 1978 when it became apparent that PCP produced highly unpredictable effects, with some patients who had been treated with PCP going into terrible psychotic fits of rage and confusion. PCP now has no legitimate medical use anywhere in the world, although some related chemicals are used as tranquilizing agents in veterinary medicine. PCP can be taken orally, smoked (often with marijuana, when it is sometimes called "killer weed" or "loveboat"), or injected.

Illegal PCP is manufactured in makeshift clandestine laboratories, often called "clan labs," with notoriously poor quality control. PCP has more slang names than any other abused drug, reflecting its complex and confusing effects. At small doses, PCP produces marijuana-like effects. As the dose rises, it produces a sense of detachment and estrangement from the surroundings. At still higher doses, PCP produces numbness, slurred or totally blocked speech, drooling, and incoordination. Characteristics of PCP intoxication are a blank stare, rapid and involuntary eye movements, and a bizarre way of walking as if the user were walking through a slush. PCP is often smoked, on tobacco or marijuana, but it can be taken orally or injected.

PCP appears to have the most complex effects on the brain of any abused drug and is therefore considered the "dirtiest" of the abused drugs. PCP affects many neurotransmitter systems, including norepinephrine (NE) and dopamine (DA). PCP affects the neuron membrane entirely separately from its effects at the synapse. PCP blocks the reuptake of monoamines (NE, DA), which accounts for some of PCP's stimulant-like effects. PCP also blocks at least one of the opiate receptors. DA excess may account for PCP's production of euphoria, stereotypical behavior, and schizophrenia-like psychotic reactions. Increased NE activity probably causes the rapid heart rate, the rise in blood pressure, and the hyperactivity seen after PCP use. The sedation caused by PCP may relate to its effects on the serotonin and gamma-aminobutyric acid (GABA) systems.

The drooling seen in PCP users may be caused by its effects on acetylcholine receptors in the brain. PCP users feel numb, like they are existing in an anesthetizing cloud. PCP users sometimes look wide-eyed and confused. Unpredictability is a hallmark of PCP intoxication, in terms of both feelings and behaviors. PCP effects last for several hours after the drug is smoked or taken orally. Long-term PCP users, like long-term inhalant abusers, described next in this chapter, seem not to return to normal as do most abstinent former nonmedical drug users. They often show persistent deadening of feelings and motivation, leading to the description of "burned out," one of the most terrible permanent outcomes of heavy drug use.

In addition to the effects PCP shares with other psychedelics, it has been tied to irrational, sometimes sustained aggressive behavior, including violence. Large doses of PCP can lead the user to fall into a coma and die. Because PCP was, and several related chemicals still are, used in veterinary medicine as tranquilizers, PCP is sometimes called "elephant tranquilizer."

Inhalants

There are dozens of inhalants that affect the brain. These substances are generally divided into two categories: organic solvents, such as paint thinner, and abusable gases, such as nitrous oxide. Solvents are usually liquids that evaporate rapidly, producing vapors with psychoactive properties. Some are glues and others are industrial solvents. Model airplane glues, paints, aerosols, and gasoline are solvents used by some drug abusers.

The physical effects on the central nervous system of volatile solvents are depressant, crudely similar to the effects of alcohol. Solvents typically are abused by teenagers and other people without ready access to alcohol. People who can obtain alcohol almost never use volatile solvents because the effects are less controlled and more bizarre. Solvent abuse is especially common and serious among poor youth in Native American and Mexican communities. Model airplane glue, aerosol paint, and typewriter correction fluid are commonly abused substances in these populations.

The abused solvents are fat soluble and appear to disrupt the neuron membrane, one of the ways that alcohol affects the brain. In low doses, volatile solvents increase nerve transmission. In high doses, volatile solvents profoundly inhibit transmission of impulses in the brain, even causing death from virtually complete brain paralysis. Solvent abuse shares with PCP abuse the reputation as the most physically debilitating of all drug abuse patterns, the dirtiest of abused drugs.

Used in moderate amounts, inhalants cause a feeling of exhilaration and lessening of inhibitions. An increased dose promotes drowsiness, memory loss, mental confusion, and physiological symptoms such as slurred speech and dizziness. Hallucinations, severe tissue damage, and coma can result from prolonged inhalant use.

Abusable Gases

Gases that have strong abuse potential are nitrous oxide, amyl nitrite, and butyl nitrite. Nitrous oxide, commonly referred to as "laughing gas," is legitimately used during minor dental surgery. It has been used less than legitimately by some academics and college students for over a century. The appeal of these gases seems to wax and wane as new generations discover their druglike effects. Unlike the solvents, the abusable gases are often used by people with easy access to other drugs, including alcohol. The gases are short-acting and share with some hallucinogens and marijuana the image of being safe and even sophisticated. The effects of abusable gases are very short-lived, seldom lasting more than a few minutes after use.

The abusable gases produce feelings of dizziness and light-headedness as they increase the heart rate and decrease the blood pressure. These symptoms may become more severe with continuous use of the inhalant until the person faints or even slips into a coma. The gases also produce irregular heartbeats, which can be fatal. The inhalant gases have sometimes been used, especially by homosexual men, to intensify and prolong sexual performance and excitement.

Look-Alikes and Act-Alikes

One of the more curious adaptations of the illicit drug traffic is the selling of fake drugs. This is relatively easy because there are no quality standards for illicit drugs, and there is no way for illicit drug users to know what they are taking. Sold as drugs by some drug dealers, these pills look like stimulants and depressants and may contain caffeine, antihistamines, and other psychoactive but not controlled substances such as ephedrine and pseudoephedrine, which are stimulants found in over-the-counter cold medicines and weight reduction remedies. The most common customers for these look-alike drugs are teenagers and other novice drug users.

Act-alike drugs, also called drugs of deception, are prescription controlled substances, but they are sold as something other than what they are. For example, diazepam (Valium) is sometimes sold as Quaalude, the wildly popular and supposedly aphrodisiac depressant that is now banned from legitimate medical use because of its wide abuse. Local anesthetics, such as procaine and novocaine, are sometimes sold as cocaine. Users will sometimes test their cocaine by putting it on their tongues. When they feel the numbing that occurs with cocaine, they assume they have gotten the drug they seek. This same local anesthetic effect is caused by other chemicals that do not produce the stimulation of the brain's DA pleasure centers that cocaine does. These tricks of drug dealers work better than most people imagine they would because many of the effects of all drugs, even for experienced users, are the result of conditioned responses that are triggered by the set and setting of the drug use. Thus, even experienced nonmedical drug users can be fooled by both look-alikes and act-alikes.

These fake drugs are not safe or benign. They serve as training drugs for youth, making the use of drugs nonmedically seem to be harmless fun. The look-alikes and act-alikes encourage nonmedical drug use. People who are used to taking these usually mild substances may get hold of the real thing and take the same huge dose of the potent drugs that they had been accustomed to taking with the fake drugs. This can produce a serious, and even fatal, overdose reaction. In addition, look-alikes and act-alikes can themselves cause serious, and even fatal, reactions because users often take huge numbers of these pills when they find that the reactions they produce are relatively mild.

Cigarettes: A Special Case of "Addiction"

Nicotine is the dependence-producing chemical in tobacco. It is a brain stimulant producing tremulousness, increased heart rate and blood pressure, and, at high doses, convulsions. It acts on the nicotinic receptors of the autonomic nervous system to increase or decrease release of acetylcholine, depending on the dose of nicotine taken. Nicotine stimulates the release in the brain of both DA and NE. Nicotine also binds directly to the brain's acetylcholine neuroreceptors. Animals will self-administer nicotine as they self-administer other abused drugs, but nicotine is far less reinforcing than amphetamine, the model synthetic stimulant.

Tolerance develops rapidly after repeated nicotine use, especially to the effects of nicotine on the heart and the gastrointestinal system. Smokers typically increase their dose of nicotine when they first begin smoking and then settle into a relatively consistent level of cigarette use over a period of many years. If smokers substitute lower nicotine cigarettes, they often increase the number of cigarettes smoked to maintain their familiar blood and brain levels of nicotine. Despite being only mildly reinforcing, nicotine is a difficult physical dependence to overcome partly because cigarettes are so available and accepted in all parts of the world, and because the negative health effects of nicotine use tend, unlike those of intoxicating drugs, to be long delayed and, for any particular individual, uncertain. Cigarette smoking is the most visible and common form of physical dependence, as typical cigarette smokers must light up about once an hour to avoid uncomfortable, but not dangerous, withdrawal symptoms.

Nicotine, especially in the form of cigarettes, is the most widely used dependence-producing substance in the world. Cigarettes produce by far the most serious health damage of any dependence-producing substance, being responsible for roughly 15% of all deaths in the United States today. This book focuses on the impairing, intoxicating, behavior-affecting drugs that are used nonmedically. When that standard is applied, nicotine is not part of the drug scene.

Even though nicotine does not produce the intoxication and impairment that are common for addicting drugs such as alcohol, marijuana, cocaine, and heroin, this chemical affects the same brain mechanisms of dependence that are involved in the addiction to alcohol and other drugs. Even more importantly, cigarette smoking is the most common cause of physical dependence and the leading cause of preventable death in the world today. Cigarettes are the only commercially available product that, when used as intended, produces cancer, heart disease, and death as predictable and common outcomes. Furthermore, cigarette smoking is highly correlated with the use of illegal drugs, especially for youth, making cigarette use an important marker for the high risk of addiction to alcohol and other drugs. For these reasons, caffeine and nicotine are covered in this book.

Dependence Without Intoxication

Cigarettes are the most serious nonintoxicating pharmacological habit. Cigarette smoking does not lead to auto accidents, lost jobs, or broken homes. Cigarettes simply kill smokers, usually at relatively older ages, mostly in the 50s and 60s. To understand why the United States has 50 million cigarette smokers is to understand the power of the brain's reward centers and the complex personal and social forces that cause and perpetuate this most common and deadly physical dependence.

Tobacco was first used in religious rites in the New World by Native Americans over 2,000 years ago. During the 17th century, tobacco use was banned in many nations of Europe and Asia because of the risk of dependence. Tolerance to nicotine develops rapidly, after only a few days of use. Withdrawal symptoms are common and obvious after repeated use of tobacco over a period of months or years. The physical effects of nicotine are to accelerate heart rate and blood pressure while depressing the appetite. Cigarette smoking irritates the lungs and causes cancer, heart disease, and many other illnesses.

In 1990 in the United States, about 420,000 deaths were attributed to cigarette smoking. In contrast, the total number of deaths connected to the use of illicit drugs in 1990 were less than 10,000. Alcohol use claimed about 125,000 lives that year. Cigarette smoking produces nicotine dependence. It kills more people than alcohol and other illegal drugs combined. It is a major health problem in all parts of the world.

Cigarettes

- Physical dependence and brain reward without intoxication
- Serious habit without impairment in everyday life
- Most lethal of all dependencies, causing more deaths than alcohol and all other drugs combined
- Cigarette smoking by youth highly correlated with nonmedical drug habits, including alcohol and other drug abuse

---

Cigarettes are the only known powerfully carcinogenic product produced and sold legally in the United States. That fact is a strong commentary for the clout of the American tobacco industry, which has lobbied long, hard, and expensively for exemption from routine public health regulations. It will be interesting to watch in the next decade how well the tobacco industry fares against the growing antismoking forces that have taken hold throughout the country.

Since 1967, when the Surgeon General mandated warning labels for cigarette packages and advertising, the public has become increasingly aware of the hazards of tobacco smoking. Yet even more impressive are the remarkable local and grassroots efforts that have gone into changing public perception and attitudes about smoking. Smoking in offices, in restaurants, and even in private homes has become prohibited formally and informally. Airlines have taken smoke out of the skies over the entire United States. From a limitation of the smoking of pipes and cigars to a total ban on all smoking, including cigarette smoking, on domestic flights, the airlines took only a few years to adopt a national trend into a universal, legally enforced industry-wide policy. Such changes reflect rapid and profound changes in American attitudes toward smoking as intolerance to tobacco smoking rises year after year. Since 73% of American adults do not smoke cigarettes, the rapid political and economic spread of the antismoking campaign is not hard to understand.

Smoking in North America is currently more prevalent among lower socioeconomic and education levels. People who are better educated and of higher economic status are less likely to smoke cigarettes. This disparity in social status is becoming even more pronounced as better educated, more affluent people become more involved in healthful lifestyles, including quitting smoking.

Yet even as public tolerance of tobacco use has dropped, the number of persons still smoking remains formidable. Most disturbing is the rise in cigarette smoking among North American teenagers that began in 1991 (see Chapter 3). The tobacco industry has shifted its advertising to appeal to population groups identified as being more apt to smoke. This tactic has resulted in

considerable backlash, from protests of athletic contests sponsored by tobacco companies to strong statements made by the secretary of the Department of Health and Human Services and the
U.S. Surgeon General, especially related to tobacco industry targets on youth and minority communities. The alcohol industry
has adopted similar targets for promotion of alcohol use, and
these efforts also have elicited spirited opposition, especially
among people concerned about health.

Labeling Nicotine as a Drug

In the United States there are increasing efforts to classify nicotine
officially as a drug, considering cigarettes to be a "drug delivery
system." Nicotine is addictive. The chronic smoker is suffering
from an addictive disorder. No illicit drug comes as close to dem-
onstrating the biology of addiction as cigarettes do in everyday
life and in highly visible ways. Smokers, more than users of alcohol, marijuana, cocaine, or even heroin, use their drug from the
first moments they wake up to the last moments before they go to
sleep, every single day. If smokers are separated from their cigarettes for even a few hours, they develop uncomfortable withdrawal symptoms.

However, officially classifying nicotine as a drug has many
disadvantages. First, although nicotine is addictive, so are caffeine
and alcohol. Are we prepared to classify those substances as
drugs? Second, if nicotine is a drug, then the appropriate response is to ban tobacco entirely. Nicotine has no therapeutic uses,
and the only reason to use it is to perpetuate a dangerous addiction. There is no historical or legal precedent for selling dangerous
drugs to the public, much less having physicians prescribe them.
The only exception to the social contract that bans the use of addicting drugs is methadone treatment for heroin addicts. It is un-
imaginable that cigarette smokers would line up each morning at
government licensed clinics to get their drugs, the way methadone patients do today. If an exception to the social contract were
made for cigarettes, it would open the process to appeals by those
who want to legalize marijuana, cocaine, LSD, and other currently illegal drugs. This would widen the doors of social accep-

tance and increase the levels of use of these drugs.

Efforts to discourage smoking, including banning cigarette advertisements, raising cigarette taxes, and reducing the accessibility of cigarette sales, deserve wide support. Nevertheless, labeling nicotine a drug and having it regulated by the Food and Drug Administration or other government agencies is not a good idea because it opens a Pandora's box for government health regulation. How much nicotine is "okay," and how can the government avoid the conclusion that cigarette smoking should be totally prohibited? Regulation implies endorsement, and that is hard to do with the leading cause of preventable death in North American today: cigarette smoking.

Prevention programs that aim to help youth should reject illicit drugs as well as help youth reject the use of both tobacco and alcohol. Alcohol and other drug treatment programs should target nicotine dependence and help their patients in every way possible to quit smoking.

It is not a good idea to pit antismoking efforts against antidrug efforts, as is sometimes done by antismoking advocates who dismiss the relative dangers of illicit drugs. A sensible public health goal is to reduce the levels of use of tobacco, alcohol, and illicit drugs. Tobacco deserves a high place in these public health priorities because of the terrible toll that nicotine takes in terms of illness and death. However, unlike alcohol and other drugs, nicotine claims the lives of older people rather than younger people. Nicotine is not intoxicating, and it does not produce the disruptive and dangerous impairments that alcohol and other drugs do in schools, in the workplace, on the highways, and in families.

The frontier in tobacco use prevention today is the roughly 1 million American teenagers who become hooked on tobacco each year. This tidal wave of new smokers is a national tragedy that reflects not only the failure of youth but, even more, the failure of adults to exercise adequate stewardship of the nation's most valuable resource, its youth. The legal smoking age should be raised from the current age of 18 to 21, and vigorous efforts should be made to enforce the smoking age, including requiring that applicants for drivers' licenses who are under 21 must pass a drug test for the recent use of cigarettes. Youth who show evidence of recent smoking should be denied drivers' licenses, as well as other benefits such as participation in extracurricular school activities. (The controversial issues of public policy are discussed in Chapter 12.)

Tobacco is in a class by itself. It should not be lumped with illicit drugs when it comes to public policy. The same is true for public policy on alcohol, which is discussed in Chapter 12. Although they are dangerous and addicting, these two substances, which are legal for adults but illegal for youth, are so widely used and so deeply rooted in the history of most of the world that they are best treated as special cases. Making that recommendation does not give a green light to either tobacco or alcohol use, but it does respect the unique biology and history of alcohol and tobacco.

We have focused on just four drugs that produce intoxication (brain impairment) and reward (stimulation of the brain's pleasure centers). These four substances—alcohol, marijuana, cocaine, and heroin—are the backbone of the addiction problem in the world today. Chapter 5 focused on alcohol, marijuana, and cocaine, and this chapter focuses on heroin and the hallucinogens. Only the hallucinogens, such as LSD, are clearly different from one of these four basic drugs, and even they are chemically related to the amphetamines, stimulants that are, in turn, quite similar to cocaine. Armed with an understanding of these four drugs and how they work, you are ready to understand old drugs and new drugs that will come along. When it comes to drugs of abuse, anything that is new is likely to fit into the patterns that have become familiar during a century of serious drug abuse problems.

Case Histories

Bill spent his adult life as one of the Washington, D.C., area's outstanding blues musicians and media personalities. I first met him when he had been recently released from the old and famous St. Elizabeth's Hospital, the public mental hospital in the nation's capital. Bill had been confined there for persistent heroin addiction. While he was incarcerated, he took many of the doctors who came through the hospital under his wing, educating a generation of them about heroin addiction. I was just one more in a long list of doctors he had helped.

Bill's greatest feat, however, was not his media or educational achievements, but his ability to figure out on his own that the only way he could survive was by going to 12-step meetings and then only by avoiding alcohol, as well as heroin and cocaine. Few of my early heroin addict patients figured that out. Most paid for this failure with their lives as they were cut down one after another in their 40s and 50s by alcoholism. Bill's story contrasts with his friend Charles, who overcame his heroin problem but did not appreciate the unity of the addiction problem, as he attempted to become a "social drinker" once he stopping using heroin. Rocky's story tells of the common, often overlooked connection of drinking to excess and dangerous, impulsive sex in the age of AIDS.

Bill and Charles

When I worked for the city government, starting the first large, city-wide addiction treatment program in 1970, I put together a group of about a dozen ex-addict advisers. We met weekly. I listened to them and learned from them. They were terrific people who had lived hard lives of considerable courage. They contributed greatly to the building of the program called the Narcotics Treatment Administration (NTA). The senior research scientist from that initial group went on to a distinguished career as a research administrator in the federal government. When he retired in 1992, many of us got together to honor his service.

The person who most interested me at the retirement gathering was Bill, who had been a member of the original group 22 years before. We had both aged, of course, but that made the renewal of our friendship all the more joyous. We reviewed the names of the others from our group. Some, like Bill, had used methadone for a while in their treatment, but most of them had not. I told Bill that the biggest change in my thinking over those two decades was that I now believed that for most people the 12-step fellowships were the only way to stay clean and sober. I did not know that in 1970. In those years, I thought psychologi-

cal, family, and vocational counseling would make a big difference. I told Bill that, in contrast to those years, I realized now
that addiction was one disease, the addiction to getting high on
alcohol and other drugs. In former days, I thought that a person
was addicted to heroin or alcohol specifically and that these
were more or less separate problems. I now saw the one disease
of addiction as progressive and lifelong, and I thought of relapse
as the likely outcome for many people over time. Preventing relapses was the primary goal of therapy. Bill told me about the
fates of many of our group members. One had died of AIDS and
a few had died of natural causes, but most group members had
died of alcoholism.

Charles was one member of the group whom Bill and I
highly respected. He never went back to the use of heroin, and
he obtained a good job with the Probation Department, working
his way up to becoming a supervisor. He had gotten married
and had quite a good life. He earned a good living and, best of
all, Charles was fulfilling his lifelong ambition to help those in
our community who needed help the most.

Although Charles had never relapsed to heroin use, his alcohol problems got worse and worse. He was arrested for driving while impaired (DWI). He took his punishment, which was
a suspended driver's license and mandatory attendance for
6 weeks at a DWI school. Then Charles went to his boss, the chief
judge who had faith in Charles, and apologized, saying he
would never do it again. Six months later he was arrested again
for DWI. This time, Charles was too ashamed to face the chief
judge or anyone else at work. He quit his job, the job of his lifetime and the only really good job he had ever had. Two years
later, his marriage in a shambles and his drinking out of control,
Charles was taken to a local university hospital in a coma from
which he never recovered. His wife asked me to visit him because he was dying of irreversible liver failure. I was busy at that
time, so I delayed visiting him until that weekend. When I called
to check on his room, I was told that I must be mistaken because
they did not have anyone by that name and suggested that perhaps Charles was in another hospital. I called Charles's wife,
who had been my secretary 20 years before. She said I had the
right hospital, but that Charles had died 4 days before. They had
already buried him, at the age of 51.

Bill told me he had seen the members of our group die one after the other and that he had figured out what he must do. He had to join AA and to stop drinking if he was to live: "I didn't beat the horse (heroin) to lose my life to cognac the way our friends have done." We agreed to go to some 12-step meetings together because Bill wanted me to see how much had changed since we had last worked together 20 years earlier: "Now there are AA and NA meetings everywhere in the city. Before it was hard to find any meetings, except in the suburbs."

Rocky

A 32-year-old successful salesman of computer software, Rocky had never been married, but he had had many girlfriends. "I never ask a girl out," he told me. "They come to me. I am always with the nicest and most beautiful women. I am still waiting for the right one to marry. I haven't met her yet." He drank with his friends, as much as six to eight drinks at a time, mostly on weekends. But he had never missed work because of his drinking, he had never had an alcohol-related accident, and he had never been arrested for driving while impaired. He rarely got drunk and did not have any alcoholics in his family. He said he was not an alcoholic, and I agreed with him.

He came to see me for public speaking anxiety, which responded well to medicines and therapy. One day he came in, visibly upset, and told me this story. "I went to Mexico for a week's vacation. I went out to the bars, as I usually do, to meet people. I was with a male friend who was a bit shy, so I was trying to set him up with a beautiful woman we met who was on vacation at the same resort. I suggested that we all go skinny dipping in the pool after midnight when no one else was there. Both my friend and the woman agreed. The next thing I knew, this woman was down at my end of the pool, and we were having sex. I just do not have unprotected sex, but this happened so fast I never even thought about protection at all. Now I am scared to death about getting AIDS. I went an AIDS clinic and talked with a counselor, who said this was not terribly high-risk behavior, but that it was definitely unwise. I will have to wait 3 to 6 months to get an AIDS test to know whether I got infected. Two minutes of fun and 6 months of fear. Every day I worry about it and kick myself for being so dumb."

I asked Rocky if he thought that his drinking had anything to do with his recklessness. He said he had never thought of that, but, once he did think about it, he realized that he would never have had sex like that if he had not been drinking. He also realized that the woman was an alcoholic whose uncontrolled sexual behavior was common for her when she was drunk. Rocky concluded, "I thought IV drug use was the only way alcohol and drug use was related to AIDS. I guess I was wrong."

These are two stories of alcohol and drug use and the ways people come to see and deal with their use of these substances. Bill, Charles, and Rocky all helped to educate me about the disease of addiction.

Section III

Overcoming Addiction

We begin this section by looking into the experience of individual addicts as they pursue what becomes an involuntary journey of personal discovery. We then look at the addict's family and the mysterious but ultimately understandable problem of codependence, the echo of addiction. We next explore the roles of family and community to investigate the various forces that promote or prevent addiction, looking in detail at the common problems of alcohol and cigarette smoking in families and communities. Next, we examine ways to drug-proof children and, failing the mission of prevention (as often happens with the best efforts), to find and use addiction treatment. We end this section with a look at the 12-step fellowships, which are modern miracles in our midst, a discussion of public policy choices to prevent addiction, and speculation about the future direction of illicit drug use throughout the world.

Chapter 7

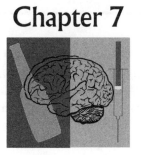

The Addict's Career

In this chapter, I describe the uniquely human process of addiction and give readers a basic vocabulary for communication about what is happening in the lives of addicts.

Addicts do not use alcohol and drugs to become addicted. Addiction is an unwanted side effect of the substance use. There are four stages to the addict's career: fooling around, getting hooked, hitting bottom, and recovery. Not everyone who

Stages of Addiction
- *Fooling around*—the honeymoon stage
- *Being hooked*—loss of control and denial
- *Hitting bottom*—paying the price for living out of control
- *Recovery*—the hard-earned, elusive gift of addiction

starts out gets to the end of the road. Some people never get out of the stage of fooling around, others never hit bottom, and many never get well. Many addicts, however, go through all four stages. The stages are the same for all drugs, but each drug has characteristic effects that distinguish it from the other drugs.

Fooling Around

Fooling around often is the honeymoon stage of addiction. It usually starts between the ages of 12 and 20, often with alcohol and/or marijuana, but occasionally with other drugs such as inhalants and hallucinogens. Like a marital honeymoon, there can be many problems at this stage of the experience.

At the age of 12, the daughter of a medical colleague of mine set two national swimming records in four-person medley relays. One of the other girls on the impressive team was my older daughter, Elizabeth. My colleague's daughter was dead at 16 because of drug use. After smoking marijuana at the home of one of her neighbors, she returned home stoned and walked into the path of a speeding car. She became a victim of marijuana, the "careless drug." She was not an addict—she never progressed past the initial stage of addiction—but she and her family paid for her drug use with her life.

In the early stages of addiction, the addict seeks euphoria, a good feeling. As the drug use continues over months and years, the low point in the feeling cycle drops so that in time the addict is no longer seeking "good" feelings as much as "better" feelings. Experienced addicts sometimes say, "I use now just to feel okay for a little while." As the disease of addiction progresses, addicts are "treating" their own drug-caused bad feelings, known as *dysphoria*. The selfish brain remembers those early highs, and it experiences the continued immediate reinforcement of the better feelings that come after each use of the drug. Fooling around is the stage in which the addict learns to ride the drug swing, the mood changes, the highs and lows, caused by repeated drug use.

The duration of the fooling around stage of addiction is determined by many factors. The higher the individual's personal genetic predisposition for addiction, the faster he or she moves through this stage toward getting hooked. This is because the drug user with a higher biological predisposition for addiction likes the drug high more than do drug users who lack this heightened risk. People who have had a malignant course of addiction, meaning that they progress rapidly from fooling around to being hooked, often say that they fell in love the first time they tried the drug, or after only a few uses of the drug. Right away, they say, they liked the feeling that the drug produced.

In contrast, many people who fool around with drugs and then drop them, without ever progressing to having a love affair with drug use, say that the drugs did little or nothing for them. Alcoholics who drink alcohol for many years without loss of control, only to lose control later in their lives, often say that the alcohol was of some interest, but not much, until they had some change in their lives that led to their turning increasingly to alcohol for pleasure.

When a person uses a substance for a long period of time without loss of control, and then later loses control of drug use, there has been an environmental change that shifted the alcohol use from benign to malignant. There was no change in the drug and no change in the brain of the user. What changed was the life of the future addict. That changed life led to changed feelings as a result of the use of alcohol or other drugs. This change in the user's life triggered the previously latent progression of the disease of addiction. A job loss or a divorce can trigger a more active phase of the illness, as can a new job, a promotion, or a new group of friends.

The first pattern—rapid and severe addiction—is most often seen in people with parents and siblings who are also addicted to alcohol or other drugs. The second two patterns—those who use a drug but drift away from it, and those who fool around with a drug for a long time without loss of control—are more often seen in people who do not have close relatives with addiction problems.

Although it is not possible at this time to test for the genetic trait associated with addiction, it is possible to determine just how much the use of the addictive substance means to the person using it by asking the person. The more important the use of alcohol and other drugs is to anyone, the more rewarding the experience of using the substance, the greater the risk of addiction. The single best way to avoid the risks of addiction, no matter what one's genetic makeup, is not to use the substance at all. Figuring out this genetic risk by trying a drug is a hazardous gamble for which many people pay high prices. Sometimes people who lose this gamble pay with their own lives or with the lives of other people.

Genetic vulnerability is not the only important influence on the relative risk of addiction among those who try drugs. The younger the person is when drug use starts, the more rapid and the more likely the progression to loss of control over drug use. Younger initiators of nonmedical drug use also tend to have more character disorders than do older initiators. Youth who are impulsive, prone to lying, and interested mostly in the present, not the future, are especially vulnerable to rapidly progressing addiction. The brains of younger users are more vulnerable to the seduction of the drug highs, just the way youth are especially vulnerable to brain-based pleasure disorders involving feeding and sex. Adolescence turns up the heat in the brain's pleasure centers.

Environments that permit and even encourage drug use at a young age tend to promote addiction. When people use drugs in settings and with people who encourage alcohol and other drug use, they are more likely to progress to full-blown addiction. Especially risky are peer groups of heavy users of alcohol and other drugs. One of the top predictors of addiction is having a best friend who is an addict. Having personal values favorable to drug use and spending time with others who have the same values increase the risk of trying drugs and, once having tried them, of progressing to loss of control over drug use.

It is said that individuals who are destined to become addicts will find alcohol and other drugs no matter how restrictive the environments in which they live. It is also said that some people will never become addicted to alcohol and other drugs no matter how permissive their environments are toward the use of alcohol and other drugs. Both statements are true but dangerously misleading.

Surely there are some people who hone in on addictive drugs the way air-to-air missiles seek out their targets. The more important reality, however, is that whereas a small percentage of people seem either utterly destined for addiction or completely impervious to it, the large majority of people lie at neither extreme. This large middle group is composed of the people who are influenced by the environment in which exposure to addictive substances exists. Thus, the size of the vulnerable population for addiction to alcohol and other drugs rises in permissive environments, and the size of the invulnerable population rises in relatively restrictive environments. This is an important perspective not only for the prevention but also for the treatment of addiction to alcohol and other drugs.

Fast and Slow on the Road of Addiction

The route of administration and the choice of a particular drug also play big roles in the speed of progression beyond the stage of fooling around with drugs. Smoking and shooting, which get drugs to one's brain rapidly at high doses, are more likely to produce rapid progression from fooling around or being hooked than is oral use of a drug. Heroin and cocaine are more likely to produce rapid progression than are alcohol and marijuana. People who use a drug more often are more likely to progress rapidly than those who use the same drug less often.

All these factors interact in powerful and sometimes mysterious ways. A rapid, malignant development of addiction usually signals a combination of many risk factors, including a high genetic risk, character disorder, early use, frequent heavy use, and an environment that is permissive for nonmedical substance use. Slow development of addiction usually means the opposite cluster: lack of genetic factors, relatively little character disorder, relatively late and infrequent drug use, and an interpersonal environment that is less tolerant of drug use.

This experimental use of addicting drugs is like playing Russian roulette, putting a gun to your head when there is a shell in one of the six chambers, spinning the chambers, and then pulling the trigger with a smile on your face. People who use drugs later in their lives and in lower amounts pull the trigger only once. Five out of six of those people survive without succumbing to addiction. People who use addicting drugs earlier and more heavily pull the trigger two or three times, so more of them are victims of their selfish brains. When people with close relatives who are addicted use drugs by smoking or injecting at young ages, they are pulling the trigger six times. Few survive that gamble without serious addiction.

In the fooling around stage, the addict is likely to become interested in using the substance because a close friend is using it and tells the neophyte user that the particular drug can be used safely and with pleasure. Use of alcohol and drugs usually begins between the ages of 12 and 20, with the most common starting age in North America today for the two principal gateway drugs of intoxication—alcohol and marijuana—being the 9th grade, or about the age 15 or 16.

Character plays an important role in addiction. In this book I use the term *character disorder* to describe a specific constellation of thoughts and behaviors. This term is commonly used by psychiatrists and others in the mental health and educational fields. More technically, the syndrome is classified as a *personality disorder*, a maladaptive pattern of behavior that appears in childhood and usually persists throughout a person's life. The specific personality disorder that most closely fits what I call character disorder is *antisocial personality disorder*. However, in the *Diagnostic and Statistical Manual of Mental Disorders*, the official diagnostic manual for mental disorders, this diagnostic term is restricted to the most se-vere cases. When I use *character disorder,* I am referring to a group of enduring characteristics that are seen in varying severity from mild to extremely severe. The severe cases are labeled as *antisocial personality disorder.*

The most prominent features of character disorder are think-ing about the present rather than the future and frequent dishon-esty. Other features include relative insensitivity to the feelings of others, rebellion against authority, and relative imperviousness to punishment. Character disorder is more commonly seen in males than in females, and it is at its peak from the ages of about 15 to 25 years, tending to diminish at older ages. It is seen in all ethnic and economic groups. (See Chapter 9 of this book for a discussion of preventing addiction among high-risk youth as well as a check-list for youth at high risk of addiction to alcohol and other drugs.) In this book, *high risk* generally refers to character disorder, be-cause character disorder creates a uniquely high risk of addiction to alcohol and other drugs.

The more the future addict suffers from character disorder, meaning the more the new drug user is focused on current pleas-ure instead of on future consequences, and the more the person lies and is reckless, the more likely the use of any particular sub-stance is to occur, and the more likely that use is to progress to addiction. The more a person suffers from character disorder, the lower the "bottom" of the addict's career is likely to be. This means that with more character disorder, the negative consequences of drug use must be terribly severe before addicts conclude that they can no longer continue their affairs with alcohol and other drugs.

This sounds more complex than it is. People, especially youth who focus on the present rather than the future, are relatively impervious to the painful consequences for using alcohol and other drugs because painful consequences, almost invariably, are delayed and uncertain for each person. That is why ever-optimis-tic character-disordered youth repeatedly engage in pleasure-producing behaviors without learning from their many negative experiences. They learn only in the present tense. In the right-now world of the selfish brain, drugs work every time they are used. Ask such people why they continue such apparently senseless behavior that produces such painful long-term consequences and they will explain that each and every time they use the drug, they think they can get away with it. They truly believe that they can have their drug fun without a painful result this time. Every time they have a painful result from their use of alcohol or other drugs, they are surprised anew. Painful results typically do not occur every time the addict uses the drug, and, when they do occur, painful results are usually delayed after the drug use and subject to excuses and explanations that hide the connection of the distressing outcome to the drug use.

Think of training a dog and rewarding or punishing the dog on an irregular basis hours or days after the behavior about which you are concerned. For example, the dog jumps up on people who come to your home, and you punish the dog for this behavior 2 days later. Would the dog ever learn? No, never. Only by pairing the reward or the punishment immediately with the behavior does the most basic form of learning take place. The human brain acts like the dog's brain when it comes to addiction, unless the human has a highly developed sense of future consequences. People with character disorder, and most youth, do not learn well under such circumstances. In truth, most of us have trouble learning from delayed and personally uncertain consequences. This is precisely the reason that laws had to be passed to make wearing seat belts mandatory in airplanes and automobiles, and to make the use of drugs, such as marijuana, cocaine, and heroin, illegal for everyone.

For addicts, the painful consequences not only have to come often and soon after alcohol and other drug use, but they have to be sufficiently painful for meaningful learning about the dangers of drug use to take place. This is true both because many addicts are relatively impervious to punishments and because the rewards of drug use are so powerful. It also helps high-risk people to learn from others who are addicted because they can more easily identify with kindred souls. They discover not only that other people learn the first time something bad happens to them as a result of alcohol or other drug use, but also that they often do not have to engage in such risky behaviors by using alcohol or other drugs in the first place.

Low-risk people learn quickly and easily when they are warned against such risky behaviors as the use of alcohol and other drugs by others, such as their teachers, parents, and the police. High-risk or character-disordered youth seldom learn this way about pleasure-producing behaviors, unfortunately for them and for everyone who cares about them. They mainly learn the hard way, through their own personal pain.

Type I and Type II Addicts

When dealing with alcohol dependence, the distinction between high and low levels of character disorder has led to distinguishing two types of alcoholics: Type I and Type II. This distinction can be extended to all forms of addiction. Type I addicts are those who begin drinking somewhat later in their lives and who progress to full-blown addiction fairly slowly, usually over many years or even over decades of drinking. These are the alcoholics who generally do well in their lives, often completing school, getting married, having children, and developing more or less solid careers.

Some Type I alcoholics are highly successful, often in part because they are relatively more comfortable taking risks than are most of their nonalcoholic peers. Type I alcoholics may or may not have close relatives who are alcoholics or drug addicts. This is the classic pattern of alcoholism of the early pioneers who founded Alcoholics Anonymous (AA). Most were middle-aged and had successful careers and families, often despite their malignant alcoholism. Some had desperate stories of their drinking problems, but they often were solid citizens except for their drinking. Type I addicts usually lie about their drinking and drug use, but they are reasonably honest about most of the remainder of their lives. Some Type I addicts are shy and dominated by severe consciences, characteristics that are uncommon in Type II addicts.

Type II addicts have severe character disorder with frequent behavioral problems, not just with their drug and alcohol use but in a wide variety of areas. They are often truant from school and rebellious against authority. They start lying at an early age. They begin drug and alcohol use early and progress rapidly into grave behavioral problems, often dropping out of school during high

Types of Addicts

Type I

- Later onset of initial use of alcohol and other drugs, usually starting use at age 16 or older
- Usually just alcohol use or alcohol and prescription medicine misuse rather than early multiple drug use
- Later onset of problems as a result of alcohol and other drug use, often in the 30s to the 60s
- Generally stable education, employment, and family life
- No arrests except possibly driving while impaired (DWI)
- Reasonably honest, except about the use of alcohol and other drugs
- High bottoms
- Better prognosis for recovery

Type II

- Early onset of problem-generating use, usually well before the age of 16
- Rapid progression to multiple illicit drug use
- Early onset of severe problems as a result of alcohol and drug use, usually in the teens
- Unstable education, employment, and family life
- Generally dishonest; frequently lie
- Low bottoms
- Poorer prognosis for recovery

school. They are frequently arrested for a wide variety of crimes, including but not limited to drug use and sale. Type II addicts lie about everything in their lives to get what they want from anyone who is foolish enough to trust them, not just about their use of alcohol and drugs.

Most addicts have some features of both types, although one pattern usually predominates. When addicts get well, most of them look like Type I addicts. When they are very ill with addiction and actively using alcohol and other drugs, they almost all look like Type II addicts. Age also plays a big role: as addicts age, they look more like Type I addicts and less like Type II addicts.

It is easier to sort out Type I from Type II addicts once addicted people are clean and sober. When that occurs, Type I addicts gradually lose most of their traits of character disorder such as impulsivity, dishonesty, and self-centeredness. In contrast, Type II addicts typically continue to demonstrate character defects to a greater or lesser degree even when they are not using alcohol and other drugs. For this reason, Type I addicts who manifest character disorder are said to have *secondary character disorder,* meaning that it was induced by their alcohol and other drug use, whereas Type II addicts are said to have *primary character disorder,* meaning that it was present before as well as after their drinking and drug-using episodes. The 12-step programs are excellent ways to overcome both addiction and character disorder. They have a way of describing the character-disordered self-centeredness of addiction: "A person wrapped up in himself is the smallest package in the world."

Whereas use usually begins during the teenage years with alcohol and marijuana, as drug users become more experienced they branch out and try many drugs depending on the current fashion of their drug-using peers. As their drug use becomes more intense and more frequent, it is likely to involve more drugs in a pattern that was once uncommon but is now typical. This is called *polydrug abuse* or multiple drug abuse. Alcohol is often, but not always, a major part of the polydrug picture today.

Being Hooked

The most remarkable of the four stages of the journey of addiction is being hooked. It is similar to falling in love, another common and magical process. Who can explain the experience of having lost control to love? I recently talked with the parents of a college freshman, a youth with a low risk of addiction. He was an honest, open young man who had suffered from moderately severe phobias as a preteen. He had been slow to get involved with his peer group, whom he considered generally to be frighteningly out of control in their lives. He fell in love, for the first time in his life, when he went to college. This was his first real girlfriend. He assumed she would be his lifelong soul mate, but she dropped him without warning and without a second thought a few weeks into his marvelous state of rapture.

He was devastated and utterly confused. "If I love her so much, how could she love me so little?" This despondent young man found it suddenly hard to stay in school, let alone study. Hard as it was, he had found it much easier to study when the brief, intense romance had been hot and heavy. Life had meaning then, even though he was preoccupied with his girlfriend to the point of distraction much of the time. Most of us have been through experiences like this. After a few such painful experiences, we gain a finely developed sense of both the delight and the despair that go with this natural "disease" of falling in love.

Although the feeling of being hopelessly, intensely in love can happen at any age, it is more likely to hit a person hard during the ages of roughly 15 to 25, precisely when alcohol and drug addictions are likely to start up. This is when users of alcohol and other drugs who have been fooling around, confident that they can handle their substance use, are most likely to get hooked. Like falling in love, being hooked on a substance can happen with lightning speed and intensity, or it can happen slowly, almost imperceptibly. The person in love looks outwardly normal. The disease can be seen only in the lover's behavior. People in love lose objectivity and rational control of their lives when it comes to the object of their love. They often hide their out-of-control behavior from others so as not to appear as bizarre as they feel on the inside.

If the object of love is a person, there are limits to the love. For one thing, the other person often does not return the love, no matter how intense it is felt to be. There are also many factors that encourage control of one's life in a human love relationship. Try as we may, we cannot control another person. As familiarity develops in any relationship, the most intense feelings of love tend to dissipate. There are, like the feelings from eating a large meal, built-in feedback loops that, to a greater or lesser degree, help people lost to love in human relationships regain their equilibrium over the course of months or years.

This does not happen with alcohol and other drugs, which have, unlike a relationship with a person, direct access to the brain's pleasure centers. Also unlike a person in love, an addict can own, possess, buy, and control alcohol and other drugs. It is possible to have your own supply and to use the substances whenever you want to, night or day. There is no natural feedback loop in the brain turning off the addiction to alcohol and other drugs, even though the search for the drug high takes the user lower and lower with each use.

Each time the drug use occurs, regardless of the sinking baseline of the feeling of well-being, there is a prompt and certain reward after drug use that is powerfully reinforcing. The brain's hardware says, "Yes, more" to the drug after every single use. The drug is a chemical lover that steals the brain's natural control mechanisms. Addiction is a perversion of brain biology and of the behavior that the brain controls, because, unlike feeding, aggression, and sex, there is no biological purpose to the use of addicting drugs. Addiction is brain stimulation devoid of biological meaning.

One of the consequences of falling in love with alcohol or other drug highs is that a subtle but profound distortion of thinking sets in which leads addicted people to deny the negative consequences of their alcohol and other drug use to themselves and to anyone who might try to come between them and their chemical lovers. These distortions of thinking are partly conscious—leading to outright lying—and partly unconscious—leading to the brains of addicts tricking themselves into thinking that their alcohol and other drug use really is perfectly fine. This characteristic distortion of thinking produces one of the most distinctive features of the addictive disease: dishonesty and deceit when it comes to the use of rewarding chemicals.

Addicts are often outgoing and gregarious before their disease, but once the addiction has taken hold, other people matter less, except as they relate to drug use. Once an addict is hooked, all that really matters is the use of the drug. Of course, that does not mean that the addict does not socialize with others, but the socialization is progressively more limited to experiences that permit, and even encourage, drug use. Absent that, there is a progressively more limited basis for human relationships and a diminishing pleasure in being around anyone. Drug-using friends are not friends; they are allies and accomplices in drug use. They help provide the drugs, and they sustain the environment in which drug use takes place. They help the addict rationalize the drug use with the view that "everyone is doing it, not just me."

The stage of being in love with the drug is of variable length, depending on many of the same factors that determine the speed of progression in the first stage of the journey of addiction, fooling around. When users of alcohol and other drugs use relatively infrequently, when they do not have character disorder (that is, if they are Type I addicts), and when their substance use is oral, the progression tends to be relatively slow. Some users can stay in this stage of being hooked for months, years, or even decades.

Addicts commonly make strenuous efforts to control or limit their substance use, especially once they experience negative consequences or if they encounter resistance to their drug use. To the extent that they succeed in limiting their use, this stage is prolonged. Hooked addicts in every case are disasters waiting to happen, because sooner or later their control over substance use will be lost, and painful, negative consequences will flood over them as a result of their use of alcohol or other drugs.

Social drinkers are not hooked on alcohol. They are people who have not fallen in love with alcohol despite recurrent alcohol use, often over many years. Usually they do not progress to become alcoholics. Social drinkers stay in the stage of fooling around with alcohol, and for them alcohol continues to be not very important. They drink moderately and never to intoxication. Social drinkers do not like the feeling of being out of control when they are intoxicated. For them, intoxication is an unwanted alcohol overdose. Once an alcohol drinker learns to drink heavily and to enjoy the experience of intoxication, then the progression of the disease of addiction takes place. The love affair takes off. The social drinker then has become an alcohol abuser, an alcoholic. (These important and practical distinctions with respect to the use of alcohol are explored in more detail in Chapter 9 of this book.)

The stage of falling in love, of being hooked, like all stages of addiction, is progressive. Over time, addicted people give up more and more of their lives that do not involve the addiction itself. Addicts first ignore and then abuse their friends, then their families, and, only at the final stages of the disease, their employers. This typical progression relates to the environment in which the addict lives. Friends are often tolerant of whatever the addict does. Families often hide behind denial, not wanting to see the alcohol and other drug use or its negative consequences. Only late in the disease do family members confront addiction and then only with great reluctance and hesitancy.

The fact that work is spared as much as possible by most addicts does not mean that serious problems cannot develop at work, even in the early stages of addiction. Addicts are not in control of their lives, so they often cause harm accidentally. Impaired workers show up at work, think they are not impaired, and cause serious accidents that may cost their own or someone else's life. Characteristically, addicts do show up at work, despite intoxication and terrible hangovers, as well as other drug-caused problems, because they do not want to be penalized for missing work. They are far less likely to meet with a friend or to honor a family obligation when they are feeling bad from their alcohol or other drug use.

All alcoholics and drug addicts are liars. Are all people who are in love also liars? Whether a person in love is a liar or not depends on the social response to their love affairs. If their love affairs are socially tolerated, then they can be openly and honestly expressed and shared with others. Lovers want to share their exuberant feelings. However, to the extent that the love affair is prohibited or discouraged, dishonesty develops. A woman need not conceal her deep love for her husband. But if she is married and having an affair outside her marriage, she surely will lie to whomever might discourage her affair, especially to her husband. As one woman having an affair told me in therapy, "I find that now the only people I can be honest with are other people who are having affairs." The literary standard of intense love is William Shakespeare's *Romeo and Juliet*. This is a story of forbidden love that leads not only to loss of control over life, but to the death of both lovers.

What turns addicts into liars is not the pharmacology of drugs, or even the psychology of love, but the societal reaction to that love. Their social environment makes them liars. Cigarette smokers who are permitted by their employers and families to smoke are reasonably honest about their behavior. But prohibit cigarette smoking and watch what happens. I recall a husband-and-wife team who were leaders in the drug abuse field. The wife was a cigarette smoker for many years but gave up the habit, encouraged by her health-conscious husband. She often talked about how she continued to dream about cigarettes, even years after she had quit the habit, as a way of dramatizing and personalizing the grip of physical dependence.

As I got to know these two brilliant people, I learned that the wife had not stopped smoking at all; she just hid it from her husband. She lied to him, she told me, to protect her self-respect and to please her husband. She later died of a heart attack, no doubt hastened by her continued smoking. After her death I learned that her husband, unbeknownst to her, had known all along that she continued to smoke. He wanted to let her believe he did not know the truth to protect her.

The more an addictive behavior is prohibited, the more it is lied about. Addiction to alcohol and other drugs always leads to lying because the negative consequences and the abnormality of the behavior caused by the addiction are inescapable. It is not possible for those who relate to an addict to make peace with an active addiction to alcohol or other drugs. Those around the addict always object sooner or later, for their own sakes and for the addict's sake. Whereas love of a person may or may not lead to dishonesty, depending on the social response to the love, addiction to alcohol and other drugs always leads to dishonesty.

Although most addicts primarily use one or another of the most commonly used drugs, they are likely simultaneously to use multiple drugs in the pattern of polydrug use. Addicts who use more than one drug are called cross-addicted to the drugs they use. Thus, a younger alcoholic today in North America is likely to be cross-addicted to marijuana and cocaine, whereas a heroin addict is commonly cross-addicted to cocaine and alcohol. The more intense the addiction, the more likely the addict is to be cross-addicted to multiple addicting substances.

This polydrug pattern is less common in alcoholics who grew up before there was widespread use of drugs other than alcohol. Thus in North America today, alcoholics under the age of about 40 are often cross-addicted to marijuana and cocaine, whereas addicts older than 40, and especially those older than 60, are seldom cross-addicted to illegal drugs. In contrast to the pattern with illegal drugs, both older and younger addicts are commonly cross-addicted to prescribed controlled substances (addicting medicines prescribed by physicians), especially the opiates, stimulants, and antianxiety medicines.

Hitting Bottom

The stage of being hooked is open-ended in the sense that addicts do not outgrow addiction or get tired of it. Addiction is not a self-curing disease. Addicts cannot learn or think their way out of it. Addiction just gets worse over time, slowly or rapidly. The next stage in the journey of addiction is hitting bottom. Addiction persists until there are painful and inescapable consequences to the alcohol or drug use. These can be negative physical or behavioral consequences. Bottoms can be medical or health problems. Often the painful consequences from addiction come from the workplace or from the law, through arrest. Today in the United States, addiction arrests are most commonly for driving while impaired (DWI), as nearly 2 million Americans are arrested each year for drunk driving.

The highest prices for addiction usually are paid in the family, but because of the workings of codependence, as described in Chapter 8, the family is seldom the place where the addict hits bottom until later in the disease. Families are, like the addict, caught up in denial, and they usually need outside help if they are to create bottoms for the addict. This is called an *intervention,* a process described in Chapter 10. Families create bottoms for addicted people when they conduct interventions. They can create bottoms for addicts that do not have the danger often seen in lower bottoms such as loss of career, accidents, health events, and arrests. This requires tough love and real determination. Simply saying, "We think you should stop using alcohol (or other drugs)" will not do the job.

The less the addict suffers from character disorder, the higher the addict's bottom, meaning that less suffering is required to reach the conclusion that further alcohol or drug use is incompatible with living a reasonable life. The more there is character disorder, the lower the bottom, meaning that more painful episodes are required to convince the drug user that the use cannot continue.

A high bottom is waking up one morning and not remembering what happened last night, or having a paranoid episode as a result of smoking pot or snorting cocaine. Some alcoholics hit bottom when their physicians tell them their liver function tests are slightly abnormal. Addicts with no character disorder, especially those without relatives who are also addicted, sometimes conclude as a result of such relatively mild experiences that they should not use alcohol or other drugs any more. For people who really like to get high, which often means people with character disorder and/or a strong family history of addiction, these mild bottoms are barely noticed. They are shrugged off as minor but inescapable costs of the intensely valued pleasures of getting high.

For dedicated addicts, bottoms are often far lower. The negative consequences have to be truly terrible to get some chemically dependent people to recognize that their lives cannot continue if they continue to use alcohol and other drugs. For many addicts, severe automobile accidents, arrests, imprisonment, life-threatening health problems, family disruption, and disastrous financial losses are not enough to convince them that they need to stop their alcohol and other drug use. For some addicts, the use of alcohol or other drugs stops only at their death. This is the lowest of all bottoms.

Never do addicts have one bottom. Bottoms, or negative consequences of the use of alcohol and other drugs, keep coming at addicts over the course of their addictive careers. Over time, bottoms get more severe, or lower, as the disease worsens. Commonly, addicts hit a painful bottom, decide to stop the use of alcohol and other drugs, and then slip back into denial and use once more, only to encounter new, lower bottoms.

The process of hitting bottoms and then making strenuous efforts to regain control of their lives—without giving up the use of alcohol and other drugs—is part of the disease of addiction. Addicts desperately try anything and everything that will let them have control of both their lives and the alcohol and/or drugs they crave. They will even give up using alcohol and other drugs for periods of time, like obese people go on calorie-restricted diets. But they continue to harbor the dream of returning to controlled, moderate, and safe use. They experience the period of abstinence the way dieters experience a strict diet, as a temporary deprivation.

Addicts "white knuckle" through the experience of willful abstinence, meaning that they mentally grit their teeth and cling desperately to their short-term resolve not to use alcohol and other drugs. They are not relaxed or happy with this deprivation, but rather they are resentful and angry. They often ask, "Other people can drink and use drugs. Why can't I?" These episodes of white-knuckle sobriety are not part of recovery, they are part of the active disease of addiction. Sometimes these episodes of sobriety are imposed by family, employers, or the courts. They are always temporary unless the process of recovery takes hold, and that comes only from the heart of the addicted person. Recovery is conversion, a spiritual rebirth. It is a sustainable state, unlike white-knuckle sobriety.

When families begin to face the addiction of one of their members, they often resist drawing clear lines and imposing tough consequences because they fear that without family support the addict will die. "How can I turn him out of the house when I know it is only my love and my nagging that keep him from using even more drugs than he does already?" Employers, judges, friends, and physicians face the same difficult dilemma and often avoid

Hitting Bottom

Examples of High Bottoms

- Having a severe hangover
- Having a single paranoid reaction to LSD or marijuana
- Having an abnormal liver function test result
- Being told you looked or acted foolish at a party
- Having an upsetting sexual experience while intoxicated
- Having a minor accident as a result of intoxication
- Being arrested for driving while impaired (DWI)

Examples of Low Bottoms

- Having multiple serious automobile accidents as a result of intoxication
- Being arrested repeatedly for drug sales or other major crimes
- Being taken to an emergency room for a drug overdose
- Having jaundice from serious liver disease
- Having a serious medical complication of drug use, such as infection of the heart valves
- Getting AIDS from intravenous drug use

confronting the addiction, using similar rationalizations. The sad truth is that such an understandable attitude feeds and prolongs addiction. Just as addicts have bottoms, so do the addicts' codependent family members, friends, and colleagues at work. All of the people around an addict are destined by the nature of the disease to continue the enabling behavior until they are convinced beyond a shadow of a doubt that to continue such behavior only prolongs and worsens the addiction, leading eventually to death.

Some codependents reach their bottoms only when the addict is dead, making the point that not only do many addicts have tragically low bottoms but so do many codependent people. One of the major objectives of this book is to help addicts and their families recognize the bottoms they experience, and to know what to do about them when they hit bottoms in their lives. Another goal, the environmental approach to prevention and treatment of addiction (see Chapter 12), is to create more and earlier bottoms for addicts and their families, to begin to pull back the disaster-producing veils of denial and enabling.

Recovery: Getting Well

Getting well, unlike hitting bottom, is not a natural or inevitable part of the progression of the disease of addiction. Fooling around, being hooked, and hitting bottom are inescapable parts of the addictive disease itself. Recovery is not part of the disease. It does not just happen; it requires a plan and hard work. Getting well requires first the painful, educational experience of hitting bottom, of realizing that to continue to use alcohol and other drugs is to incur the certain repetition of the intolerable pain of hitting bottom after bottom after bottom. Getting well usually means learning about the disease concept of addiction. It usually means that the addict and the addict's family go to a treatment program for initial education, and that they go to 12-step fellowship meetings for many years to support recovery.

The first three phases of addiction—fooling around, being hooked, and hitting bottom—usually take their own natural and virtually irresistible course. The selfish brain experiences the drug high and wants more of it, blocking out contrary forces with the iron curtain of denial. To some extent, addicts can cover up their secret chemical love affairs, but over time they all hit one bottom after another. Addicts and their families simply do what comes naturally throughout these first three stages of addiction. This is like a plane flying on automatic pilot; no thought from the pilot is necessary.

The heart of the addict's job and the family's job is the getting well stage of the process. This stage requires a true dedication from both the addicted person and everyone in the addict's family. It requires stripping away the denial and fully accepting the role each member of the family has played in the addiction. Often the denial of the addict is no more intense or resistant to change than the denial of the codependent. They both are frighteningly difficult. The stage of recovery, if it occurs at all, requires taking the controls of one's life and flying with skill and courage. The growing recovery movement is an expression of the plan needed to get well from addiction.

Almost all addicts and families of addicts need to stay in a program of recovery, since the return to denial and the return to active addiction and codependence are seductively common. The payoff for recovery is nothing short of miraculous for both addicts and their family members. But the gains, important as they are, have to be earned one person at a time by sustained hard work. The gains of recovery are elusive. The process of getting well often includes many false starts, slips (relatively short reversions to alcohol and drug use), and relapses (more prolonged reversions to alcohol and other drug use). Getting well is hard because it requires overcoming the powerful direction of the addicted selfish brain. Getting well means saying to one's own brain, "I know where that road leads and I will not go down it." Getting well is almost never successfully done alone; it requires help and a plan.

Addiction, like character disorder, diabetes mellitus, and bronchial asthma, is not all-or-nothing. It exists in a spectrum from relatively mild to malignant. In milder cases it is hard to even call it a disease or addiction. Some people in the fooling around stage use alcohol and other drugs to reckless excess, especially in permissive environments, only to conclude that they are better off without using alcohol or other drugs. They simply stop or limit such use to occasional episodes without intoxication, as is typical of social drinkers. I do not see people like this in my practice because of their use of alcohol and other drugs, but I have met such people in many settings, including when they seek professional help for problems other than addiction. Such people do not need addiction treatment, drug tests, or 12-step meetings to limit or stop their use of alcohol and other drugs. For such people, the pattern of nonuse, or very occasional use, of alcohol and other drugs is stable with little or no effort.

How can this pattern be related to the disease concept of addiction and the belief that once an alcoholic, a person can never again use alcohol safely? Although it is admittedly a retrospective way of thinking, in my view such people never were alcoholics. Their addiction switches never got turned on, even though they may have used a lot of alcohol and other drugs, and even though they may have had serious problems as a result of that use. They never fell in love with the alcohol or drug high. Such people are not rare. They give an appearance of legitimacy to the hope of many addicted people that they, too, can return to the controlled use of alcohol and other drugs. That hope, in my experience, is invariably both false and dangerous.

Would anyone ever suggest that a heavy smoker could return to the use of cigarettes, perhaps smoking only three cigarettes a week? I have never seen that happen. If heavy smokers are to get over their dependence on nicotine, they must stop smoking. Zero is the only stable number for addicted smokers. On the other hand, there are a few people who do smoke only three cigarettes a week over many years. These people have never been addicted smokers. They are people who did not get out of the fooling around stage with cigarettes, and their addiction switches were never turned on.

Almost every alcoholic and drug addict I see wants to go back to the long-ago time when they believed that they could use alcohol and other drugs relatively under control. That simply cannot work. That futile hope, sometimes fostered by well-meaning but ill-informed physicians and critics of the disease concept of addiction, is a major cause of relapse into the depths of addiction.

Just as there are some people whose addiction switches have not been turned on and who can stabilize with occasional use of alcohol and other drugs, so there is a range of efforts that need to be made by addicted people to get well. Some can do it fairly easily after a single episode of treatment and a year or so of attendance at 12-step meetings, whereas others have repeated relapses and require virtually everyday 12-step meetings throughout their lives. I do not see many people like those in the first group. The people I see are those who are deeply caught in the denial of their disease and who are struggling to hold on to their secret chemical lovers by any means they can, including doing their best to deceive themselves, their families, and me. When I hear a user of alcohol or other drugs who bargains to use alcohol and other drugs socially, or to limit their involvement with treatment and 12-step programs, I am sure I am seeing the full-blown, hard-core disease of addiction yet one more time.

Relapses: Remedial Work on Addiction

Recovery from addiction often includes one or more returns to the active use of alcohol and other drugs as the grip of the disease tightens. Typically, relapses occur when the addicted person begins to think, "Maybe I was not really addicted at all," or "I was not as bad as many of the people I met in treatment and at meetings." Once the addict's life has stabilized in the beginning phases of recovery, the pain of addiction recedes from the addict's thinking. Denial reappears. Usually, attendance at meetings stops long before the return to the active use of alcohol and other drugs.

Relapse has nothing to do with withdrawal symptoms and everything to do with the selfish brain's selective memory of the good times associated with the use of alcohol and other drugs, and its selective forgetting of the bad times associated with addictive substance use. A return to use of alcohol and other drugs may be prolonged, lasting many years, or so brief that it is called a "slip" rather than a "relapse."

Relapses are learning opportunities for everyone involved. The saddest part of a relapse is to see the disease come back in full force as it reclaims its victim. Dishonesty reappears, as do the character traits associated with active use of alcohol and other drugs. It is always hard to get out of a relapse. The addict may face a new bottom that is even lower than the one that preceded the previous episode of sobriety. Looked at rationally, a relapse is not so bad, it is just further research into the process of addiction. But addiction is not rational. Observers of the addicted person in a relapse often cannot believe the rapidity of the fall and the depths to which the addict falls as the disease once again takes over the addict's thinking.

Sooner or later, if the addict does not die first, the relapse ends with a new bottom and a new period of sobriety, often initiated by a readmission to addiction treatment or a resumption of attendance at 12-step meetings. At that point, it is important for everyone involved to take advantage of the new opportunity for recovery, including fixing in everyone's memory, as best they can, the pain and humiliation of the renewed period of addiction. Most of all, however, it is important to understand that relapse prevention is not a logical process, and recovery is not prolonged deprivation of pleasure. Recovery is rooted in continuous participation in one or more of the 12-step fellowships and the determination to keep coming back to work the program, including daily involvement with a personal sponsor.

Addiction and Pseudoaddiction

Much behavior that looks addictive is not addiction and, paradoxically, some behavior that does not look addictive actually is addiction. Drinking 3 or 4 drinks in an evening—or even 6 or 10 drinks—does not define a person as an alcoholic. A person can be arrested for DWI with a high blood alcohol concentration (BAC) without being an alcoholic, even though the use of alcohol caused the impaired driving.

Addiction is a deeper disorder than simply using, or even having problems as a result of using, addictive drugs. Addiction involves the repetition of behaviors that produce pleasure and/or reduce discomfort, but much behavior that is not addictive also involves pleasure and the relief of discomfort. Addiction has two key features. The first feature is loss of control over the addictive behavior. This involves the persistence of the addictive behaviors despite problems and despite repeated efforts to stop the behaviors by the addicted person and by other people. The second feature of addiction is denial and dishonesty.

Many people smoke cigarettes and even experience withdrawal when they first stop smoking. Nonetheless, they are able to stop smoking without a treatment program or participation in a long-term recovery fellowship such as AA. Many people drink too much or use illicit drugs for a while and then stop. They have no problem either stopping or staying stopped for years, and even for lifetimes, without treatment or recovery fellowships.

A friend told me about his experiences with drinking and overeating. He habitually drank two or three martinis at night, almost every night. His family did not like this behavior and labeled it alcoholic drinking. They tried to get him to stop drinking. He liked alcohol and saw no reason to stop, reasoning that, other than the fact that his family did not like it, he had no problems of any sort because of his drinking. He had struggled with his weight for decades, having an especially intense and enduring relationship with ice cream. In his family, obesity was common, but none of this man's blood relatives had been an alcoholic or a drug addict.

Late in his life he was diagnosed as suffering from diabetes mellitus. His physician advised him to stop using both alcohol and ice cream. My friend told me that he stopped drinking the day the doctor asked him to stop, without any effort. He had not had a drop of alcohol in the following 4 years. On the other hand, he continued to struggle with his ice cream habit, alternating periods of white-knuckle abstinence with periods of relapse to ice cream use despite his belief that both alcohol and ice cream were harmful to his health and despite his resolve to stop both behaviors.

From the outside, pseudoaddiction looks like addiction to people who have different behaviors. My friend's family did not drink much, and they thought that his alcohol use was an addiction. Pseudoaddiction does not have the two central features of addiction: there is no loss of control with continued use despite problems, and there is no denial or dishonesty. It is common to see people engage in behaviors involving potentially addicting substances that do not involve either loss of control or denial. Once such people believe that they have a sufficient reason to stop their behaviors, they do so without treatment or 12-step fellowships, and they usually do not relapse.

This is a common pattern in the workplace where the initiation of drug tests leads many illicit drug users simply to stop illicit drug use so their jobs are not at risk. The same sort of positive change is taking place in North America today as the DWI programs linked to alcohol tests curb drinking and driving. People who routinely drank, sometimes heavily, and then drove now have a reason not to drink and drive, so they stop the behavior. Dietary advice to limit fat consumption and to maintain weight within healthy ranges has a similar effect, as the people who have not lost control of their eating have a relatively easy time changing their behaviors once they are convinced it is in their interest to do so. However, other people, who are equally motivated by their desire to be healthy, simply cannot change their eating patterns or, if they do change them, they are unable to sustain the new and more healthy pattern.

True addiction does not end with a simple decision to quit a particular behavior. The grip of addiction on the addict's brain is too firm for that to happen. Addicts and pseudoaddicts look alike until they are confronted with a reason to quit, until they face serious consequences as a result of their addictive behavior, or until they try to stop. Then the two groups separate, with the pseudoaddicts simply quitting and the addicts either not being able to stop or relapsing to addictive behaviors again, often at an even greater intensity than before they attempted to stop these pleasure-producing behaviors. It is the behavior of the addicts that is both irrational and puzzling. Such addictive behavior is the behavior from which this book seeks to learn.

The distinction between addiction and pseudoaddiction is slippery, and it can be dangerous. Many addicts claim that they can stop their behaviors any time they want to. They say that they continue because they do not want to stop. Sometimes pseudoaddicts, confronted by social disapproval, perceive themselves to be addicted despite the fact that they have never tried to stop the addictive behavior. We have seen in this book that addiction is a disorder of the entire self, and that both loss of control and denial are central features of this disorder. Only when the environment sends a strong message to quit is the person who is engaged in pleasure-producing, potentially addicting behavior likely to quit. And only when the person tries to stop and stay stopped can the distinction be clearly made between addiction and pseudoaddiction.

In the example I gave of my friend who stopped drinking alcohol easily but could not stop eating ice cream, we see the distinction between addiction and pseudoaddiction, a distinction that even this smart and self-aware man would have had a hard time making until he came up with a good reason to try to stop those two pleasure-producing behaviors. It is important to realize that potentially addictive behaviors, including the use of alcohol and other drugs, can have serious consequences for the person engaging in the behaviors, and for others, even in the absence of addiction. Furthermore, people cannot get addicted unless they engage in addictive behaviors. The powerful role of the environment in both promoting and curbing potentially addicting behaviors is hard to overemphasize.

Why was it that my friend found his doctor's advice so convincing and his family's concerns so unpersuasive? There are many mysteries in addiction that are close to the human heart. Could it be that this man was genuinely fearful of his own potential death, especially as he was aging and the inevitability of his death became more palpable? In contrast, why was the unhappiness of his family less important to him? Perhaps he retained a streak of rebelliousness from his own childhood that prevented him from accepting the good advice of his family, whereas his physician escaped this link with his childhood. Which bottoms lead to changed behaviors and which do not is hard to predict. One thing is clear, however. In real addictive behaviors the bottoms keep coming, ever deeper, until the addicted person dies or figures out that life cannot go on without real change.

The distinction between addiction and pseudoaddiction helps explain a disturbing problem. Some critics of addiction treatment and of the 12-step recovery programs point out correctly that many people stop drinking and stop using drugs with little effort and no expense at all. They label addictive behaviors as "simple bad habits." Complaining about people like me who encourage the wider use of both addiction treatment and the 12-step programs, they have a point. All of the follow-up studies of potentially addicting behavior do show that many people who engage in these behaviors, even some who have serious problems as a result of these behaviors, do stop—and staystopped—once they have good reasons to stop.

My answer to these critics of the disease concept of addiction is that they have mixed up addicts and pseudoaddicts. It is true that many pseudoaddicts do not need addiction treatment or 12-step programs because they do suffer from simple bad habits. However, it is also true that virtually all addicts need real and sustained help if they are to stop and stay stopped. Addicts have fallen in love. They are hooked on their addictive behaviors. Pseudoaddicts are still fooling around. They have not lost control of their potentially addicting behavior.

People in Alcoholics Anonymous and Narcotics Anonymous are amazed at the claim that alcoholics and addicts can simply stop using alcohol and other drugs. They have never seen such an occurrence. They are right. They are describing the experience of true addicts, people who, despite having plenty of good reasons to stop, nevertheless continue to use alcohol and other drugs, doing no end of harm to themselves and to those around them.

When it comes to treatment and the use of the 12-step fellowships, the right course of action is to do whatever is necessary to help the particular person stop using alcohol and other drugs. Less is more. This means that it is both unnecessary and wasteful of scarce resources to do more than is necessary to achieve sobriety, just as it is wasteful of resources to do less than is necessary to achieve that goal. For true addiction, less is not likely to do the job. For addicts, recovery is an inside job, a matter of changing thinking as well as changing behavior. For most addicts, getting well and staying well means regular attendance at 12-step meetings, probably for a lifetime. For many pseudoaddicts, all it takes to get well is a reason to stop.

Confusing addicts and pseudoaddicts can muddle thinking on individual, family, and community levels. When it comes to alcohol use that produces problems, including family problems, and all illicit drug use, whether that use is addictive or not, it is important that the environment shift to make it clear that the behavior must stop whether the person using alcohol or other drugs is an addict or a pseudoaddict. The difference between these two groups is not the value of the environmental pressure to stop, it is in how much effort needs to be put into achieving that important personal and public health goal once the environmental message is clear. Pseudoaddicts get the message once it is clear. Addicts do not. They do not get the message because their disease whispers in their ears that they are fine and that they do not have a problem. This is the disease of addiction.

When I visit cancer patients and their families in a hospital, I think about what a joy it would be if I could tell them that all they had to do to get well and stay well was to go to meetings once a day for an hour or so and do a few things differently in their lives. With that approach, they could be free of the ill effects of their disease. When I go to an alcohol or drug unit in the same hospital and see someone equally close to death's door, I can deliver that message. The cancer patient and the patient's family would leap at the opportunity. They are desperate for any help.

On the other hand, the polite addicted person in response to my offer says, "No thanks, Doc. I can handle this myself." Addicted patients who are less polite simply say, "Get lost. I've heard that before, and I don't need it." The difference between the cancer patients and the addicts, who are both suffering from potentially fatal diseases, is that the disease of addiction tells the addicts they are okay. The cancer patients know they are seriously ill. When I see a person in stable recovery from addiction, I see a person who is as grateful for recovery, and the means for recovery, as I would see if I could offer that opportunity to a cancer patient. That is what it means to get well: the disease is held at bay, and the addicted person can get on with his or her life with sobriety and gratitude. Denial has also been held at bay, but it remains ready to return and cause a relapse at any time.

The *Diagnostic and Statistical Manual of Mental Disorders,* 4th Edition (DSM-IV), distinguishes between *abuse,* a relatively mild form of recurrent use of alcohol and other drugs, and *dependence,* a more severe form, which is often labeled *addiction.* The distinction between abuse and dependence is similar to my distinction between pseudoaddiction and addiction in the sense that one is less severe and the other more severe. However, the distinctions in DSM-IV are more symptomatic and less focused on the natural history of addiction than is my distinction. I have invented the term *pseudoaddiction* to describe a commonly observed phenomenon of heavy use of alcohol and other drugs that persists over time (often producing serious problems) but vanishes at later stages of the users' lives without benefit of treatment and without relapse. Such people do not appear to suffer from the "disease" of addiction.

Although understanding the nature of the disease of addiction cannot cure addiction, it can set the stage for recovery. Having words to describe the intensely personal experiences of addiction that are otherwise confusing and overwhelming can help both understanding and communication.

Case Histories

In the other chapters of this book, the case histories are drawn from my practice and my life. In contrast, here are two case histories condensed from the pages of *The New York Times,* in the words of the reporters who wrote the stories. Here you see the varied faces of addiction, one involving a woman, the other a man; one a youth, the other a person of middle age; one from a family of poverty, the other from a family of wealth; one an apparent story of failure, the other a story of success. Both are clearly unfinished stories of continuing struggles with the disease of addiction. Stories like these have become common in the media in North America. They are becoming more common throughout the world as the media plays a valuable role in public education. My patients tell their stories privately to their doctor. Here, in the media, are public stories easily accessible to everyone.

Linda Marrero[1]

It is going on a month since Linda Marrero went home again. On a weekend visit, she swore to stay out of trouble for good and begged her parents to let her stay. And despite advice from counselors at the residential school for drug users where Linda had spent the last 2 years, Maria and Eliezer Marrero could not resist their 17-year-old daughter's pleas. They wanted their baby back.

---

[1] Copyright 1994/95 by The New York Times Company. Reprinted by permission.

About 2½ years have passed since Mr. and Mrs. Marrero landed in jail for chaining Linda to a radiator to keep her away from crack and riotous living. They had no way to help her, they said, and did not know what else to do with a daughter who had been running wild for years. She would take off for days, only to come back drugged up and sometimes beaten. Soon she would leave again, repeating the pattern. The headlines about the Marreros' desperate attempt to wrestle with the consequences of drug addiction helped to get Linda into treatment. Although the family has faced a series of crises since then, life with Linda back seemed to be going smoothly.

Then, on March 24, Linda got into a fist fight at her new school. . . . Linda was arrested and spent two nights . . . [in jail] while her family scraped together her $500 bail. She is due in court . . . to answer a felony charge of assault. For Mr. and Mrs. Marrero, this is the worst crisis yet. Even if all charges are dropped and Linda returns home, they must grapple with the same question that has plagued them for years: what to do next? They moved to this . . . village 65 miles away from . . . [where] they had lived for 20 years, . . . for Linda's sake. The sacrifice has proved worthless. "With all the problems, Linda had never been arrested before," Mrs. Marrero said. "I think we should move somewhere else."

Over the weekend, the Marreros' . . . house was full of friends and relatives who had come to show their support. But despite idle chitchat and trips to the local malls, the mood was glum. Only Linda seemed undaunted. Sitting with a visiting school friend, she giddily told stories about her jail experience, discussing everything from the stale cheese sandwiches ("No way was I going to eat that!") to other inmates. Until the fist fight, Linda, who is in the 11th grade, was dutifully . . . going to school. . . . Then Linda would spend the evening in the frilly white room her parents had decorated for her, fussing over her clothes and school supplies. She had new friends, a boyfriend.

"I never thought this would happen to Linda, thrown in jail like a criminal," Mrs. Marrero said. Still, the Marreros had not presumed they were about to live happily ever after. Their other daughter . . . [aged 24], is entering a treatment center next week, after turning to drugs as a teenager. Linda had been playing hooky and hanging out with the wrong crowd since elementary school. There have been many ups and downs since. Linda was scheduled to come home from the treatment program in New Hampshire last December. The week before the move, on a 4-day visit home, she ran off and plunged back into using drugs. Her parents say she was lured by her sister, then in the full throes of a crack binge. . . . As her two brothers scoured the streets for her, she stayed in a notorious crack house . . . .

The family has barely scraped by since moving around the end of 1991. . . . Even before Linda's arrest, the Marreros considered moving on. The place lost its innocence once their daughters found where to go for drugs. Mrs. Marrero, unable to drive, felt isolated from her relatives. . . . And she could no longer pretend that the place was anything like her rural hometown in Puerto Rico. . . . Her main entertainment, Mrs. Marrero said, is staring out the living room window overlooking a dirt driveway. "Sometimes I stare out the windows, I'm thinking I want to kill myself," she said. "I loved my apartment," she added. "I had a lot of friends. When we moved, I cried. We were going to be all alone."

. . . Besides Linda, the Marreros live with their two sons, Jose, 22, and Junior, 21, and their sons' girlfriends, who are both 6 months pregnant. The Marreros have custody of their older daughter's three children, all under 6, and Jose's girlfriend's two toddlers also live in the four-bedroom house. The sons work, and Junior . . . also goes to school. But the family lives mostly on Social Security disability checks. Mrs. Marrero worked for a time as a housekeeper, . . . but found it impossible to keep the job and manage the house.

Despite their money problems and shortage of space, they managed to save a bedroom just for Linda. They filled it with everything a teenager could want—stereo equipment, telephone, television, Nintendo. Stuffed animals dangle from the ceiling. Linda, her parents concede, has always been babied. She was still drinking out of a bottle when she was 15 and was showered with presents for no particular occasion. "Whatever Linda wanted, all her life, her father would buy for her," Mrs. Marrero said. "If she say, 'I want new sneakers,' he would work a job to buy the sneakers." Mr. Marrero said, "I don't know what happened."

There was a time, last July, when they had hope for the future. Linda came home for 2 weeks, her longest stay since she entered the treatment center. The only bit of mischief she stirred was persuading her brother to give her a haircut, scalped on the bottom half of her head with a pony tail piled high on top. She had blossomed from the emaciated girl of 15 seen in photographs around the world into a muscular 150-pound athlete proud of her skills on the basketball court . . . .

The Marreros say they have never been able to figure out what to do when it comes to courts and agencies. They are not sure . . . whether the state ever gave them back custody of Linda after they were arrested, because they have never been told. (A spokeswoman for the city's Human Resources Administration . . . said the department could not comment on the case.) . . .

The Marreros are suing the city for the humiliating treatment they received after their arrest, Mrs. Marrero said. When they had chained Linda to a radiator at night, for 3 months, she said, police officers knew and said they didn't blame them. "They said, 'Good for you,'" Mrs. Marrero said, adding she still believed she and her husband did nothing wrong. Nor do the Marreros regret allowing Linda to come home this time. "How long were they going to keep my daughter away?" she said. "It wasn't doing any good."

Pondering Linda's long history of troubles, she recalled a 3-day group therapy session she and her husband attended with other parents of troubled teenagers. "They had cars and money and everything they wanted," she said. "I said I had to explain chaining my daughter to the radiator because I had no money to get her help. How come your children are doing the same thing? If it's not the money, then what makes these kids do all these things they do?"

—Evelyn Nieves
The New York Times
April 2, 1994

Larry Kudlow[2]

Larry Kudlow seemed a master of the universe. Being a top Wall Street economist was not the half of it. Mr. Kudlow had been a prominent member of President Reagan's economic team. He helped conceive and fight for the tax-cut proposal that helped Christine Todd Whitman become Governor of New Jersey. One of the nation's most articulate and charismatic commentators on financial issues, he has become the economic guru of Jack Kemp and of the conservative radio host Rush Limbaugh, as well as a regular on television interview programs and a speaker commanding hefty fees. He even starred in Cadillac ads. To hear some leading Republicans, the 46-year-old Mr. Kudlow has nowhere to go but up. They consider him a hot political property, a potential challenger for the Senate seat of Daniel Patrick Moynihan in New York, or, should a right-leaning Republican like Mr. Kemp win the White House in 1996, a shoo-in for a Cabinet position . . . .

But last week, in an interview with The New York Times, Larry Kudlow had a confession to make: behind the polished facade lived a troubled and deeply unhappy man who has been battling an addiction to drugs and alcohol. Swiveling in his chair in the offices of his new employer, National Review magazine, Mr. Kudlow . . . began an explanation that many others would not summon the courage to make: 15 months ago he took a four-week medical leave of absence from his Wall Street firm, Bear Stearns. "I went into drug rehab," Mr. Kudlow said, deciding to discuss his problem after being told he was the subject of a profile. "I had an alcohol and substance-abuse problem that needed to be taken care of." He said that for 15 months he has been attending twice daily a self-help program for recovering addicts. "I am willing to share with you my problem," he said, following the example of many people in programs like Alcoholics Anonymous. . . . Then this dapper man, . . . a man sometimes described as poker-faced, began to cry. Sounding scared, not at all like the suave raconteur and deft name dropper of 2 hours earlier, Mr. Kudlow said he lived in fear of sliding backward. "I live my life day to day," he said. Mr. Kudlow said he was talking largely because he wanted to be honest and because his story might benefit other families with alcohol and drug problems. "I'm on top of this thing, God bless," he said. "Maybe somebody reading about this somewhere will be helped."

Mr. Kudlow is still striving to understand what drove him to depend on drugs and alcohol, and the elaborate lying and dodging that are required to conceal such habits from friends, family and colleagues. Whatever the reasons, it is clear that there are many Larry Kudlows. One in 10 Americans has some form of alcohol or drug-abuse problem, recent studies show. America's success-conscious society is full of people who are less afraid to snort a line or put away a fifth than they are of letting someone else see that they are not all they appear to be. Everyone knows someone talented, ambitious and magnetic who has a serious problem but chooses to ignore it for a long time, hoping that other people will look the other way because he's so valuable.

. . . Mr. Kudlow refused to say what drug he used or to be specific about how his drug use began. He did say that he began drinking regularly in the second half of the 1970s and that his drinking led to drugs. Mr. Kudlow attributes his slide partly to pure pressure. On Wall Street there are producers and then there's everyone else, and the pressure to produce helped drive Mr. Kudlow to drink and drugs. Then there was the exhausting travel and entertaining. . . . "I felt invincible and that there were no limits as to how late I could stay up or how much I could travel. Today, I can see how tough it was." There was also the easy availability and acceptability of alcohol and drugs, especially in the 1980s, combined with having plenty of money to throw around. And he had no children to ground him.

Another problem was that when he felt down, he didn't know how to turn to a friend. He described himself, for all his gregariousness and bonhomie, as a man who spent much of his life isolated, ashamed to let others know him well enough to share his failings and embarrassments along with the successes. "I never had any friends beyond a certain superficial level," he said. "We hate to admit weaknesses. We were raised to want to get ahead, to be good and clever and successful. You're just ashamed to open up." . . .

[**Author's note.** Mr. Kudlow, who at one time was a member of the left-wing organization, Students for a Democratic Society, had a meteoric rise in the world of finance to the pinnacles of fame and power. Initially a junior economist at the New York Federal Reserve, he became chief economist at the brokerage house of Paine Webber. Soon thereafter, he joined Bear Stearns, a prosperous Wall Street firm that "liked his outspoken free-market ideas." For a time in the Reagan Administration, he was chief economist of the Office of Management and Budget. He subsequently founded a consulting firm and then returned to Bear Stearns. He is now with the National Review magazine.]

As he tells it, Mr. Kudlow hid his problems well. . . . But colleagues did notice that Mr. Kudlow was losing weight . . . and [one remarked that], "There's been a lot of last-minute cancellations. After a while there was a certain exasperation level. People always wanted to know, where is Larry?" . . . Mr. Kudlow's personal problems worsened in 1992. "All of a sudden I could not face the 3-day road trips," he said. "The two or three plane flights in a day. I was having trouble facing it. I was dreading it. So here I am in Salt Lake City, Indianapolis, Chicago, Paris, Frankfurt, Buenos Aires, Budapest. Not only am I tired, dragging my feet, but I've got responsibility and the show's gotta go on." On top of the demands of the firm and its clients, Mr. Kudlow had a full plate of extracurricular activities. "If the producer of 'Cross-Fire' called me to go that night to Washington, I'd go," he said. "If Jack Kemp called, I'd go. I'm a person who has a hard time saying no." . . . It was on the road . . . where Mr. Kudlow lost control. "I'll give you an example," he said. "One drink over dinner turns into two and pretty soon your problem becomes a bigger problem."

Mr. Kudlow said no one at the firm complained about his performance at the time . . . "Ironically, the last few years have been the best performance years for me." . . . But "my personal life was getting bumped," he added. "I valued my marriage." By autumn 1992, things were spiraling out of control. Judy Kudlow . . . says that it was her husband who decided that he had to act. "He's the one who knew he needed to get help," she said. "And I was behind him. I was aware that he had a problem. We're devoted to each other. We did it together, but he is the one leading the way." In mid-December 1992 Mr. Kudlow . . . took a leave of absence in order to enter a treatment program. The treatment program involved spiritual counseling, introspection and group therapy. Since his release, Mr. Kudlow has been attending a self-help program for recovering addicts—as often as every morning before work and every evening after work— where people, some of whom have been sober for years, help each other struggle with their demons . . . .

Mr. Kudlow . . . returned toward the end of January last year. Around that time, Christine Todd Whitman came to him for advice at the urging of their mutual friend, Forbes magazine's publisher, Steve Forbes, Jr. Armed with facts showing that New Jersey's economy had become hopelessly noncompetitive, Mr. Kudlow argued for a state version of the original Reagan tax-cut plan. Ten months later, Mr. Kudlow stood behind Mrs. Whitman as she proclaimed her upset victory over Jim Florio in the governor's race.

Then this year, on Tuesday, March 1, Mr. Kudlow was scheduled to speak to a large group of institutional investors in Boston. Two hundred people turned up for lunch. But Mr. Kudlow, the featured speaker, failed to show. Given Mr. Kudlow's recent troubles, a lot of people were suspicious. But Mr. Kudlow said, "I was sick. It was not a relapse. I know there were rumors." Why would he not have called to say he didn't feel well and wasn't coming? "Unfortunately, there was a communications gap," he said. "I wish I could make amends to every person who was there." . . . Mr. Kudlow said "the explosion hit" when he went into the office the next day. "Being unreachable was a fairly high-level sin" said [a retired company official]. . . . Mr. Kudlow handed his resignation . . . [in] that day. The decision was his, Mr. Kudlow said, though the firm made it clear, in an unusual news release, that it felt Mr. Kudlow's departure was also in its best interest. Bear Stearns officials refused to discuss Mr. Kudlow's departure but the firm described it as a "voluntary termination" in mandatory public filings made with securities regulators. Missing the luncheon, Mr. Kudlow said, "reinforced to me the notion that I needed a less stressful and less energy-consuming job. It's as if you had cancer, or a heart attack, or had your hip replaced. You've got to make changes in order to live a healthy life." . . .

Within 2 days Mr. Kudlow became economics editor of National Review, for perhaps a tenth of his former income of nearly $1 million. He was soon crowing, "You know, this is a real job," and preparing for tapings of "Firing Line," the television program hosted by his new boss, William F. Buckley.

Mr. Kudlow says that he has been in recovery . . . for more than 15 months. One thing helping him now, he said, is sharing his experiences with younger men and women in the program who are struggling to take the first steps to help themselves. He has also turned to the spiritual counsel of . . . a Roman Catholic priest and a former Wall Streeter who now counsels high-powered people.

Sitting in the couple's Upper East Side apartment, . . . Judy Kudlow says: "He is better than he's ever been. He's stronger." Mr. Kudlow . . . said he has put any political plans on hold. But he doesn't rule anything out. Punditry, politics and the lay priesthood—and more remotely, a return to Wall Street—are all possibilities. Can he still make it in politics? The decision by the media-wise Mr. Kudlow, whose wife was once a Reagan press official, to go public with his problems may be the best way to put the problem behind him and preserve some chance. Indeed, some politicians who admitted such problems have gone on to victory. Ann Richards, one of Mr. Kudlow's idols, became Governor of Texas even after acknowledging she was a recovering alcoholic. . . . A spokesman from Richards' 1990 campaign said voters might be less forgiving about drugs. But "you can overcome anything if people believe you've changed your ways. He's got to get some time on his side and some years of sobriety under his belt." . . . Mr. Kudlow certainly hopes so: "In our society there are a lot of people who have suffered from alcohol or substance abuse—you name it—and society has been understanding. Listen, I have a lot of faith and a lot of hope."

—Sylvia Nasar with Alison Leigh Cowan
The New York Times
April 3, 1994

Chapter 8

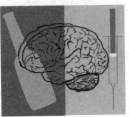

Codependence
The Mirror of Addiction

In this chapter, we explore the specific nature of the disease of addiction as it is seen in family members.

As long as addiction is equated with physical dependence, all the addict appears to need to get well is to stop using the drug. The popular view of addiction is almost that simple: the reason addicts continue using their drugs, despite the inevitable painful consequences of their drug use, is that they experience withdrawal symptoms when they stop using their drugs. In this view, the problem for drugs addicts is that they are physically dependent on their drugs.

This picture not only is wrong, but it commonly perpetuates addiction. The addict's problem is not physical dependence but the crippling loss of control resulting from having fallen in love with the drug-caused high. This loss of control is the result of the chemical stimulation of the brain's pleasure centers. The addict's downfall is the reward the addict's brain has found in drug use. This love affair leads the selfish brain to send out a cry for more of the drug, no matter what the costs. Once drug use stops for any reason, although physical dependence quickly ends, the addict's brain never forgets the pleasure of getting high. That is why addicted people are never free of the risk of relapse, no matter how long they have been drug free and no matter how far behind them they put their physical withdrawal symptoms. Addiction is unrelated to any problem of physical dependence or withdrawal. The cries for more drug are as loud, or louder, after detoxification, after the experience of withdrawal is ended, as before.

Behind the brain disease of addiction lie two problems that set the stage for addiction: the character of the addict and the environment in which the drug use occurs. Now we focus on the most personal, the most controversial, and the most important aspect of the addict's environment: the addict's family.

The Family's Own Disease

The modern understanding of the disease of addiction to alcohol and other drugs includes the recognition that the addict's family members are more than passive victims of the addict's bad and sick behavior. The addict's family typically suffers from *codependence*. Codependence comes in two forms: primary codependence, which has existed from childhood exposure to addiction, usually the addiction of a parent; and secondary codependence, which develops only after close personal exposure as an adult to an addicted person, often to a spouse or a child who is addicted

Codependence

Primary Codependence

- Grew up as a child in family dominated by addiction
- Usually need extensive participation in Al-Anon and sometimes psychotherapy
- Worse prognosis for recovery

Secondary Codependence

- Childhood generally free of addiction
- Involved with addict, usually spouse or child, only as an adult
- Usually need less therapy and/or Al-Anon participation
- Better prognosis for recovery

---

to alcohol or other drugs. Both forms of codependence mirror the addict.

Addicts are characteristically self-centered and irresponsible. They also often appear to be outgoing and self-confident. Codependents, in contrast, commonly appear to be self-deprecating and sometimes even shy. They typically try extremely hard to do the right thing and to please others. This behavior of codependent people contrasts with the outward behavior of active addicts, who often recklessly disregard the feelings of others. Codependents are typically unusually concerned with how they appear to others. They highly value their good reputations for hard work and selflessness. Nevertheless, they are locked into a malignant synergy with the addict. The codependent is the mirror of the addict and is equally the suffering hostage of the selfish brain. The self-centeredness of codependents is more deeply hidden but no less fundamental or troublesome than is the self-centeredness of the addict.

Many physicians, health care workers, and other human service professionals, including teachers, are codependent people who are living out their family-based roles as caregivers in their work lives. Often they found that they were unable, despite their most heroic efforts, to save their own addicted family members. Later they, usually unconsciously, try to save others through self-less, dedicated, and tireless human service work. Although this is not a bad reason to enter into a life of social responsibility, it is wise to understand our own motives and to anticipate the ways in which they can distort relationships with those being served. For example, when the best efforts of the codependent caregiver are rejected or ignored, this can repeat earlier traumatic experiences and lead to inappropriate and sometimes dangerous responses from the frustrated, overstressed codependent human service professional.

Codependence is a disease of lost selfhood, of having one's self and self-esteem defined by someone else's behavior. The codependent person is as hooked on the addict as the addict is hooked on the alcohol or other drug. Codependents neglect their own inner, deeper needs as they try tirelessly but futilely to fix themselves by fixing the addicted person in their lives. Codependent people have trouble thinking of themselves without thinking of their addicts. Their lives and self-concepts, to a large extent, are defined by their relationships with their addicts.

Codependence is relatively easy to see, once you recognize the disorder. When people come to me announcing that their problems are someone else's behavior, be it addiction or something else, I am alert to this diagnosis. When people say that they would be just fine if only someone else changed, I am all but certain of the diagnosis. When people seeking my help continue talking for a long time and never mention their own needs or feelings, except as they relate to the troublesome people in their lives, I know that I am dealing with codependence, the disease of the lost self.

Codependents are in a trap from which they cannot escape. The harder codependents struggle to free themselves by trying to control the behavior of an addicted person, the more deeply they are enslaved in this family disease. Love itself pushes them ever deeper into this trap. Their behavior calls out, "I cannot let this go on. It is too painful to watch this person I love destroy himself (or herself). I must act. I must save him (or her), and you must help me do it right now. We haven't a minute to spare!"

Learning From Suffering

The 12-step programs, based on Alcoholics Anonymous (AA), have faced the problems of the addict's family for more than 50 years. These fellowships, described in Chapter 11, have developed a time-tested approach to the family problems of addiction. The approach is built on the mutual-aid program Al-Anon, the fellowship program that helps families of alcoholics. The central idea behind this approach is the concept of codependence. Addicts are often strong personalities. Their addictive behaviors outwardly dominate their families. Because such awful things happen to addicts over time, it is inescapable for families to center their lives around the addicts and the destructive dramas they create in family life. Family members come to believe that almost all of their problems can be traced to the addicted person. They think that if the addict would only get well, would only stop drinking and using drugs, then the other members of the family would be well also. Salvation, it appears, is just around the next corner. All that is needed is for the alcoholic or drug addict to become alcohol free or drug free.

Addiction is a far larger problem than the reward caused by the drug high. Addiction is a disease of the entire self. It is a disease of values. Addictive disease afflicts not only the addict but the addict's family. It is not merely a disease of the addicted person but a disease of those who care for the addicted person.

As people in Al-Anon have learned more about how to help the families of alcoholics, they have learned that alcoholism is often a multigenerational disease. Many of the spouses of alcoholics and addicts themselves grew up in families that were dominated by alcoholism and other addictions. This may seem puzzling. If people grew up in families dominated by the pain of alcoholism or addiction, why did they not learn from their experiences and be sure not to repeat them? Why would the child from such a family marry someone who repeated the same painful pattern? Some early psychiatrists observing this common pattern of repetition concluded that the spouses of alcoholics were inherently masochistic, that they found perverse satisfaction in being victimized by alcoholics.

Later, a better understanding of this mysterious repetition developed. People who grew up in families dominated by addiction and other dysfunctional behaviors developed their own characters around the deeply held belief that if they could live their lives right in their own marriages, by controlling the addict's behavior, then the addict would not be an addict at all. By their work and their love in their own marital families, they thought they could solve this deadly problem that they had not been able to solve in the family in which they grew up. As children growing up, they often felt a hidden shame about their parents, their homes, and, ultimately, themselves. Codependents concluded, unconsciously, that they could overcome their hidden shame by finally solving the problem of addiction in their spouses or their children.

Many children, destined to become codependent adults, could not bring their friends into their homes because of the embarrassment they felt when their friends saw their alcoholic parents. When they went out to find a mate, they sought, usually without being aware of the process, someone who had many of the characteristics of their alcoholic parent. They loved that parent especially, and wanted as children to be able to make life right for that addicted parent, to live out the family romance they dreamed of with a happy home for both parents and children.

The future codependents acted as if they believed that this time, in their own marriages and with their own children, it would all work out the right way. They would work it so that their own spouses and children would not become alcoholics or addicts, and in doing that they could overcome the shame that they felt, first in relation to their addicted parent and then as a deeply rooted part of themselves as failures at the most important challenge of their lives, their efforts to save an addicted parent or sibling. The underlying belief of these budding codependent people was that their self-worth, their self-esteem, was dependent on what their addicted spouse or child did or did not do. Further, they believed that through selfless work and love, and whatever else it took, they could control their spouse's or their child's addictive behavior.

Sometimes the spouse was an active alcoholic, but more often, the spouse was, at the time of courtship, a budding addicted person who had characteristics of the addicted parent but who had not yet developed the full syndrome of addiction to alcohol and other drugs. In some cases it appeared as if the codependent spouse acted in ways that unwittingly promoted the developing of addiction, for example, by making drug or alcohol use easy or by making excuses for early problems that arose from the excessive use of drugs or alcohol. Another all-too-common pattern was for the person who grew up in an alcoholic or drug-addicted family to develop his or her own addiction to alcohol and other drugs, thus repeating the role of both parents simultaneously—the addicted spouse and the enabling spouse.

This story of codependence in the family life cycle seldom had a happy ending. The most common pattern was for the development of addiction in the spouse of the codependent person. As the addiction worsened, the codependent spouse sought to improve the addict's behavior in an anxious, ever-worsening cycle of failed control. First the codependent worked to control the addict with love and, when this failed, with bribery and manipulation, and finally with anger, resentment, and ultimately a punishing withdrawal of affection. The codependent spouses acted as if they could feel good about themselves only if their addicts got well. Usually, the addiction just got worse. Family life progressively deteriorated into recriminations, wounded pride, and anger, deepening the codependent person's shame and feelings of failure. The codependent person became isolated and demoralized as his or her greatest childhood pain was repeated as an adult.

The addicted family member felt victimized by this progressively more extreme behavior of the codependent spouse. He or she felt that the spouse was trying to control him or her and that the spouse did not understand or respect the addict. The addicted family member felt that he or she was being hounded by a mean spouse who had become a parole officer bent on shaping his or her life to meet the spouse's own excessive needs. The addict used the anger and resentment he or she felt as one more good excuse to drink alcohol and use other drugs. The addict's behavior, and often his or her words, said, "You made me do it by your nagging and by your suspicions." The same process often has been played out by parents of addicted children, sometimes when the children were teenagers, sometimes when they were adults. In these cases, the codependent parents sought to control their addicted children in fruitless, self-defeating ways.

Many professionals working in the field of addiction have recognized this pattern in families and have developed techniques for helping families afflicted by alcohol and drugs to get well through use of the Al-Anon program. The first step on the road to recovery is to recognize that addiction in the addict is not simply physical dependence or even merely a result of alcohol or drug use. The addict's disease is a disease of the self, rooted in the addict's self-centered sensitivity, and sustained by dishonesty. Getting well for the alcoholic or drug addict means genuinely caring about others and becoming honest. The same is true for the codependent person, whose dishonesty, like his or her own self-centeredness, is usually deeply hidden.

Narcissus and Echo

Echo was a mythological Greek goddess condemned by Hera, the jealous wife of Zeus, never to speak except to repeat what was spoken to her. Echo fell in love with Narcissus, a young man with beauty to match her own. Because Narcissus scorned those who loved him and never returned their love, Nemesis, the goddess of righteous anger, condemned Narcissus to fall in love with his own reflection, which he saw in a pool of still water. When he fell, literally, for the face he saw in the pool, he drowned. The story goes that out of grief after the death of Narcissus, Echo lost her physical substance so that all that is left today of this wounded, grief-stricken beauty is the sound of her voice in caves and canyons endlessly repeating sounds made by others.

This story, related to codependence by Timmen L. Cermak, M.D., captures the horribly common, mutually destructive relationship of the addict and the codependent. The narcissist is locked in a fatally flawed affair of the heart with an echo who is unable to speak his or her own mind. What is the key to release the lock that binds these two doomed, ancient lovers? The most powerful antidote is for both the addict and the codependent to disengage, to let go of the other, and to focus honestly and openly on their own unique and personal needs. Paradoxically, the way toward real closeness for families dominated by addiction lies through the neglected door to independence for all of the trapped, pathologically entangled parties.

For the codependent person, recovery means giving up on the dream of fixing the addict and, instead, going about his or her own life, whether or not the addict gets well. It means "detaching with love." Anger and resentment are not appropriate or helpful, although they are certainly understandable, and, at some stages of the process, they are inescapable. The simple understanding that the codependent person cannot be responsible for the addict is the start to recovery. Codependents can manage only their own lives with effort, but they cannot manage their addicts' lives, no matter how hard they try. In working with codependent people, I encourage them to find and develop themselves. They need to restructure their views of themselves and their whole lives in ways that do not reflect the behavior or character of their addicted family members. They need to figure out what to do to become themselves, and to give up on fixing the addict. If they focus on fixing the addict, they are continuing in their codependence. Unlike Echo, they need to find their own voices and stop repeating the sounds of others.

Many codependents see this goal of having a good life for themselves to be insufficient to make the changes that need to be made. It seems to them to be selfish, a very serious, negative charge for most codependent people. After years of false starts, I have found an effective suggestion for these basically good but trapped people: "You need to be independent and to live your own life to save your addict. By continuing what you have been doing, you make his (or her) life worse." At least in the early stages of recovery from codependence, this goal is more appealing to

---

Characteristics of a Codependent Person

- Focuses on the family addict
- Is hardworking and selfless
- Wants to please and do the right thing
- Believes personal success and happiness lie in stopping the addict's alcohol and drug use

---

many codependents than the goal of living a good life for themselves no matter what the consequences for the addict. Ultimately, of course, codependent people have to become their own selves to meet their genuine needs, not to save their addicts, if they are to recover from this tragically crippling disease.

For the addict, detachment with love means "first things first." This means doing what the addict has to do to achieve and then to maintain sobriety. It means that the addict must stop trying to either please or manipulate codependent family members. It means letting go of a destructive, magical dream of people living for and through one another, for both the addict and the codependent. For codependent people, first things first means letting go of the lifelong dream of fixing the addicts and settling down to the far less exciting, but far more achievable, goal of living their own lives.

Stick Together or Fall Apart

These ideas sound both paradoxical and easy. They are paradoxical, but they are not easy. It is rarely, if ever, possible for codependent people to manage their feelings and their lives unless they go to Al-Anon meetings to understand the disease concept of addiction and to find support and specific techniques to get well by becoming themselves. Remember the saying, "You alone can do it, but you cannot do it alone." This is as true for overcoming codependence as it is for overcoming addiction. Alone, the addict and the codependent are helplessly in the grip of the disease of addiction. Releasing each other, they can begin the long, hard, wonderful road to recovery.

Primary codependent people are more likely to need long-term treatment as well as long-term attendance at 12-step meetings, usually Al-Anon. Many codependent people themselves become addicts, if not to alcohol or drugs then to other addictive behaviors, as they have become addicted to the addict in their relationship. Thus, in addition to attending Al-Anon meetings, many codependent people find it useful, in their efforts to meet their own needs, to go to meetings dealing with whatever addictions from which they personally suffer. Because most primary codependent people grew up in homes dominated by alcohol and drugs, they often benefit from attending Adult Children of Alcoholics (ACOA) meetings. These additional meetings are often essential to the development of a stable life, but it is also important that codependent people, like addicts, keep in mind the rule, "First things first." That means keeping attendance at Al-Anon meetings high on the priority list, as it means for addicts and alcoholics keeping their attendance at Narcotics Anonymous and Alcoholics Anonymous at the top of their priorities.

For secondary codependents, people whose codependence developed when they were adults in relationship to alcoholic or drug-addicted spouses or children, the treatment of codependence is usually less intensive and less prolonged. It may be enough to go to Al-Anon meetings for a period of time without any intensive therapy. For people suffering from secondary codependence, finding out what is wrong (the syndrome of addiction and the central role of the codependent person), along with what to do about it (detach with love), is sometimes all that is needed to get moving in the direction of real and lasting recovery.

Addiction is an old diagnostic label. *Codependence* is a new word and a new idea. Addiction, following the lead of AA and consistent with a rapidly growing body of neurophysiological research, has been redefined in recent years. When addiction was thought to be simple pharmacology, the family was irrelevant. Once addiction was understood to be an enduring way of living, rooted in biology and shaped by the characters of addicts interacting with their specific environments, it suddenly became clear that the family was the most important environment for addiction. The family was also the most important engine of change for addiction. Just as recovery was a great gift for the addict, so was recovery a great gift for the codependent. Recovery for the codependent means finding, and fulfilling, the lost self.

Case Histories

These two faces of addiction show the role of codependence, the family side of the addiction coin. Jane came to her role with an addicted husband from the childhood training program of a painful relationship with an alcoholic father. With regard to Earl, I know little about his family except that they failed totally to help him. In fact, the "help" they offered appeared to him only to make his disease worse.

Jane

Jane, at 75, lamented her sad state after having lived with an alcoholic husband for over 50 years. When he was dying of cancer, he needed her as much as he did in every other phase of their relationship. At the end, he had not had a drop of alcohol for over a decade. He found himself terribly afraid to die and deeply in need of his wife's constant attention. They did not have a lot of money, but what they had was tied up in her husband's insurance and his personal savings, about which he told Jane very little except that he would always see that she was well cared for. He assured her that he would meet her needs even after he was gone. She was a saint in caring for him, giving up her own children's needs, as she had all of their lives, to be with her emotionally very needy husband. When he died and his will was read to his family, Jane was overcome with shock: The limited sum of money they had accumulated was placed in a trust she could not touch, to be passed at her death to their children. She could live on the interest from these funds, a sum so meager that her life was crippled. "He did it to me again. Even in death he robbed me of my independence and my dignity," she said.

Why did Jane stay with her alcoholic husband for 50 years? Why did she not develop her own career and an independent income? Why did she not insist on seeing the will while her husband lived so that she could change it as she saw fit while her husband was still competent to change it? Members of Al-Anon understand Jane, and they can guess that she had an alcoholic father on whom she doted, a man who never gave her the respect she earned by her selfless love. When she married her husband at the age of 25, he had never had a drink in his life, having grown up in a strict family at the end of Prohibition. He found alcohol in her family's home and quickly became the family alcoholic, modeling himself in this way on Jane's father. To understand this multigenerational pattern and its painful, humiliating persistence over 5 decades is to understand codependence.

Earl

At an NA meeting, Earl, a young black student at the local community college, talked about how he used the NA program: "I did everything wrong in my life, it seemed to me. I was tossed out of my parents' home, and I was arrested three times and sent to prison twice. I was in two long-term addiction treatment programs, and each time I just blew it all off, figuring I was a whole lot smarter than those fools. I came from a good family. The more everyone tried to help me, the worse I got.

"Then I met Jesse, a home boy I had used dope with for years, and he looked happy and healthy. I was amazed because I looked and felt so terrible. He told me it was not so hard to stay straight if he went to an NA meeting every single day and worked the program. He took me along with him. At first I didn't say anything at meetings, but then I started to talk up a little. I saw a guy I liked and I talked to him, but I couldn't seem to get my words out. So he asked me, 'Hey, man, are you asking me to be your sponsor, or what?' I said I guessed I was, and he said 'yes.' That was the smartest move I ever made. That guy understood me because he had done all the dumb things I had done. All of a sudden, a lot of things people had been telling me for years sort of fell into place, and I understood what they meant. I could understand things like getting up in the morning and getting to work on time, being honest, and thinking about other people instead of just feeling sorry for myself.

"So now I have 7 months of clean time. I feel better than I ever thought I could feel. People see me and they say, 'Hey, man, you are looking strong,' and that makes me feel good."

Family members cannot make addicts well by their caring or their love. As these cases show, family love that includes codependence usually lowers the bottoms of addicts, inadvertently and paradoxically, but completely understandably, creating more suffering for both the addict and the family. The release from this trap lies in a creative disengagement based on an understanding of the complementary relationships of the addicted person and the echo of that person in the codependent family members.

Chapter 9

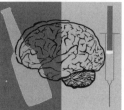

Preventing Addiction

In this chapter, we explore the best ways to prevent addiction from starting, focusing on the relationships of adults and teenagers.

Prevention of addiction is everyone's responsibility, one that is never finished. The most critical time for prevention is before youth reach the ages of 12 to 20, when nonmedical drug use usually begins. The key to preventing addiction to alcohol and other drugs is the family team, parents and children working together to achieve shared goals. Families should begin at the earliest ages, certainly before children reach the age of 8 or 10, talking about the family team and its goals. The family goal that transcends all others is to help the children grow up to become healthy, productive, and independent adults. To do that they must be free of addiction to alcohol and other drugs.

In this chapter, I emphasize family-based prevention of addiction. There is an important environmental role for prevention that is more fully explored in the Preface and in Chapter 12 of this book, where we consider policy options for prevention. In this chapter, we explore the role of character disorder in addiction and the boundaries for social drinking of alcohol. When it comes to prevention of addiction, there are no guarantees. A family can do everything right and still have problems with addiction. Equally remarkably, families can do everything wrong and still avoid addiction in some family members. Prevention is a process of reducing, not eliminating, the risk of addiction. The risk of addiction to alcohol and other drugs cannot be eliminated completely because it is part of our shared human vulnerability.

The family that wants to prevent addiction must talk with and listen to each other with the clear understanding that the children will be in the parental home for a relatively brief time, until about the ages of 18 to 25, when they will leave the parental home and go off to make their own homes. The children's position in the world as adults, including their economic status, will be determined by their own choices and achievements, not by those of their parents. While the children are at home, they need to work with their parents to have good childhoods and to prepare themselves for their own long life of self-support. While the children are in the parental home, their parents provide for their needs as best they can.

Both parents and children owe each other love and respect. Families do not work well if the children do not respect their parents and if the parents do not care for their children. Families do not work well without open communication and honesty. Families need clear rules about the behavior of the children, especially when it comes to respect for adults, work around the house and at school, and the use of alcohol and other drugs. A successful family can come in a variety of structures and at any income level, but success in the prevention of addiction is unlikely without clear-cut rules rejecting youthful use of alcohol and other drugs.

To achieve the primary goal of preventing addiction, the family team must develop working processes for everyday life that take into consideration the unique characteristics of the family and of each individual family member. Like any other team activity, this involves sustained practice and effort over time. It involves people working to help each family member achieve his or her unique potentials.

Each family will approach the process of prevention of addiction differently. My suggestion, however, is that whatever approach your family takes be put into words in ways that everyone understands so that the roles of each family member are clear. There needs to be plenty of room for both pleasure and hard work for all family members, for time alone as well as for time together. Preventing addiction means tough love about drug and alcohol use, but it also means using solid principles to live good lives. There is more to preventing addiction than simply "saying 'no'" to drugs and alcohol, although that is a fundamental part of a successful addiction prevention program.

Making prevention work in the family means playing the game of life within life-sustaining rules, which are often found in values that transcend the family. For many families, this means religious values and an active, personal relationship to God or a Higher Power. It certainly means living within the law and being honest. Children are most likely to prosper if they work with their parents, accepting parental authority, and if they make the best use of their childhoods to prepare themselves to leave their parents' home after their teenage years and support themselves financially.

Pseudoadults and Pseudochildren

In North America in recent decades, the boundaries between childhood and adulthood have become blurred. Youth are given freedoms and choices during childhood that are best restricted to adults, such as the use of alcohol and other drugs and choices about sexual activity. This downward movement of previously adult choices has disastrously eroded the experience of childhood, a time formerly protected from such choices by adults so as to promote the development of young people. Children who use alcohol and other drugs, and who are sexually active, are pseudoadults. They exercise the choices of adults without the responsibilities of adults. When pseudoadults get into trouble as a result of their choices, their parents rescue them, thus depriving them of the painful but valuable lessons that life provides to adults.

When people enter their 20s, 30s, or 40s without becoming financially and emotionally independent of their parents, they often continue to act as if they were children, expecting their parents to rescue them from the negative consequences of their own choices, choices that often involve the use of alcohol and other drugs. Such people are pseudochildren. They act like adults, but they do not carry adult responsibilities, and they expect protections from their parents that in the past were usually restricted to children.

A 37-year-old businessman whose cocaine use led to the loss of his business and his marriage, as well as to criminal charges, returned home to live with his mother and father. He had no car to get to work and no money to pay for a lawyer to fight his entanglements with the law. His parents provided a home, a car, and a lawyer. They struggled with his repeated relapses to cocaine use and his dishonesty, but most of all they struggled with his anger at them and his frustrated sense of entitlement. They were terrified that if they did not help him, he would die of his disease. This man was a pseudochild, locked in a relationship with his codependent parents. Although this is a tragically common picture in North America today, it is not as common as teenagers being treated by their parents as adults. Both pseudoadults and pseudochildren are at high risk of addiction to alcohol and other drugs. Both are primary targets of addiction prevention, and both represent common failings of the modern family.

All too often, families do not clearly define a teamwork pro-

Pseudoadults and Pseudochildren

- *Pseudoadults.* Young people, usually under the age of 19, supported financially by their parents, but who make adult choices, for example, with respect to sex, alcohol, and drugs.
- *Pseudochildren.* People 19 and older who should be supporting themselves, but who are supported by their parents. They act like adults, but do not pay their own bills, often living in their parents' home.
- Both pseudoadults and pseudochildren are angry and resentful of their parents. They are unhappy people who are at high risk of addiction to alcohol and other drugs.

cess or family goals. Prevention is subverted by seductive assumptions and misunderstandings. Many children come to think of their childhood as a time to "have fun." They see work and adult responsibilities as their enemies, to be postponed as long as possible. Surprisingly, the parents often share these crippling assumptions. When high-risk teenagers do work, they think only of the current wage, not of the larger potential of the job to provide experience and future rewards for themselves and for their communities. For pseudoadults, childhood appears to be freedom; self-supporting adulthood looks like prison. At-risk children, often with the active but unwitting connivance of their parents, attempt to postpone the real independence of adulthood as long as possible. They act as though they will never need to support themselves or as though they can take care of their problems and begin to work hard once they are adults, at some vague, far away future time.

Parents may be so caught up in their own problems and needs that they do not help their children face what has to be faced if the children are to fulfill their personal potentials. If the parents or the children have disabilities, it is often all the more difficult for parents and children to keep their focus on the need for hard work and on their roles on the family team. Both parents and children can use disabilities and hardships as excuses for poor performances rather than as incentives for greater, better focused efforts. The plain truth is that the only solution to any disability is to work harder. No other approach has ever worked. Anyone who does not tell this truth to disabled people is not doing them a favor. Hard work is not the enemy of either children or parents; it is their friend. A good life is not an easy life, but a life of fulfilling personal potentials and of helping others. A good life is a life in balance with time both for work and for healthy play.

Young people who use alcohol and other drugs frequently blame others, especially their parents, for their problems. Many adults, often those most dedicated to the welfare of youth, agree. This is unfortunate. The point of this book is that all of us are responsible for our own lives and for our own choices. This includes young people. Many drug-using youth come to my office, brought by worried parents, saying that their problems are "my parents." Complaints are legion from drug-using youth, but mostly they relate to parents being too strict or having expectations that are too high.

Young people, whether or not their parents have serious failings, need to recognize, and adults need to help them recognize, that they are almost always better off working with their parents than against them and that parents deserve respect, whatever their imperfections in the eyes of their children. I remind young people that in the rest of their lives no one will ever again give them what their parents are giving them: unearned financial support, including food on the table, a roof over their heads, and an opportunity to learn and grow into their own unique independent and adult selves. Bosses will insist that they work long and hard for their paychecks. Spouses will require tremendous work to support the family. Friends will not provide the financial support that parents do.

Even the most difficult parents have something positive to offer their children, and, in any event, there are plenty of positive role models around for young people to emulate: teachers, coaches, neighbors, friends, religious leaders, and others. If children are to make the best of the opportunities they have, they need help in focusing on their primary work, which is school, and on their major goals, which are to develop their skills and their intellectual and moral lives. Complaints and excuses do not help young people grow up to become happy and healthy adults. A genuine respect for parents and other adults in authority, including teachers, is a good place to start for all young people.

The 10-Point Plan for Prevention

Here, based on the principles outlined in this book, are 10 practical ways to drug-proof your child:

1. **Set a family standard on drug and alcohol use.** Tell your children the family rules about the use of alcohol, tobacco, and illicit drugs early, when they are in grade school or even before. Let your children know what your expectations are for their use of alcohol and other drugs, including marijuana and cocaine. Take a stand on smoking cigarettes. No use usually is the best rule for children, including teenagers, for cigarettes, alcohol, and other drugs, but whatever your family rules, make them clear to everyone in the family. It may help to remember that both drinking alcohol and smoking cigarettes are illegal for teenagers. Remind everyone often of the family rules on the use of addicting drugs. Here is an important fact: all of the terrible problems caused by alcohol and other drugs can be prevented completely by not using alcohol and other drugs.

2. **Establish reasonable consequences for violations of the family rules.** Examples of effective punishments include loss of privileges such as driving a car or being with friends away from the family's supervision. Make the consequences for violation of the family rules clear in advance and impose them without exception every time there is a violation of the family rules about the use of alcohol, tobacco, and other drugs. The

best punishments usually are those that are swift and painful but fairly brief. Not being permitted to use the family car for the next 2 weeks is better than not being permitted to go out with friends for the next 6 months, for example. Make punishments that are enforceable. Do not make punishments so painful for the children or for the parents that they are unendurable.

3. **Set aside a time every day to talk with your kids about what is happening in their lives, how they feel, and what they think.**   Starting from infancy and continuing through teenage years, let them talk while you listen, giving them your full attention. Actively listen, respecting your children's experiences and feelings. Kids grow up fast. Make time every day to listen to your children, to let them know that you value them just the way they are, and that you want to know what they think and what they feel. You do not have to solve their problems or give them advice. Just listen and care. That is a great gift to anyone. It is especially important to give that gift to your children every day, even if only for a few minutes. Do not reinterpret your children's experiences into those of your own life or give them high-flown lectures on what they should do or feel. Respect their feelings and experiences as their own. Love your kids and appreciate their troubles as well as their triumphs, without attempting to take over their feelings and experiences.

4. **Help your children establish personal goals.**   Define with your children simple, practical goals that can be reached, and help your children reach them. These should include academic, athletic, and social goals. The goals should be both short term (the next day or two) and long term (the next month or two). Help your children accept and learn from their inevitable failures. Failures are growth opportunities and not reasons for giving up. Do not set goals so high that your children often fail. If you do that, the children will feel it is hopeless to try. Set small goals that are relatively easy to achieve. Feel good about your children when they achieve their goals.

5. **Know your children's friends and spend time with them.** Know your children's friends and the parents of your chil-

dren's friends. Both your children's friends and their parents can enrich your life as well as help you to be a better parent. Your kids are part of your family, and you are part of their family. Socialize together; share your lives. This does not mean that there is no time for privacy or separateness for adults or children, but it does mean that the common ground, the shared experiences and relationships, are important to the health of the entire family. When common emotional ground shared by parents and children in the family is lost, then both parents and children lose, with children's drug and alcohol use being more likely to start and more likely to progress to bad outcomes.

6. **Help your children feel good about themselves and their achievements, large and small.** Get excited about what your kids care about. Life is an adventure. Share the adventure with your kids; you will not have them with you for long. Parents too often feel either disengaged from the lives of their children or as if they have to run their children's lives. It is important that parents learn to enjoy their children's lives, to share with their children so that the children understand what is going on in the parents' lives, and the parents learn what is going on in the children's lives. This means that sadness and joy, and other human feelings, get communicated between parents and children in an open, direct, and respectful way.

   It is fun to care about someone else. It is fun for people to care about you. Friends come and go, but families are for a lifetime. For family life to be a positive experience, it is important that children and parents openly and honestly share their lives regularly, respecting both what links them and what separates them. Know what mountains your children are climbing in their lives' adventures. Share the tough journey up, the view from the peaks, and the pain and frustrations of the falls and disappointments.

7. **Have a system for conflict resolution.** Your kids will not agree with you about all the family rules of the house. Parents are in charge, and their decisions are the rules. Parents carry their authority best when they are open to appeals from their

children. Establish a process for review, such as seeing a religious adviser, a mutually respected family member, a neighbor, or a counselor if conflicts develop. Parents need to be open to challenges from their children to their authority. Parents also disagree with each other about how to handle their children, especially when the children have problems. The more serious the children's problems, the more likely the conflicts between parents, and between the parents and the children. Parents can use the same system for conflict resolution for conflicts between themselves. The strong parent is open to new learning and adapts to new challenges, many of which are unforeseen.

8. **Talk about your children's futures early and often.**   What do you expect from your kids? What can they expect from you? Children need to know that they will be with their parents for a relatively short time until they are grown up and leave home. Help your children know that they will *soon* be out of the parental home, paying their own bills and making their own rules. This change from childhood to adulthood comes at various ages but usually between 18 and 25. Children become adults when they leave their parents' homes and financially support themselves, not when they get a driver's license, turn 18, or go to college. Until children are adults who support themselves financially, they need to accept parental authority. That authority needs to be exercised by the parents as a trust for the children's welfare.

9. **Enjoy your kids.**   One of life's greatest joys is having children in your home. Work with your children to make your home a positive place for everyone. That means family teamwork and mutual respect. It also means accepting, and appreciating, that your children are each unique human beings with interests, abilities, and goals that are different from you and anyone else. This diversity and uniqueness needs to be respected and even celebrated, not suppressed or frustrated.

10. **Be a nosy parent.**   Ask your children questions; know where they are and who they are with. This information is necessary for you to be an effective parent. As a parent, you cannot fly blind while piloting a family and avoid crashing. Let your chil-

10 Ways to Drug-Proof Your Children

1. Set family rules on drug and alcohol use.
2. Establish consequences for violations of these rules.
3. Set aside a time every day to talk with your kids about what is happening in their lives, how they feel, and what they think.
4. Help your children establish personal goals.
5. Know your children's friends, and spend time with them and their parents.
6. Help your children feel good about themselves and their achievements, large and small.
7. Have a system for family conflict resolution.
8. Talk about your children's futures early and often.
9. Enjoy your kids.
10. Be a nosy parent.

dren know that you are being nosy because it is your job as their parent and because you love them.

These prevention techniques work best when they are put in place early in children's lives so that they are familiar with the operation of the family team and have a clear understanding of the healthy, realistic roles of parents and children. It is difficult to confront a drug or alcohol problem in a teenager and try, at that point, to establish parental authority for the first time. By then, typically, the youth has been making his or her own often impulsive and irresponsible decisions for many years and has spent time with other youths who are living with uninvolved and/or dangerously permissive parents. It is far harder then to regain parental control than it is to start when the children are infants so that they can grow up with this understanding of their roles and goals as part of the family team.

Character Disorder: A Distinguishing Feature of High-Risk Youth

Prevention of addiction is easier with some youth than with others. Families with children at low risk of addiction have a relatively easy time following this 10-point plan for family-based prevention. When these families fail in their efforts to live wisely, they often suffer no adverse consequences. They often think of addiction prevention as fairly easy. On the other hand, families who have children at high risk of addiction will read this 10-point list and see that, despite their best efforts, their children dive into the use of alcohol and other drugs the way young ducklings dive into water. Families with low-risk children can afford the velvet glove approach to addiction prevention. Families with high-risk children need to take out the iron fist of parental authority, keeping their children under tight supervision.

Families with high-risk children deserve and need support, which often is best found through a parent-support network with other families coping with similar problems. Many junior and senior high schools now have active parent-support programs. Another good place to find support for families dealing with high-risk youth is at an Al-Anon meeting, as described in Chapter 11. Many parents who are concerned about preventing alcohol and other drug problems in their children also can find help at an Employee Assistance Program (EAP) at their places of work. Larger employers are likely to have EAPs, which can discuss concerns and help parents find support, including treatment for their children or for the entire family, when that is needed.

The toughest challenges are youth who suffer from character disorder, which is a common and relatively mild form of antisocial personality disorder. At its simplest definition, this means that youth who are at high risk of addiction to alcohol and other drugs are willing to be dishonest with anyone who may get in their way, including their parents, their teachers, and anyone else in authority. High-risk youth are the true test of any addiction prevention effort. High-risk youth are attracted to alcohol and other drugs. No effort to stop their headlong dive into addiction will stop all

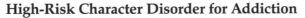

High-Risk Character Disorder for Addiction
- Act on the basis of immediate consequences only
- Are impulsive, extroverted, and dishonest
- Lack religious or moral values
- Lack concern for the feelings of others
- Lack respect for the law
- Are relatively impervious to punishment
- Seldom do homework
- Do not save money
- Are often dishonest

such youth from doing their own personal exploration of addiction. (See Chapter 7 for more information about character disorder and Type I and Type II addicts.)

Dishonesty: Addiction's Essential Requirement

Active addiction requires lying and dishonesty, the willingness to live outside the conventional boundaries of family and community values. To repeatedly take an addicting drug despite social disapproval requires that one value highly personal and immediate pleasure (the drug high) above responsibility to others or even one's own long-term self-interest.

Lying is like drug use in that it produces pleasure now, even though it almost always produces eventual pain. In working with addicts and teenage drug abusers, I have learned a lot about lying. I have learned that the more a person loves the drug abuser the easier it is for the drug abuser to lie, because lying is simply a matter of telling the caring person what that person wants to hear. The more the person loves the addict, the more eager the person is to hear the lie and the easier it is for the addict to get away with the lie in the short run. I have also learned that lying does not work in the long run, although it sometimes works in the short run.

Lying to someone who cares for you is like avoiding homework or spending money you do not have. It comes to a bad ending, usually in a big hurry. But because high-risk people typically do not think ahead, they are blind to the inevitable outcomes of their dishonesty and shortsightedness. In contrast, most anxious people are compulsive truth tellers. They find it hard to lie, even about trivial things. I asked an anxious teenager why he did not lie. He told me, "It is not because I am moral or religious. I can't lie because I am sure I will be caught and punished." This attitude of an anxious person could not be more different from the attitudes of character-disordered drug addicts and alcoholics.

The Good and Bad Effects of Fear and Fearlessness

When I see this distinction between character disorder and anxiety disorder in teenagers, as I often do, I see a simple distinction in their attitude toward homework. High-risk kids do not do homework because it is pain now, pleasure later. If the teenager is thinking only of the next 10 minutes, homework is not an attractive activity. In contrast, anxious kids often do their homework to the exclusion of other important activities, including spending time with peers, as they worry excessively about the next test or even about what college they will get into in a few years.

As a psychiatrist, I find myself saying to high-risk kids, "Think about the future," "Think about what is likely to happen to you if you do this or that," and "Worry more!" Alcoholics Anonymous puts it this way: "Think through the drink." In other words, do not just think about the good feelings of using alcohol or other drugs, but think about what comes after the high and then think about what comes after that. This calculation of future consequences, as one of my drug-abusing patients told me, wrecks the fun of drug use. Right, that is reality.

With anxious teenagers, I often say, "Stay in the present; let the future take care of itself," and "Worry less about tomorrow; have fun now." High-risk kids think primarily of positive future outcomes. Anxious kids think mostly of negative future outcomes. "A" students worry about exams. "F" students rarely worry about tests or grades. When "A" students come out of exams, they often feel as if they have flunked. High-risk kids come out of exams feeling that the exams were easy and that they did well, even when they actually failed the tests. These fundamental differences in character can be seen in all ages, not just in kids. People who worry a lot are less likely to use drugs; people who do not worry enough are more likely to use drugs.

When I talk with high-risk youth in my practice about dangerous behaviors, I can say, "Three out of four people who do what you are doing are dead within a year." My high-risk patients typically reply, "Those are the best odds I have had in a long time. I am not worried at all. I know that I will be in the 25% who make it just fine." For high-risk people, the future holds limitless prospects for happy, lucky outcomes. On the other hand, when I tell my anxious low-risk young patients, "One in a thousand people who do what you are doing may have a relatively minor illness as a result," they are frightened by the danger. They are sure that they will be the one person in a thousand who has the problem. For characterologically low-risk people, the future is scary.

High-risk people may ride motorcycles, and anxious people may be afraid to drive on freeways or fly on commercial airplanes. Most high-risk people, especially high-risk youth, are not interested in exciting or risky activities that take a lot of work. They like passive, quick, intense pleasurable rewards. They do not seek risks; they seek rewards. For them, risk is a by-product of reward, not the goal in itself. Mountain climbing or white-water rafting are not usually preferred activities by character-disordered drug abusers; neither is a pleasure-producing activity that has a delayed payoff and that takes a lot of self-control or social control, such as organized sports. Drug use does not compete with wilderness backpacking in the minds of most drug addicts. Wilderness survival training, mountain climbing, scuba diving, and skiing all take planning and sustained effort. These activities are subject to authority and rules, making them unappealing activities to many drug addicts who are not attracted by the rewards of delayed gratification. Drug highs are quick, easy, and personally controlled. Drug highs fit the character of high-risk people like a glove fits a hand.

Rewards: Now and Later

High-risk people are said not to learn from their mistakes. That is not true. They do learn from their short-term successes—they believe that what works right now is good. Most high-risk people cannot see into the probable negative future, so they repeatedly do things that get them in trouble. Each time, when asked why they did the dumb thing that got them in trouble again, they say simply that they thought they could get away with it or, even more commonly, that they never thought at all about what would happen after they acted as they did. People have called this the illusion of invincibility, but, more accurately, it is blindness to the likely future consequences of pleasure-driven behaviors.

There are some other obvious correlates of these opposite character styles. High-risk people lack empathy, a respectful sense for the feelings of others. High-risk people are aware of other people's feelings, but they do not feel pain when they hurt others. High-risk people think of other people's feelings mainly in terms of what they can do to manipulate those feelings to get their own way. High-risk people are relatively unconcerned about punishment. When anxious people are punished, they feel devastated for long periods of time even by mild disapproval. In contrast, high-risk people are relatively oblivious to punishments. As one teenager said when he had been punished by his parents, "Is that all there is to it?" A typical high-risk response to a problem, such as being found out in a lie or drug use despite solemn promises not to use, is "I said I'm sorry. What more do you want from me?" or "I don't know why I did it."

Most addicted people expect that by simply saying they are sorry all will be forgiven. Here is what one member of Narcotics Anonymous said at a meeting I attended, when the topic of the meeting was making amends for the harm that addicts had done to other people:

> When I was using drugs I always said I was sorry when I got caught, but I knew all along that saying I was sorry meant I was just going to do it again. Other people seemed to think I meant that I would not do it again. I never meant that. They kept expecting me to act that way, even though I never did. They said I

didn't learn from my experiences, but they didn't learn from their experiences either. I never figured them out, and I guess they never figured me out.

Future Thinking

High-risk people do not save money. When I work with people with a character disorder, I can watch their savings balances and see how they are doing in therapy and in their lives. If they live financially in the red, their character disorder is continuing; if they live financially in the black, they are getting better. Growing debt reflects more character disorder, saving money reflects less of it. When high-risk people have money, and they sometimes do, they put it at risk with investments that hold out the promise of quick gains, or they simply spend it on something they want right away. Such investments seldom work out, which is why they are called "high risk." This pattern of being unrealistically optimistic about the future creates some truly phenomenal debts for those relatively rare, financially successful high-risk people.

High-risk behavior is not all or nothing, so some high-risk people have this potentially destructive character trait under fairly good control, with the result that they can do well in life, often because they are congenitally optimistic and willing to take big risks. This concept of a "little bit of character disorder" helps to explain the people who succeed in many areas of life but then have serious addiction problems. Some of these people have a smaller dose of high-risk characteristics. They win some of their high-risk gambles.

Anxious friends, family members, and associates often marvel at the seemingly magical fates of mildly character-disordered people. When anxious people do gamble and take other risks and lose, as they commonly do because people who take risks lose sometimes, they rapidly become "risk averse." When high-risk people take risks and lose, they habitually pick themselves up and do it all over again. Just as high-risk people are relatively impervious to punishment, so too are they relatively impervious to failures. The other side of that coin is that many worried people find that even when they succeed, they still have trouble believing they will succeed the next time, feeling they were merely "lucky" and that surely the next time their luck will fail.

Life is not fair. This is nowhere more true than with character disorder. Some people have a lot of it, and some have a little. There are some obvious correlates of character disorder. Age is one. The character disorder syndrome is most intense between the ages of about 15 and 25. People with character disorder can get well with help, especially help from the 12-step programs. Character-disordered people mature out of their problem for many reasons. They get well partly because they learn, however slowly, from the pain they cause themselves and partly from changes in their nervous systems as the biological fires that fuel their high-risk behavior dampen with age. When people get well from character disorders, they often continue to show interest and ability in two areas, both related to their underlying character traits. On the one hand, they are often risk taking and entrepreneurial, and, on the other hand, they are interested in human relations and human service activities because they are often extroverted.

Males are more likely to suffer from the character disorder syndrome than females, again for both biological and social reasons. Some environments foster this sort of behavior more than others. Irresponsible, neglectful, permissive, or indulgent families tend to produce more high-risk kids than do other families. But whether a person has character disorder or not is often observed at an early age and apparently biologically determined. I see many families with several children, only one of whom has this high-risk character even though all the children have been raised more or less similarly. Many of these families are quite exemplary. Conversely, I also see some very dysfunctional families that produce healthy children. In this, as in most human behaviors, it is not just nature (the genetics) or just nurture (the environment) but it is both that cause the patterns of behavior we see in ourselves and those around us.

Coping With High-Risk Children

There is no simple solution to the problems created by high-risk children for themselves and for those who care for them. The

10-point prevention plan is a good starting point in the family and in social institutions dealing with children. It is helpful to talk directly with high-risk children about the difficulties they create for themselves thinking unrealistically about present rewards rather than about probable future consequences of their choices. It also helps to state clearly the family rules and to enforce them consistently with love. High-risk children who are still supported financially by their parents need to be held to the standard of respecting their parents and others in authority. High-risk youth who have left their parents' homes need to be held to the standard that their parents will not rescue them from the bad choices that they make.

Drawing clear lines between childhood and adulthood is essential in dealing with a character-disordered child of any age. Psychotherapy can sometimes be helpful, but high-risk people themselves are seldom interested in psychotherapy because it is experienced by them as a barrier to their being able to do what they want when they want to do it. Psychotherapy is more likely to be useful for family members who must deal with high-risk people because they create dilemmas for those who love them.

When all looks dark and hope is hard to hold on to, recall that time is on the side of recovery because many character-disordered youth mature out of the worst aspects of their problems, although this can take until they are into their 20s, 30s, or even beyond in especially difficult cases. Parents need to keep up hope and to work with other parents of high-risk youth to find the best ways of helping their children stay on course for a good life as adults, supporting themselves.

Four Simple Boundaries for Social Drinking

Prevention of addiction requires a clear understanding of the place of alcohol in family and community life. Although alcohol use by adults is legal, and although many adult alcohol drinkers have no health or behavioral problems as a result of their alcohol use (unlike cigarette smokers), alcohol poses a significant health risk for adults. Underage drinking is even more likely to generate serious health risks, from driving accidents and suicide to AIDS and academic failure. Although the decision not to drink alcohol removes all of these health risks, many North Americans choose to drink. Although most drinkers are convinced that their own drinking is safe, the new and growing intolerance for cigarette and alcohol use, by adults as well as by youth, raises important questions for social drinkers. Is my drinking safe? How can I tell if I have a drinking problem, since denial is a hallmark of alcoholism? There are four understandable and uncontroversial ways to prevent alcohol-caused problems:

1. Don't drink alcohol if you are under the legal drinking age of 21.
2. Don't drink alcohol while pregnant.
3. Don't drink alcohol within 4 hours of driving a car or going to work, because of possible impairment and associated safety and performance risks.
4. Don't drink alcohol at all if you have a personal history of drug or alcohol addiction. Abstinence from alcohol use also may be prudent for people who have parents or siblings who are alcoholics or drug addicts.

Drinking alcohol in pregnancy deserves special attention because of the concern for the health of the unborn child. The best and simplest rule is not to drink alcohol at all while pregnant. Drinking up to two or three drinks of alcohol a week during pregnancy may not harm the mother or the unborn baby. However, because there is no absolutely safe level of alcohol for the unborn baby, zero is the safest number when it comes to drinking alcohol during pregnancy. Many women today take this clearly safe course, and they do not drink alcohol at all when pregnant.

Some women are concerned about calories during pregnancy, as well as about their baby's health. Because alcohol is the emptiest of calories at about 150 calories a drink, this fact alone is enough to convince many pregnant women to stop drinking alcohol altogether while pregnant. Maternal alcohol use in excess of two drinks a day on a regular basis, and even repeated but not daily consumption of five drinks or more a day, are serious risk factors for the unborn child, as is maternal nonmedical use of other drugs such as cocaine and marijuana. Lower levels of alcohol use may also become problems for either the mother or the unborn baby. Abstinence from drinking alcohol during pregnancy is the simplest and the safest course to follow.

Traffic Signals for Social Use of Alcohol

For adults who choose to drink alcohol, I use a "stoplight" system. This is a recommendation that is both personal and controversial, unlike the four boundaries described above. To understand the stoplight system, a drink is defined as 12 ounces of beer, 5 ounces of wine, or 1.5 ounces (a standard jigger) of distilled spirits. Each of these amounts contains about the same quantity of pure ethyl alcohol, about one-half ounce. Drinking up to two drinks in any 24-hour period and up to four drinks in any week falls into the green light zone. This is a generally safe drinking level for everyone over the legal drinking age who is not pregnant and who does not have a personal history of drug or alcohol dependence. Most American social drinkers stay within this green light zone without making any effort to control their drinking. Few, if any, alcoholics drink alcohol at this low level except occasionally, and usually briefly, when they begin to drink for the first time in their lives or during periods when they make great efforts to cut down their use of alcohol.

Drinking up to four drinks in any 24-hour period and up to 10 drinks a week is the yellow light zone. This is more alcohol than most social drinkers choose to drink and is potentially dangerous. Apparent drinking at the yellow light level is often the result of problem drinkers making a big and usually temporary effort to control their drinking. Yellow light drinking may also be a temporary stage in a progressive increase of drinking leading to higher levels of alcohol use. Drinking in the yellow light zone is seldom a stable, long-term drinking pattern in North America, although it is in some wine-drinking countries where widely accepted, traditional social controls restrain many drinkers from further escalation of their alcohol use. Most social drinkers in North America find that drinking the amount of alcohol in the yellow light zone is unpleasant. Those North Americans whose drinking puts them in the yellow light zone need to recognize that they are at risk for serious alcohol problems.

Worrying about your drinking is generally a good reason to stop drinking entirely or to reduce your drinking permanently to the green light zone of four drinks a week or less. Healthy social drinkers do not worry about their drinking and they do not count their drinks because they drink so little, usually less than four drinks a week. If the green light goal is not easily reached and maintained without effort, then it is wise to seek help from Alcoholics Anonymous and/or from a professional in the treatment of addiction. Many drinkers who report drinking in the yellow light zone are alcoholics in denial (that is, they claim this amount of drinking but they actually drink more).

Drinking more than four drinks in any 24-hour period, even on New Year's Eve, and drinking more than 10 drinks a week in

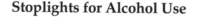

Stoplights for Alcohol Use

Green Zone

- Not drinking more than 2 drinks in 24 hours or 4 drinks in a week

Yellow Zone

- Not drinking more than 4 drinks in 24 hours or 10 drinks in a week

Red Zone

- Occasionally or frequently drinking 5 or more drinks in 24 hours or more than 10 drinks in a week
- Drinking under the age of 21
- Drinking more than 3 drinks in a week if pregnant
- Drinking within 4 hours of driving

any week puts a person in the red light zone. This level of alcohol use is presumptive evidence of a serious alcohol problem. This is not a normal or healthy pattern of drinking. Alcoholics usually socialize with others who have problems with their drinking, which gives a social camouflage to their denial of their alcohol problems.

People with drinking problems find the green light boundaries extremely restrictive and cannot stay within them, except for short periods of time, with great effort. This attitude of heavy drinkers toward alcohol use is an expression of their addiction, of their loss of control over their drinking.

Is Drinking a Little Good for Your Health?

Recently the media has highlighted the claim that drinking a little—up to two drinks a day—may reduce the risk of heart disease as a result of the effect of low levels of alcohol on fat metabolism. These arguments, often promoted by the alcohol industry, are potentially dangerous because they encourage people to drink alcohol. Although a few scientific studies show that moderate drinking has some health value, an important factor is disregarded in this calculation of benefit. Many people who intend to drink no more than two drinks a day lose control of their drinking and drink more than that. For these people, alcohol has profoundly negative effects on their bodies and on their lives. When groups of people who succeed in limiting their drinking are added to those who do not limit their drinking, the net health effect of alcohol use is clearly negative.

Calculating the health benefit of moderate drinking while excluding the costs of heavy drinking is similar to calculating the benefits of speeding (more fun driving, quicker arrival at a destination) while excluding the costs of crashes from the minority of speeders who kill themselves and others. For this reason I do not encourage adults to drink alcohol. However, if you never drink more than two drinks a day, and feel no urge to drink more, it may be that you will have a health benefit from alcohol use, or at least you will suffer no harm. In my experience, most people who say they routinely drink two drinks a day actually drink far more than that amount. The scientific research is clear that drinking more than two drinks a day is definitely unhealthy. Heavy drinking is dangerous to the drinker's health and to people who come in contact with the drinker.

The CAGE Test for Alcoholism

Another simple screening test for alcoholism is the CAGE test. You can take it yourself. Physicians often use it, but it is equally useful for teachers, ministers, and others who want to do a better job of identifying alcohol problems. Here are the four CAGE questions:

1. Have you ever tried to Cut down on your drinking?
2. Are you ever Annoyed when people ask you about your drinking?
3. Do you ever feel Guilty about your drinking?
4. Do you ever take a morning Eye-opener?

The key CAGE words to make this screening tool easy to remember are Cut down, Annoyed, Guilty, and Eye-opener.

Research has shown that even a single positive response to any of the CAGE questions suggests the presence of alcohol problems, that two or three positive responses create a high suspicion of alcoholism, and that four positive responses are confirmatory of alcoholism.

Strategies for Parenting:
The Hazards of Solving the
Problems of the Next Generation

Many parents do not instinctively develop a sense of the family team, or of the central role of parental authority, because when they were growing up either they had parents who were intrusive and negative, or as children they themselves were so self-motivated that they did not need much guidance or structure from their parents. Successful parents often have a hard time with the guidelines I am proposing for families because as children they were self-starters. Their hard work produced success, which began early in their lives. Such successful parents have achieved a great deal in their lives as adults as a result of their hard work over many years, although most such successful people came from families that had relatively few financial resources. Their success was usually based on sustained hard work and, most successful parents are quick to admit, a lot of good luck. These parents want to share their success with their children "so that they don't have as hard a time as I did," or "so that they can have the fun in childhood that I was not permitted to have because I had to work so hard from such an early age."

Parents who come from modest circumstances and had, from an early age, the understanding that whatever success they were to have would be the result of their own efforts had an advantage that they cannot give to their children. This advantage was the incentive to work hard and the tremendous boost to their self-esteem that came from breaking new ground of success in their families. Children of successful parents typically have the opposite experience, which is much more difficult. They live an easy life of relative affluence that they have not earned. They are often indulged by their well-meaning, generous parents. Many successful parents, mistaking their children for themselves at their age, keep waiting for their growing children to manage their lives productively, a wait that can last forever.

Successful parents often fall into another easy trap. They expect too much of their children, figuring that because their children have had so many advantages that they themselves lacked, their children will be all the more successful. This simple logic is flawed in two important ways. First, having unsuccessful parents is a far better incentive to success than having successful parents. Second, successful parents frequently underestimate the uniqueness and difficulties of their personal achievements. They think, and they lead their children to think, that their success was fairly easy.

Both of these errors, commonly made by successful parents, put children at high risk of serious problems as children and as adults, including addiction to alcohol and other drugs. It is better by far for successful parents to share what wisdom they have achieved and to let their kids know what a tremendous challenge there is ahead of them, one only they can manage, in developing their own self-supporting lives. The children's ultimate situation in life, including their economic standard of living, will be determined by their own work as youth and as adults, not by the status of their parents. Successful parents should honestly tell their children that the parents' own success is a real impediment for their children, potentially undermining their motivation for hard work and personal achievement.

Parental success commonly leads to lazy children. Plain, realistic talk about this fact is seldom heard in successful families, which is one of the reasons why rich men's sons are rarely rich men's fathers. Most successful families have success for only one generation because of this repetitive pattern of family life. Families with substantial wealth face this problem over many generations. It is rare for them to succeed in subsequent generations. Most of the major achievements in the world, and the world's fortunes, are made by people who come from modest circumstances. This is as true today as it was 100 years ago. It is certain to be true 100 years from today. Few people who are successful themselves ever consider the consequences of their success for their children, that is, the prices that will be paid by their children for the advantages they as parents have given to their children. Even fewer children of unsuccessful parents recognize the tremendous advantages their families have given to them as children, the advantages of needing to work hard if they are to have much in their lives.

Parents who are themselves impoverished and troubled by drugs and alcohol or other problems are often so preoccupied with their own painful lives that they are unable to give much to their children. Some of these parents are harsh with their children; others are neglectful. Neither harshness nor neglect is likely to help children. Children do best with parents who encourage them to solve their own problems, parents who are involved with them on a daily basis but who do not soften the often painful blows of reality for them. Parents help their children when they celebrate their children's successes, but they also help their children grow from their failures. This is not easy, but it is the most rewarding way to be a parent. It is also the most likely to lead to a happy outcome of family life for both parents and children regardless of the level of parental success.

Families with disabilities in the parents, and especially families with high-risk teenagers, will have the most difficulty with parental authority and family goals. Nevertheless, such families have, paradoxically, a great opportunity for raising healthy and strong children by helping them to see how the family team copes with adversity. Children in families that have few problems do not necessarily have an easier time than those in families with more problems, because the children are likely, sooner or later, to confront many serious problems in their own lives. The sooner children learn that the measure of their characters is their ability to deal with adversity and failure, the better off they will be. On the contrary, families that are closed (humiliated, frightened, or in denial), families that pull apart rather than together when they encounter adversity, and families that lie and deceive each other are unlikely to thrive. They are especially likely to be tormented by addiction, which is a disease of spiritual impoverishment as much as it is a disease of disordered brain chemistry.

Families need to help their children face the fact that having great abilities is of little value unless those abilities are harnessed in productive ways in the children's lives. All too often, children who are performing poorly in school and elsewhere are told that they have high IQs and other exceptional innate talents. Telling failing children that they have great abilities may help them maintain their self-esteem in the short run, but it will hurt them in the long run if they come to believe their talents will automatically lead to success. This sort of reassurance misleads children about what they need to do to succeed.

Life is scored on performance, not on ability. The biggest determinant of success in life is the ability to do hard and goal-oriented work over a long period. If people, including youth, are not able to work hard and to maintain their efforts, they are unlikely to prosper no matter how great their talents. Many people with modest talents do extremely well in life because of their good work habits. Adults need to explain these facts to children and to help children develop sound work habits. There is plenty of room in life for a highly diverse range of interests and talents, but success in any area of activity, from music to mathematics and from creative writing to athletics, is impossible without steady, hard, and productive work.

Strength in Weakness

It helps children if parents talk openly about their own failures, mistakes, and deficiencies, and the ways that the parents worked to cope with their difficulties. Parents should talk about both their successes and their failures with the children. For many parents, such discussions are disturbing because they seem to undermine the children's view of the parents as having the answers and of being strong. The opposite is more often the case. Although it is not desirable for parents to harp on their heroic exploits in overcoming problems, it is nonetheless generally useful to children to know of the more serious problems their parents have confronted and what the results of those confrontations have been. Failures in school or at work, health problems, divorce, financial failure, and personal rejection are the typical problems that most families must confront. Each of these problems is a growth opportunity for all family members. Parents can also say that while the kids are at home (that is, still in a child's role), they will do their best to offer guidance to the children, including setting appropriate limits when health and safety are at stake. On the other hand, once the child leaves the parents' home and is self-supporting, this parental safety net will be removed and the child will be free (or burdened!) by independence from parental authority.

Preventing addiction to alcohol and other drugs is a shared family project that fits well in the overall family goal of raising children who pursue their own destinies, independent of their parents. Families that have a history of addiction and families with high-risk children are those most likely to be put to the test in preventing their children from having serious problems with addiction to alcohol and other drugs, especially during their children's teens and 20s. Families that have little or no history of addiction, and who have children who lack high-risk character traits, usually escape the pain of children who are addicted to in-toxicating drugs. Often these families attribute their success to their skillful parenting and other supposed superiorities. Such a happy outcome usually reflects the fact that the family was not put to the test with high-risk children.

Typically, families that have serious addiction problems in their children are not inferior in their functioning, but they have been confronted by difficult problems that many other families have escaped. It ill behooves families that do not have addiction problems to feel superior to families that do have these problems. Confronting problems is a source of strength. The guidelines of-fered in this chapter can help to reduce the risk of addiction. They cannot eliminate that risk. These guidelines are also helpful to families that do not face addiction by helping the family team function better regardless of the problems it confronts.

Parents, working together if there is more than one parent car-ing for children, need to define clearly what the family's expecta-tions are for the children with respect to certain vital behaviors in adolescence. First and foremost, the parents need to deal with the issues of alcohol and other drug use by their children. When, if ever, is the use of alcohol and other drugs permitted? What about the use of tobacco? What are the consequences for violation of the family rules about alcohol and other drugs? How will the rules be enforced? The reasons for the rules, whatever they are, need to be clearly spelled out so that the child knows, from an early age, that the rules are not arbitrary or mean-spirited.

Family rules also need to be defined for other behaviors re-lated to health and safety, including sex. Many other health-re-lated behaviors also should be discussed openly in the family, with the clear understanding that the ultimate, personal respon-sibility for each of them rests with the maturing child. The family rules should be designed not only to make the family function better, but to help the child grow up to be a healthy, productive, reasonably happy, and independent adult living outside the parents' home. All too often these issues of rules and goals are not discussed within the family. The child is left in the dark about parental expectations until there is a problem, and only then are the "rules" defined, usually in negative terms. That is too late for the good functioning of the family.

Family rules and parental authority are deeply rooted traditions in all cultures. In the last few decades in North America, there has been a potentially dangerous shift of values in many families. There is a lessened parental commitment to putting the children's welfare first and a matching greater commitment to letting children have their own way running their own lives as they see fit, from young ages.

It is not hard to see where these changes in North American culture have come from. They reflect the general movement toward each person, including children, being more responsible for himself or herself and toward greater immediate personal pleasure rather than delayed gratification. At the same time, behaviors and decisions previously limited to adults have been shifted to children at ever younger ages. These trends in values are characteristic of modern society. North America has been in the forefront of these developments. Although there is much to recommend in some aspects of this change of values—for example, it not only encourages diversity but gives a far larger scope for individual choices—it has a steep downside cost when it comes to addiction because of the specific vulnerability of the selfish brain to the lure of addicting drugs. The price is most often paid by vulnerable youth. Prudent families and communities recognize this risk in modern life and take appropriate actions to remove the choices of addicting drugs from the menu offered to young people. This includes alcohol and tobacco, the use of which is legal for adults but not for youth. We have laws governing these behaviors for youth, but the laws against teenage drinking and smoking continue to be haphazardly enforced and widely flouted. Families need to reassert their authority and to use the current laws against youthful drinking and smoking to support them in these important prevention efforts.

The same prevention guidelines should be used in other social institutions that deal with children and youth. These institutions should review their policies and procedures to ensure that they systematically and routinely reinforce the community-wide values of nonuse of addicting drugs. The most difficult case is the modern college, which has become a breeding ground for alcohol

Places to Practice Prevention

The Community

Social institutions such as schools, religious institutions, and the criminal justice system

The Family

Extended family, parents, siblings

The Individual

Personal responsibility and values

and drug abuse, as vulnerable youth are concentrated in environments that are permissive or even encouraging of drug and alcohol use. Middle schools and high schools are other institutions that need to be clear on these values.

The discussion of prevention in this chapter has focused on family roles in preventing addiction. It has also dealt with the environment in which decisions are made to use or not to use alcohol and other drugs. Typically, drug use of all kinds begins during the teenage years, when the most serious addictions have their onsets. Because the toughest cases of addiction are youth with character disorder who are impulsive and irresponsible and who live in environments that are tolerant about the use of alcohol and other drugs, the guts of any serious addiction prevention program must focus on high-risk youth between the ages of about 12 and 16. Education and assistance are vital for these youth. Readers of this book know that the only way that most high-risk youths will be discouraged from the continuing abuse of alcohol and other drugs is if their use is promptly and positively identified, and if that use leads to immediate painful consequences. If young victims of addictive disease are permitted to play out the addicts' career, they will progress deeper and deeper into addiction as they become older teenagers, with desperately destructive consequences for them, their families, and their communities.

The true test of any serious prevention effort is what it does for high-risk youths. As I make clear in Chapter 12, I am convinced—only reluctantly and only after years of resisting this conclusion—that it will be necessary to develop drug testing programs for high-risk youth that are linked to swift and certain painful consequences if they are to be deterred from full-blown careers of addiction. Addiction, if ignored, is the cultural and biological destiny of high-risk youth today in North America and, increasingly, in all parts of the world. Schools and other social institutions can help, but the primary responsibility for raising a drug-free youth rests squarely on the parents' shoulders. When it comes to addiction prevention, the central problems in North America today are teenage use of beer and cigarettes. (See Table 9–1 for a checklist for identifying high-risk youth.)

Effective prevention requires information and knowledge. It is important that everyone, especially vulnerable youth, know the hazards of nonmedical drug use and the consequences for violation of the prohibition in their families and in their communities against the use of alcohol and other drugs. Prevention also benefits from loving, supportive human relationships in the family, at school, and in the community. Compassion and respect are essential for prevention of addiction to work over the long haul. There is no reason to be hostile or rejecting of drug abusers, including drug-abusing youth. They need real help. High-risk youth need to be held tightly in their communities to find meaningful support, not to be cast out of their communities. In this way they are like preschoolers having a temper tantrum. They need to be held close so they do not harm themselves by their out-of-control behaviors.

Prevention means not buying into enabling and denial, two central elements of the addictive disease. *Enabling* is the behavior of those around an addicted person who wittingly or, more often, unwittingly permit the addictive behavior to continue. Parents who hire attorneys to get their alcohol- and drug-using teenage kids out of trouble with the law, and people who call the office to say their spouses are sick when they are actually hung over from drinking are enabling. *Denial* is to be consciously or unconsciously

Table 9–1. Identification of high-risk youth

1. Has parents or siblings who are (or were) addicted to alcohol or other drugs.
2. Has good friends who are addicted to alcohol or other drugs.
3. Holds values that are sympathetic to the use of alcohol and other drugs by youth.
4. Thinks of right now. Is impulsive rather than using delayed gratification.
5. Is dishonest. Lies easily and often.
6. Is frequently in conflict with adults, especially those in authority. Is close to rebellious peers.
7. Does not do homework.
8. Does not save money.
9. Smokes cigarettes.
10. Uses alcohol and other drugs early (often by fifth to seventh grades).
11. Has no religious beliefs and no attendance at religious services.
12. Lacks empathy; lacks sensitivity to hurt feelings of other people and animals.
13. Has home and/or school environment tolerant of teenage use of cigarettes, alcohol, and other drugs.
14. Is pessimistic.
15. Is extroverted.
16. Is disorganized.
17. Lacks long-term personal goals.
18. Receives grades in school below the student's intellectual ability.
19. Has frequent conflicts with teachers, parents, and others in authority.
20. Is often late for school and/or truant from school.

Note. In rating a child, one must have an idea of how other children of similar age in the same community behave so that the rated child's behavior can be compared to that standard. A child with fewer than four of these characteristics is a low-risk child. A child with more than seven of these characteristics is a high-risk child. A child with five or six of these characteristics is at borderline risk of addiction to alcohol and other drugs.

Note that as children grow older, they have more of these risk factors. That reality is reflected in the increasing risk of addiction children face as they grow older in their teenage years. Some children appear to be at high risk by the third or fourth grade; others do not appear to be at high risk until late in high school. Many youth never score more than four on this checklist.

Source. Office for Substance Abuse Prevention: *Stopping Alcohol and Other Drug Use Before it Starts: The Future of Prevention,* OSAP Prevention Monograph-1 (DHHS Publ No ADM-89-1645). Rockville, MD, U.S. Department of Health and Human Services, 1989.

unaware of the addictive behavior even though the behavior is plainly there. When alcoholics lie about their drinking, and when parents ignore their children's drug use, this is denial.

Prevention requires knowing when youth are using alcohol and other drugs and taking active steps, called *interventions*, to deal with youthful alcohol and other drug use. Prevention is not simple and not singular. Prevention requires a continuum of responses based on a thoughtful blend of elements into a coherent and comprehensive community-wide effort to stop the use of alcohol and other drugs by youth before it begins, and, failing that, to detect it at an early stage and to intervene decisively to see that it stops. Nothing less fulfills the community's urgent need to end the tragic modern drug epidemic. Nothing less is worthy of the name *prevention*.

Effective prevention of addiction has many dimensions, some of which are within the family and some of which are within the youth culture itself. Many productive addiction prevention efforts are best conducted in schools and in other community settings involving youth. Prevention of addiction to alcohol and other drugs means helping young people fulfill their personal destinies, to become all that they can each become to better serve their own long-term interests and the interests of their families and their communities.

This discussion of the environmental approach to the prevention of alcohol and other drug use by youth should not, however, distract from the recognition that the primary defensive line in all high-risk behaviors is the family. No change in the environment can make up fully for failed family performance, and even with terrible environmental situations, strong families committed to antiaddiction values can often raise drug- and alcohol-free children. However, even with both a healthy environment and a strong family taking forceful stands against alcohol and drug use by youth, some high-risk youth will still succumb to the siren call of addicting drugs. Failure to recognize this fact reflects failure to face the power of addiction and the widespread vulnerability to that risk.

In the final analysis, the responsibility for the use or nonuse of addicting drugs falls on the individual. That is why the bedrock of all addiction prevention and all addiction treatment approaches must be personal responsibility. The benefits from getting these issues right are great; the costs of miscalculation are often devastating.

The disease of addiction knows no pity and no generosity. Addiction to alcohol and other drugs is a cruel, relentless, and often devious slave driver. However, by confronting and overcoming this dreadful disease there is a great gift. Families and individuals dealing with addiction can find new and better ways to live as individuals and as families. For most people there is an important spiritual dimension to recovery from addiction. There is often a deeply spiritual dimension to prevention of alcohol and drug problems as well. To say "no" to drugs for many people requires a clear understanding of the purpose of their lives.

The following chapter helps to organize the family when prevention efforts fail and addiction to alcohol and other drugs has to be confronted directly in an addiction treatment program.

Case Histories

Dan is a challenge for prevention both because of his own character and because of the environment in which he grew up. His parents' successes set standards that were beyond Dan's reach. Rather than using this to motivate him to do his best, in many ways he simply quit before he got started, at least on the surface. Look a little deeper and you will see that Dan had plenty of ambition and that he was not without his achievements. Today, to finish college in 4 years is quite an achievement, as many young people with troubles like Dan's stretch out their college careers as long as possible to avoid what is to them the terribly threatening step into independence. Maria shows the face of addiction in modern North American colleges, one of the most addiction-promoting environments ever created.

Dan

Dan, at age 22, is graduating from college. He is uncertain about what he will do next year. His father is a law professor who has been successful, financially as well as professionally. Dan's older sister is married to a successful young physician and is herself raising their first child and completing a Ph.D. from an Ivy League university. Dan had wanted to go into law. He graduated after 4 years in college, but he took a minimal load and lacks the requirements for law school or the grades to get in. His father suggested that he could help Dan gain entrance into the school at which he teaches if Dan could take tough prelaw courses for a year and raise both his grades and his law aptitude scores. Mostly, he told Dan, "You have to show the admissions committee that you can do hard work over a period of time. If you do that, they will let you in. If not, there is no way you can get into any law school, no matter how much influence I exert."

Dan was not a hard worker. He and his friends, also from wealthy families, were not the winners in their age group. They liked the easy life—living in elegant homes, driving expensive cars, and traveling to exotic locations for frequent vacations. After college graduation, Dan planned to live at home and take courses at the local community college. The immediate issue for his parents was which course he would take. Dan wanted to take off altogether for the summer after his graduation, "for a much-needed vacation," and to take only two prelaw courses at a time in college, even though he was not planning to get a paying job. His parents wanted him to start in summer school and to take the difficult courses first so that he would discover sooner rather than later whether he was prepared to work hard.

Never discussed by Dan and his parents were the alternatives to law school for Dan. His parents never explained to him that his status in life, including his income, would be determined by his earnings, not by theirs. They did not tell him that they would not subsidize his lifestyle and that he could not live with them once he finished his schooling. As his mother asked me, "How can we have so much and he have so little? How can I let him suffer like that?" His father, who had been a relatively late bloomer himself, was waiting for Dan to find himself. He remarked, "He has so many opportunities that I never had. I just don't understand it. Why doesn't he take advantage of them?"

Dan's problems are surely his own, and it is wrong to attribute them to his parents or to society. Yet it is impossible not to see that Dan's view of reality has been distorted by his parents' success and that his parents have never explained the facts of life to him. Equally difficult, how can anyone imagine that Dan's parents would let him live on minimum wage jobs when they had such affluence? What are they going to do with their wealth when they die, since they cannot take it with them? When and how will all that family money fall to Dan and his sister? When should his parents talk with him about these important facts?

Dan's parents do not want to have this discussion because they do not want to further undermine his incentives. Dan drinks a lot but denies the use of other drugs. Dan's sister, growing up in the same family, was always academically more successful and was driven by the success of her parents to find areas in which she could excel that were unmistakably different from those chosen by her parents.

Dan's environment has compounded his own personal failures. He, like many children of affluence, especially of self-made parents, lives a life strikingly similar to that of children of poverty: he sees few reasons to work hard and simply lives for the moment, with truly frightening disregard for his own or his community's long-term welfare.

Maria

Maria announced at a meeting of Narcotics Anonymous, "This is my first meeting in this town. I'm from Charlotte, North Carolina. I moved up here to finish college. I had to leave Charlotte because the drugs and alcohol were so bad in my school, and I had a horrible time with my own use. I worked the NA program, and I got my life back under control.

"You can already guess what happened next. When I got to my new school, my roommates were both addicts, of course. Is everyone addicted, or is it just my bad luck? Anyway, I procrastinate about everything, so I procrastinated for 3 months after I got to town before I came to an NA meeting here. I was hoping, I guess, that I might not need to go to meetings, since I have so much studying to do as a premed student.

"But tonight one roommate was passed out by 6 P.M., and the other one has friends over to smoke dope. I just couldn't take it any more. The worst part was that I almost used drugs again with that stuff all around. So here I am. I feel at home already, even though I don't know any of you. Can I get some names and phone numbers after the meeting?"

These are two stories of hope as well as danger. I do not know what became of either Dan or Maria, but when I knew them they were both resourceful young people. It seemed likely to me that both would do well as they took their giant steps into their own adult roles. Often I see young people paralyzed by their own fears of adulthood. I wish that their parents and other adults had spoken more directly and openly with them about this big step from childhood to adulthood. It is hard because life is hard.

Children's positions in life will be determined by their own achievements, not by the achievements of their parents. For poor children, this simple, timeless fact can be a relief. For rich children, growing up can be terrifying. For children from all parts of the economic spectrum, this fact must be faced directly as a great opportunity, one that they need not face alone if they will simply reach out to others, both inside and outside of their families, who can help them with this incredible transition. There is one more truth that is seldom spoken to young people who are growing up and getting ready to go out on their own: life is scored on one's actual performance and not on one's ability. This simple truth can be disturbing to children who have been told for years, "Don't worry about your grades. You are a smart person with lots of ability."

Chapter 10

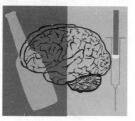

Intervention and Treatment

*In this chapter, we explore the treatment of addictive
disease, what it is and how to use it.*

ere is the chapter that many readers will turn to first when

they pick up this book because they are confronting a crisis, and

they need to know what to do about it. If that is you, welcome

aboard! If you are curious about the mysterious disease of addiction to alcohol and other drugs, the source of so much of your current suffering, I hope you will take the time to explore other sections of this book. They are written not only to help you cope better with this disease, but also to help you understand it.

We need to start with definitions and to draw lines so that we can build treatment on a firm foundation. Addiction to alcohol and other drugs is the malignant disease of the entire self. It has two central features: first, the loss of control over the use of alcohol or other drugs, and second, dishonesty about that use and the problems caused by that use. This disease is progressive and potentially fatal. It is not self-curing. The disease of addiction involves the family and not just the alcohol- or drug-using family member. Getting well or, as it is known today, recovery, involves more than not drinking or using drugs. Recovery from addiction means a new way of living for the addicted person and for the codependent people in the addict's family.

Addiction treatment is a long-term, difficult, and uncertain process. It is not a magic bullet for addictive disease. Formal addiction treatment, whether inpatient or outpatient, can help addicted people and their families begin the long and hopeful road to recovery. When people come out of treatment programs, they are not remade even if they have stopped using alcohol and other drugs. The deeper aspects of addiction, aspects that involve the character of addicted people and of their families, take months and years to fulfill the promise of recovery. Not only is tough love needed, but so are patience, persistence, and a sense of humor. Relapses are common in recovery. Failures also are common, even after the best efforts of all concerned. Addiction to alcohol and other drugs is a dreadful disease from which recovery is possible but by no means certain. Recovery from addiction is never swift, certain, or easy. Recovery is possible, however, for everyone facing addiction, and it is worth the effort it requires.

Identification

There are five stages in the process of getting well: identification, intervention, treatment, aftercare, and recovery. The first, and usually the hardest, is identification. This is the step in which the family, and sometimes the addicted person or the social institution such as the school, comes to recognize that they are dealing with a serious disease and that someone's life is out of control or, in the language of recovery, "unmanageable." The family must identify and name the problem that afflicts them. Identification grows out of a painful and usually long process in which the alcohol and drug use of the addicted person grows progressively worse and more troublesome. The family or community interactions become increasingly dysfunctional because of addiction. Denial is a powerful and crippling feature of the disease for everyone involved. The alcohol or drug user defines the problem as everything but the alcohol or drug use. The family avoids facing the alcohol and drug use and refuses to accept their own self-defeating roles in the process of addiction.

Recall the simple boundaries suggested in Chapter 9. Alcohol use by anyone under the legal drinking age of 21 and any use of an illicit drug are evidence of an addiction problem that needs to be solved. Life on the other sides of these boundaries often reflects addiction if the behaviors persist. Use of a prescription controlled substance without fully and openly informing the prescribing physician is illegal and dangerous, especially if such use causes problems and is used in association with alcohol or other nonmedical drugs.

When is adult drinking a problem? There are no easy answers, but I find it useful to consider adult drinking in terms of the "stoplight" system described in Chapter 9. The green light zone is use of alcohol by people 21 years of age and older when these adults do not drink more than 2 drinks in any 24-hour period and not more than 4 drinks in any week. In the yellow light zone are people who drink more than 2 drinks occasionally, but never more than 4 drinks in a day, and who drink more than 4 drinks in a week but not more than 10. The red light zone is where most of the serious alcohol problems are found. These are people who drink 5 or more drinks in any 24-hour period and who drink more than 10 drinks a week. Anyone who misses work, has an accident, or is arrested because of alcohol use has a serious alcohol problem, as does anyone whose family is concerned about their drinking.

These boundaries to addiction are meant as initial guidelines.

The real definition of alcoholism lies deeper than how many drinks a person takes in a day or a week. The definition of alcoholism rests in the relationship of the drinking person to the drink: Is that person in love with the effects that alcohol produces? What are the effects of drinking on that person's life? One of my patients told me, after years of denying that he was an alcoholic, "I'm still not sure what that word *alcoholism* means, since it seems to mean so many things to so many people. But I have learned that when I drink, bad things happen to me and to the people I love. So, at AA meetings, when I say I am an alcoholic, what I mean is that I know that when I drink bad things happen. That is all I need to know about alcoholism in my life." If you or any member of your family fits any of these definitions of addiction to alcohol and other drugs, I suggest you define the drinking and/or drug use as a serious problem for the whole family.

As the North American attitudes and laws toward nonmedical drug use, including the use of alcohol, become more restrictive, behaviors that a few years ago seemed normal are now increasingly defined as serious problems. Repeated marijuana use by adults was seen by many people in the mid-1970s as normal, whereas it is now seen by most Americans as both a serious health problem and a crime. Similarly, people who more or less routinely drink three or four drinks a day, and far more on occasion, were defined as social drinkers a decade ago if they held a steady job. Today that level of drinking increasingly is seen as

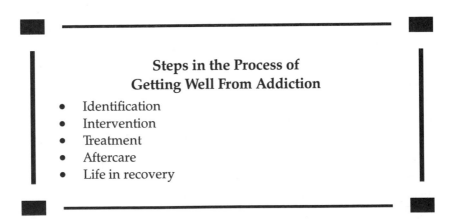

**Steps in the Process of
Getting Well From Addiction**
- Identification
- Intervention
- Treatment
- Aftercare
- Life in recovery

probably reflecting a serious alcohol problem.

Given these changing boundaries, what is the danger today of "overlabeling" someone as addicted? The worst possibility of such an error, in my experience, is that the person would be advised to stop nonmedical drug use, including the use of alcohol, and to go to meetings of a 12-step fellowship. Because I do not consider either of these two outcomes to be negative for anyone, I am not concerned that a small percentage of people who are labeled (by themselves and others) as addicted would not have been so labeled some years ago, or that such people might unnecessarily stop drinking and go to 12-step meetings. The basic cure for the disease of addiction is downright healthy in its own right, so one need not be worried about the overdiagnosis of addiction. The major danger is not overlabeling but "underlabeling," as most people suffering from addiction to alcohol and other drugs continue to use denial to perpetuate their diseases. Underlabeling is a manifestation of denial.

One problem of overlabeling of addiction is when medical patients take prescribed controlled substances, and other people, including physicians as well as regulatory or legal authorities, mislabel this appropriate medical use as "addiction," even though the use does not generate problems and is not associated with dishonesty. Such nonaddicted patients are no more addicted to their medicines than I am to my use of glasses to see more clearly. They have not "fallen in love" with their medicines or lost control of their lives, although they often make strenuous efforts to continue the use of the medicines, the way I would if someone were to take my glasses away from me.

Some medical patients who fit this description because their use of prescribed controlled substances is not characterized by an unmanageable life or dishonesty are nonetheless sent to detoxification and long-term addiction treatment programs on the mistaken assumption that they suffer from addiction. When they have trouble stopping their use of medicines, or reject the label of "drug addiction," they are said to be showing further evidence of the seriousness of their addiction. Addiction means loss of control over the use of alcohol and other drugs, it means continued use despite the problems caused by that use, and it means dishonesty about both the use and the problems that use causes. If the behavior of a particular person does not have those characteristics, it is not addiction, and it is unlikely that the person with the behavior in question needs or will benefit from addiction treatment or attendance at 12-step meetings.

Intervention

The second step, once the problem of addiction has been clearly identified, is intervention. This means that the entire family comes together and focuses on what they have each observed about a family member that leads them individually to the conclusion that this person is facing addiction to alcohol and other drugs. Sometimes the addicted family member will accept this judgment quickly and without resistance. More often, the addicted person is in denial and resists facing this conclusion. In these cases it is useful to find a trained intervention specialist to help the family plan and conduct a formal intervention. An interventionist can be found by calling local drug abuse or alcoholism treatment programs and asking for recommendations or by locating the names of addiction specialists in the phone book. You also will find many useful books in your library or bookstore devoted to intervention and addiction treatment. You can go to an Al-Anon meeting, the 12-step mutual-aid program for family members, to find help.

Successful interventions are planned and structured. An intervention is a formal meeting of family members with the addicted person, often led by a trained professional. Interventions last an hour or longer. The intervention is designed to break through denial. During the intervention, family members should remain calm and focus on what they have personally observed and not on hearsay. Emphasis should be put on love and concern, not on anger or punishment. Before the intervention, family members need to figure out what they want as a result of the intervention. This usually means the admission of the addicted family member to a specific inpatient or outpatient addiction treatment program.

The process of admission to addiction treatment is best worked out in detail before the intervention, including the costs of treatment, so that the addicted person can go directly from the intervention into a treatment program chosen by the family. Recruiting family members for regular attendance at Al-Anon meetings to help them deal with their codependence is another important objective of the intervention. Usually the family members are as handicapped by denial of their self-defeating roles as is the addicted person. Family members may be more than willing for the addicted person to enter treatment but quite resistant to the idea that they need help to overcome their part of the disease of addiction.

Treatment

The third stage in the process of recovery is intensive treatment. This is the step in the process of getting better that you read about and see on television. Formal addiction treatment is a central step on the road to recovery for both the addicted person and for the codependent family members. But, surprisingly, it is not the hardest part of the process for most families. Usually the toughest steps are the first two, identification and intervention. By the time the family has gotten to addiction treatment, the healing process from addiction is well under way. The treatment phase is almost a relief compared with the less structured and uncertain first two steps on the road to getting well from addiction to alcohol and other drugs.

Two basic forms of treatment for addiction are available in North America today: inpatient and outpatient. Inpatient addiction treatment involves a more or less prolonged stay in an addiction treatment program, often in a hospital or in what is called a *residential treatment center.* The typical private sector addiction treatment program has been the 28-day residential program pioneered in Minnesota in the 1950s and 1960s, known as the *Minnesota model* or the abstinence model of treatment. Increasingly, residential treatment for addictive disease has evolved into diverse structures, from relatively brief (a few days) to quite long (a year or longer), reflecting a program or a continuum of care appropriate to individual needs and financial limitations.

Because addiction is a lifelong disease for which there is no quick fix, regardless of how long or short the residential phase of care, addiction treatment almost always includes prolonged and intensive outpatient aftercare. Recovery is possible, but it is never brief. Relapse to addiction remains a possibility long after even the most successful treatment.

These new forms of addiction treatment are sometimes called *recovery-based* treatment because of their commitment to the 12-step model of addiction and recovery. The term *abstinence*, when used to describe a model of treatment, emphasizes that the treatment is committed to the nonuse of alcohol and other drugs as part of the process of getting well. This approach is the antithesis of treatment models that focus on a single substance and those that encourage controlled or moderate use of the substance as part of the process of getting well. For example, some earlier addiction treatment programs dealt with only one drug, such as alcohol, cocaine, or heroin, and attempted to help patients stop the use of that substance while permitting or even encouraging continued use of other intoxicating substances.

Many early programs designed to combat heroin addiction permitted the continued use of marijuana or alcohol as long as that use was not deemed to be excessive. Similarly, some alcohol treatment programs attempted to teach alcoholics to drink moderately, as social drinkers do. Although these earlier approaches to addiction recovery can still be found today, they are becoming less common as they are more widely seen to be ineffective. I am skeptical of addiction treatment approaches that define only one substance as the patient's problem, permitting other alcohol and/or drug use, and approaches that encourage alcoholics to learn to become social drinkers.

Detoxification, the structured treatment to overcome the withdrawal symptoms of physical dependence to become drug free, was once the heart of inpatient treatment for addiction to alcohol and other drugs. Today detoxification, if needed at all, is usually a brief part of the first few days of either inpatient or outpatient treatment for most alcoholics and drug addicts. Many addicts have no withdrawal symptoms when they stop use or, if they do, their withdrawal symptoms are handled with routine medical treatment, depending on the specific drug that the addict had been using.

Some people who are physically dependent on alcohol, barbiturates, and opiates such as heroin face more difficult experiences when they detoxify from drugs. Their detoxification requires medical skill because there are potentially serious risks if the detoxification is not managed well. The transition from intensive nonmedical drug use to becoming drug free can be painful and distressing. Nevertheless, this period of detoxification is usually brief, meaning it lasts for a few days to a week or so, and it is relatively easily handled in an appropriate setting. With good medical care, detoxification is usually neither painful nor dangerous, although it is sometimes distressing. The biggest danger during the detoxification period is not that the addicted person will flee from treatment because of distressing withdrawal symptoms, because once addicted patients are medically managed the withdrawal symptoms are not severe. The biggest danger during this period is that the addicted person will terminate the treatment prematurely to resume the abusive chemical love affair with alcohol and other drugs. Because of the powerful grip that physical dependence and the fear of withdrawal have on the public, the detoxification period of addiction is exaggerated in most discussions about treatment.

The core of contemporary addiction treatment is education about the disease concept of addiction and long-term participation in the 12-step fellowships based on Alcoholics Anonymous (AA). Modern addiction treatment also involves the family. The disease concept holds that not only is the addict sick but so is the addict's family. Typically, the abstinence model programs have 5 to 7 days for "Family Week," when family members are brought into the treatment process and helped to understand their role in both the disease and the recovery, including the importance of the family attending Al-Anon meetings frequently and for a long time.

Although addiction treatment used to mean a 28-day inpatient stay for people with health insurance or the ability to pay for their treatment, this was seldom the model in publicly funded addiction treatment. In public settings, methadone treatment, an outpatient approach to heroin addiction, was teamed with therapeutic community programs (year-long intensive residential programs, mostly for criminal offenders), and outpatient drug-free counseling programs.

The abstinence model addiction treatment program has many innovative elements, including the multidisciplinary treatment team (meaning that the patient receives help from doctors and social workers as well as from addiction specialists, many of whom are themselves recovering people). The abstinence model also involves an individualized treatment plan, which outlines the specific goals for each patient, and family involvement in the process of getting well. Underlying this treatment model is the disease concept of addiction and a strong, lifelong commitment to the 12-step fellowships.

This new model revolutionized drug abuse treatment in the private sector. More recently, and to a more limited extent, similar changes are taking place in publicly funded addiction treatment. The therapeutic communities have been the first publicly funded treatment programs to grasp the 12-step philosophy and to integrate it into every aspect of their programs. The 12-step approach to lifelong recovery is also making increasing inroads into both methadone treatment and outpatient drug-free treatment in the public sector.

Meanwhile, cost consciousness in health care has promoted a new generation of addiction treatment programs that use shorter and more flexible inpatient stays as well as intensive outpatient treatment, which may involve participation in treatment from about 5 P.M. to 11 P.M., 5 days a week, and for 10 hours or more each day of the weekend. This new intensive outpatient addiction treatment approach permits addicted patients to continue to live at home and to work while in treatment. Intensive outpatient treatment lowers the cost of addiction treatment. It is not yet clear whether patients accept the intensive outpatient approach as well as they do the 28-day inpatient approach. When addiction treatment is mandated by an employer or the court, patient preference is not a critically important variable. Patients who complete intensive outpatient addiction treatment do as well as those who complete inpatient treatment.

These newer, more flexible models of treatment all contain the basic elements as the original abstinence-based model, but these elements come in a lower cost package. A similar evolution is beginning to take place in publicly funded addiction treatment for the same reasons of cost consciousness. The newer approaches are more effective in helping addicted people regain control of their lives, and they are less expensive than the alternatives, including the most expensive alternative of all, doing nothing to help addicts.

The central goal of addiction treatment used to be to get the addicted person off drugs. That simple-sounding goal proved relatively easy to achieve for a few weeks but futile to maintain, as patients left the treatment programs and rapidly relapsed to addictive drug use. Today, the primary goal of addiction treatment is to break through denial and to help addicted people and their families accept the reality of the disease concept of addiction. It is vital that addicted people and their families understand the essential role of a lifelong program of recovery based on abstinence from the use of alcohol and other drugs and, usually, long-term use of 12-step programs.

Aftercare

Following intensive inpatient or outpatient addiction treatment comes aftercare. This is a structured outpatient treatment involving urine testing to ensure that drug and alcohol use do not continue, plus regular attendance at 12-step meetings and psychotherapy group sessions, with or without individual or family counseling. The formal aftercare period lasts 6 weeks or longer. Aftercare is a continuation of the professional care that is found in formal addiction treatment and a bridge to lifelong 12-step fellowship attendance. At the start of aftercare, the therapy sessions may be daily or several times a week. Later in the aftercare process, the therapy sessions may be once a week or even once a month. Throughout the aftercare period, 12-step meetingsareattended three to seven times a week, or more often. Aftercare may be combined with individual or family psychotherapy or counseling.

Recovery

The fifth and final step is recovery. This usually means going to meetings of 12-step fellowships two to seven times a week for many years, often for a lifetime. In this stage of getting well, the addict has a personal sponsor and works the 12-step program daily. The recovering addict finds a new road map for life and new, better ways to think, feel, and grow as a person. Daily life comes to have positive meaning, and the addict experiences serenity with self-respect and stability. This new life in recovery replaces the addict's old life of chaos and self-loathing. Healthy ways are used to have fun and to deal with painful feelings such as anger, fear, and rejection.

Relapse Prevention

Addiction is a lifetime disease. A "cure" does not mean that addicted people no longer have the problem of addiction. Getting well starts with not using any drugs nonmedically and not using alcohol. Being "clean and sober" was almost always impossible for addicts to imagine before they got into treatment. Because the idea of life without alcohol and other drugs is overwhelming and even frightening, the 12-step fellowships break the goal down into living clean and sober "one day at a time." Because relapse is a common experience in the treatment of addiction, one of the central goals of both aftercare and life in recovery is the prevention of relapse, and when relapse does occur, it means managing that relapse. This requires finding ways to solve problems, including dealing with painful feelings, without resorting to the old, bad habits of drug and alcohol use.

Key triggers for relapse include feeling Hungry, Angry, Lonely, and Tired. These common and dangerous feelings are captured in the acronym HALT to help addicted people recognize these common danger signs in their own feelings. Recovering addicts learn that feeling hungry, angry, lonely, or tired is a trigger to relapse to substance abuse. They learn what to do to prevent relapse, including how to manage these and other feelings. The best way for addicted people to deal with high-risk feelings on the edge of a relapse is to go to meetings of the 12-step fellowships right then and/or to call their sponsors.

In addition to the integration of the 12-step programs into addiction treatment, the other powerful new feature of addiction treatment is cognitive-behavior therapy. This approach to self-management has been pioneered by a new and more practical breed of psychologists and, less often, psychiatrists. Cognitive-behavior therapy, which means that therapists use techniques to help their clients learn new ways of thinking and behaving, is playing an increasingly positive role in addiction treatment, especially in relapse prevention. This is the single most important focus of cognitive-behavior therapy addiction treatment because relapse is such an important part of the lifelong disease of addiction.

The cognitive-behavioral approach to addiction treatment is based on a social learning theory that views addiction as related to major psychological problems in the addicted person's life. The therapy helps the addicted person learn better techniques to address a broad spectrum of problems that led to the addictive use of alcohol and other drugs. Cognitive-behavior therapy teaches skills to overcome the addicted person's problem-solving deficits rather than having a single-minded focus on drinking and drug use.

The goal of cognitive-behavior therapy is to increase the addicted person's ability to cope with high-risk situations that commonly precipitate relapse, including problems in both relationships and feelings. The therapy trains addicted people to identify their personal triggers for drinking and drug use and to learn new techniques to cope with these problems. The new skills involve obtaining the social support that is needed to maintain sobriety.

A cognitive technique is one that changes the meaning of a behavior or a feeling. For example, the addicted person learns to identify anger and to see it as an inevitable and even a healthy part of his or her life. The behavioral dimension of cognitive-behavior therapy means changing behaviors. For example, the addicted person learns to manage anger in ways that are constructive and that do not involve resumption of drinking or drug use. An effective anger management technique is to put the angry feelings into words and to seek direct or indirect resolution of the problem that led to the anger. Other anger management techniques are to let time pass before acting on the anger and to talk the feeling over with friends or therapists. Cognitive-behavior therapy is not in conflict with the 12-step approach to addiction treatment. Many modern treatment programs integrate these two promising approaches into their everyday programs.

Preventing relapse means, in addition to handling feelings that can trigger relapses, finding new friends who are clean and sober and who live their lives in positive, unselfish, and honest ways. Relapse prevention has an environmental dimension requiring staying away from the places and situations that were associated with drug and alcohol use. In other words, "If you don't want to slip, don't get into slippery places." A *slip* is a brief return to drug and alcohol use on the road to recovery. In contrast to a slip, a *relapse* is a more sustained and problem-generating return to substance abuse. For example, a slip may be a single use of alcohol or other drugs by a recovering person, or it may last a day or two. A relapse may last for as little as a few days or for as long as many years.

Addiction treatment is a hopeful, long-term project. The road to recovery is often marked by relapses of longer and shorter periods of time when the person who has been in treatment returns to the addictive use of alcohol and other drugs. Sometimes relapses lead to readmission to the original treatment addiction program or to admission to a different treatment program. Relapse may come soon after release from treatment, or it may come many years later after a long period of sobriety.

Because relapses after treatment are both so common and so frustrating for all involved, a great deal of study has gone into identifying the factors that are likely to lead to relapse. These factors range from psychological changes, such as the emergence of depression or other mental illness, to environmental factors, such as the loss of a job or family distress. Relapse is not a simple, singular event. It is a long process that usually begins with distancing from aftercare and from participation in 12-step fellowships with a reemergence of denial. Addicts who are at high risk of relapse come to believe that they can use alcohol or some other drug in a controlled fashion, or they give up caring about their own well-being as the sense of loss they feel in giving up their addictive substance comes to outweigh their feeling of benefit from being clean and sober.

A relapse leads to a worsening of the addiction and a heightening of the pain caused by addiction. It ends with a new, and often a lower, bottom. Research shows that the best way to reduce the risk of relapse is to remain active in aftercare treatment and/or to continue to attend meetings of one or more of the 12-step fellowships. Families can help to reduce the risk of relapse by actively continuing participation in Al-Anon.

Finding a Personal Springboard

This general picture of recovery has limitless variations and alternatives. Many people find their ways to addiction treatment as a result of a confrontation with a judge or an employer rather than through a family intervention. Often the legal system gets ahold of addicts and alcoholics through the driving while impaired (DWI) programs, which funnel nearly 2 million Americans each year into educational programs involving once-a-week films and discussions, plus 12-step meetings once or twice a week for many months.

In the workplace, the initial confrontation with addiction can involve a supervisor's intervention or a routine drug test that indicates a violation of the company's drug-free standard. This may trigger the employee being sent to an Employee Assistance Program for evaluation, and then, if indicated based on that evaluation, going on to formal addiction treatment. All addicted people need to find their own personal springboards into a new life of recovery.

The Costs of Treatment and Recovery

Take a look at these five stages of overcoming addiction: identification, intervention, treatment, aftercare, and recovery. Think money. A family can do an intervention on its own; it can use Al-Anon and books from a library to learn about addiction and intervention; or the family can use the services of a professional intervention expert, which may cost several hundred dollars. Neither identification nor intervention is expensive. This cannot be said for the next two steps, treatment and aftercare. A 28-day residential treatment program usually costs between $6,000 and $30,000. The low end is an AA-model residential program with relatively few professional staff members. The high end of the cost scale is a psychiatric hospital addiction treatment program with abundant highly trained mental health professionals, including psychiatrists. Health insurance often pays for part or all of the costs of addiction treatment for people who have generous coverage, so the out-of-pocket cost may be zero for these relatively expensive treatment programs.

If the family has to pay directly, however, this phase of treatment is quite expensive. Because of the explosive growth of the inpatient treatment program, especially the most expensive ones in psychiatric hospitals, many employers and health insurance companies are restricting the use of this form of treatment. Addiction treatment has been one of the fastest growing elements of health care over the last decade, so these reactions are not difficult to understand as the government and health insurers seek ways to slow the growth of health care costs. Intensive outpatient treatment, the modern alternative to the 28-day inpatient program, typically lasts 6 weeks or longer and costs from about $1,500 to $4,000, substantially less than the cost of even an economical 28-day inpatient program.

The professionalized hospital-based treatment of addiction is probably best restricted to the treatment of addicts with major mental illnesses that preceded their first drug or alcohol abuse and for addicted people who will not attend outpatient addiction treatment. When addiction is combined with another mental illness it is called *dual diagnosis* or *dual disorder*, meaning that the patient has both a substance use disorder and another mental health disorder (such as panic disorder, bipolar disorder, or schizophrenia). Most addicts seem mentally ill or "crazy" when they are actively using drugs or alcohol. All addicts appear to be dual-diagnosis patients when their addiction is active. Once they are clean and sober for 6 months, the symptoms of mental illness disappear for most addicted people. The symptoms of serious mental disorders are real enough in active addicts, but they are caused by the toxic effects of the drugs and alcohol on the addict's brain and by the stress of the addict's lifestyle, not by an underlying mental disorder separate from addiction itself. On the other hand, some severely mentally ill people develop serious secondary problems with addiction to alcohol and other drugs. These dual-disordered people usually need specialized treatment provided by professional mental health workers as well as addiction treatment and the 12-step fellowships.

Outpatient aftercare can also be expensive. It may or may not be covered by health insurance. A typical cost is $100 to $500 a week for 6 weeks or more. The cost of addiction treatment needs to be considered not only in the context of all health care costs but in the context of not providing treatment for the addicted person. Untreated addiction generates terrible costs for addicts, their families, their health insurers, and society. Even a $50,000 course of treatment for an addicted person is a bargain for all concerned if it succeeds in transforming an addicted person into a person who is in a stable, long-term recovery.

The fifth and final stage of recovery, life in recovery, costs no money. In fact, you cannot pay for what you get at Alcoholics Anonymous, Narcotics Anonymous (NA), and Al-Anon meetings. These 12-step programs do not accept government grants, health insurance payments, or gifts from anyone, except for small ($1–$2) donations taken at meetings to support the costs of the local chapters.

Some recovering addicts choose, if they can afford it, to participate in some form of mental health treatment once they are clean and sober. That also can be relatively expensive. Professional psychotherapy costs from about $70 to about $150 or more for each session. These sessions can be scheduled as often as two or three times a week or as infrequently as once a month or less often and may continue for many years.

What are addicted people to do if they lack health insurance and if they are not wealthy? Remember the rule, "The only solution to any disability is to work harder." This is as true for addiction as it is for life in general. The key to getting well from addiction cannot be found in a doctor's office or in a drug treatment program, no matter how expensive and prestigious they are. There is no surgery and no medicine that can cure addiction. At best, professional addiction treatments help addicts to find their ways to the 12-step fellowships for the long haul.

All too commonly, active addicts under external pressure to quit the use of alcohol and other drugs choose professional treatment as an alternative to joining a 12-step program for the explicit or implicit purpose of being able to say to themselves and others, "Look, I am getting help. Leave me alone." Sadly, sometimes professional treatment, expensive as it is, perpetuates the active addiction to alcohol or other drugs when addicted people hide their addictive behaviors behind a veil of getting help. Worst of all, medical treatment of addicted people who continue to use alcohol and other drugs can add prescribed controlled substances to the already poisonous chemicals that active addicts put in their brains.

As one alcoholic told me after he got into full addiction treatment and then joined Alcoholics Anonymous: "I came to see you for 5 years in individual psychotherapy so that I could continue to drink, not to stop drinking. You never seemed to figure that out. Neither did my wife or my business partners. They knew you were an expert in this field, and they thought I was doing fine as long as I saw you." This man wasted my time and his money for all those years. He taught me a valuable lesson, one of many I have learned from my patients.

Seeing a Mental Health Professional

When professional mental health treatment works for addicted people and their families, and it sometimes does, it can be tremendously valuable in helping addicts stay well, often by helping them find and use 12-step programs. Mental health and other health and educational professionals not only can legitimize the 12-step fellowships for addicts, but they also can educate addicts about how to find and use 12-step fellowships. I am not one to quarrel with the cost of either intensive drug treatment or outpatient psychotherapy or counseling, because I know both can work. But I know that professionals do not have the answers to the problems of addiction.

No one can buy recovery. Neither wealth nor health insurance can buy it. Recovery can be earned only by the work of the addict and the addict's family. In the end, recovery from addiction is not a matter of money, but a matter of sustained personal effort over time. Addiction is a disease of personal character. Recovery also is, at root, a matter of personal character.

The Smart Shopper's Secret

So what is the low-cost way to get well from addiction? Go to 12-step meetings. The simple standard, developed over many decades by the AA program, is "90/90." Go to at least 90 12-step meetings in 90 days. For many newly recovering addicts, the beginning stages of recovery involve two or three meetings a day. The meetings are free and open to everyone. You do not need a psychiatrist or a counselor to get you in. You do not need health insurance. You simply need to take your body there and stay for the entire meeting at least once a day for 90 days. Take the body, and the mind (as well as the heart) will follow. Go to meetings before you or your family member enters professional addiction treatment. Go to meetings during addiction treatment. Go to meetings after addiction treatment. Go to meetings. The 12-step programs work. Keep coming back!

You do not need to be drug or alcohol free to benefit from 12-step meetings. You can join any fellowship by simply expressing a desire to be clean and sober. That is the sole criterion for membership (see Chapter 11, Appendix 1, and Appendix 2 in this book).

Having said that, however, for most Americans the most effective and accessible door into recovery for the last decade has been the residential addiction treatment program or one of the new alternative intensive outpatient addiction treatment programs. Recognizing that, how can you find the best treatment program for you and your family? Below is a simple 10-point checklist to help you make wise choices.

10-Point Checklist for Addiction Treatment

In your telephone directory under "Alcoholism Information and Treatment" or "Drug Abuse and Addiction—Information and Treatment," you will find a list of many of the addiction treatment programs in your community. You can also contact your local medical or psychiatric society and ask for addiction treatment programs they recommend. You can call your state, county, or city alcohol or drug abuse treatment agency to get their suggestions. If you live near a medical school, call them and ask for their addiction program to get recommendations. Once you have compiled a list of the two or three programs you are most interested in, use the following 10 checklist items to help you make your decision:

1. What is the nature of the treatment for addiction (inpatient or outpatient, residential or hospital), and how long does it usually last?
2. Is there an adequate evaluation of the addicted person and the family at the outset to identify particular problems, including medical and psychiatric problems that may complicate the treatment of the addicted person, and to establish that the person needs formal addiction treatment?
3. How much does the treatment cost? How much of that cost will be paid for by your insurance, and how much will you have to pay out of your own pocket? The treatment program staff can help you figure out how much of their costs your insurance will cover. Often the best addiction treatment costs less than the not-so-good treatment. Do not let high price convince you that a particular addiction treatment program is the best.

4. What is the aftercare for the treatment program? Is it built into the treatment? Is aftercare both intensive and prolonged? Six weeks or longer is typical.
5. What is the family involvement in the addiction treatment program? If the family is not actively involved in all stages of the treatment, then the treatment program is not likely to work because addiction is a family disease and recovery is a family affair. Good residential addiction treatment programs include 1 week of intensive treatment for family members during the 3 to 6 weeks the addicted person is in treatment.
6. Does the entire addiction treatment program, including both the intensive treatment and aftercare phases, integrate the 12-step programs and their principles, including the disease concept, into all aspects of the treatment? Is the program an abstinence model treatment?
7. Go to local open meetings of Al-Anon, Alcoholics Anonymous, and Narcotics Anonymous and ask the people there what they think of the addiction treatment programs in your area, including the specific ones in which you are interested. This is where you will find a consumer's view of the local addiction treatment programs. This is where you will get the best assessment of which programs are good and which are not, because you will find in these 12-step meetings the people who have been through all the treatment programs in your community.
8. Go to the addiction treatment programs you are considering. Talk to the staff. Do people, staff, and patients appear to be glad to be there and busy at all times of the day? You may not be able to go into the unit because of concerns about confidentiality, but get as close as the staff will let you. You can often feel the difference between a good and a poor addiction treatment program simply on the basis of the atmosphere of the place. Good programs are happy, active places. Poor programs are often morbid places where not much is happening, where patients and staff mostly just let time pass.
9. Even if you are sure where you want to go for addiction treatment, consider alternatives. Make a list of at least two or three different addiction treatment programs, and get the facts

about each before you decide on one program. This is too important a decision to be made without careful consideration of all of the facts. Consider at least one intensive outpatient program.

10. Talk with physicians specializing in the treatment of addiction in your community. You can obtain a list of specialists in your area from the American Society of Addiction Medicine (see Appendix 2). Find out what addiction specialists in your area think of the addiction treatment programs you are considering, especially those specialists who do not work for the program in which you are interested. Here you will find out what the competition thinks about the programs you have selected. If the doctors with whom you are speaking work for the particular treatment program in which you are interested, ask them which other programs in your area they would pick if they, or a member of their family, needed treatment for an alcohol or drug problem and they could not use their own treatment program.

You should also consider nationally recognized addiction treatment programs such as the Betty Ford Center in Rancho Mirage, CA, and Hazelden Foundation in Center City, MN, which has both a main campus and Pioneer House, its youth and adolescent treatment program (see Appendix 2). The programs at the Betty Ford Center and Hazelden are the standards against which other addiction treatment programs all over the country measure themselves. They are not expensive programs. They are both residential treatment programs, not psychiatric hospitals.

Although the justly famous programs at the Betty Ford Center and Hazelden may be at some distance from where you live, airfare is often a lot less expensive than the difference in cost between these benchmark programs and many other addiction treatment programs that are not as good and that often cost more. Both of these nationally recognized addiction treatment programs have local programs in many communities to which they refer patients. Ask the Betty Ford Center and Hazelden where they send people for aftercare in your community. Those will often be good local addiction treatment programs for you to con-

The 10-Point Treatment Selection Checklist

1. Find out the nature of the treatment offered.
2. Determine if there is adequate evaluation of the addicted person.
3. Find out the costs of treatment.
4. Ask about aftercare.
5. Determine the extent of family involvement.
6. Ask whether the program integrates the 12-step programs into the treatment.
7. Go to open meetings of Al-Anon, Alcoholics Anonymous, and Narcotics Anonymous for advice.
8. Visit the addiction treatment programs.
9. Consider alternatives, including outpatient treatment.
10. Talk with physicians specializing in the treatment of addiction.

sider. Many North American communities today have excellent inpatient and outpatient addiction treatment programs close to home. Look closely at your local options for treatment before you decide to go a long way to find help.

Finally, what if you and your family cannot afford any of the organized addiction treatment programs because you do not have health insurance and the resources needed to pay for this expensive treatment? You can go directly to 12-step meetings. The richest people in the country go to those same meetings. They just go to an expensive treatment program first, usually for only 4 weeks. Simply short-circuit that step and get on with your own recovery. You can put an effective lifelong recovery plan together yourself if you have the toughness to do it.

Be an informed consumer. Ask questions. Use all the resources you have available to you in making a decision about which addiction treatment program your family will use. This is one of the most important decisions you will make in your lifetime.

Once you and your family have chosen an addiction treatment program, put aside whatever misgivings you had before starting treatment and put your whole heart and soul into the recovery process. Make full use of your addiction treatment program and your counselors. Addicts and their families became sick and stayed sick by trying to run their own lives in their own ways. Do not do that with your addiction treatment. Work the program and do what the program staff tells you to do. The people in your 12-step fellowship and in your addiction treatment program are the experts you have chosen to help you and your family.

Formal addiction treatment takes a short time in anyone's life; give it everything you have from the first day to the last. Be open and honest with the staff, and participate in all of the program's activities. When I see people resisting the recommendations of their counselors and pulling out of some portions of, or even all of, addiction treatment, I see people who are headed back to the pain and suffering of addiction, people who are continuing to run their own make-believe programs of recovery, right into disaster.

Most addiction treatment programs now have a similar structure and do a reasonably good job, unlike many other forms of mental health and medical treatments today, where there is a huge range of treatment quality from great to truly awful. For this reason, you can be confident that the treatment program you picked is a good one. The biggest factor determining whether you and your family get well using any particular treatment is not the character of the program, it is the character of the effort you and your family make. Do not let the precious—and expensive and brief—opportunity of recovery provided by addiction treatment slip away from you. Seize it and use it to the maximum.

A Look Inside Addiction Treatment

In this chapter, I have focused on the important external aspects of the experience of addiction treatment: the options for treatment, how to find and use treatment, and the costs of treatment. Professional addiction treatment, the most publicized and the most expensive part of the lifelong, never-complete process of recovery from addiction to alcohol and other drugs, is, at best, an introduction to a community of dedicated people who have been there and seen the problems of addicted people and their families many times before. Treatment often is an introduction to the 12-step programs.

The helping people in addiction treatment have real answers to difficult, highly personal questions. They can give effective help to addicted people and their families at a time of crisis. Addiction treatment is a profound personal education; it is an exercise in learning by immersion in the process of recovery. Addiction treatment, when it works, is a door into a new, better, and drug-free life for addicted people and their families.

Modern addiction treatment has been developed within the last 20 years. Although it was introduced in the 1950s and 1960s, addiction treatment became common throughout North America only in the 1980s. It started with a state hospital program and grew to become the 28-day residential private addiction treatment program. Later it came to include the closely related intensive outpatient treatment programs that have sprung up in all parts of North America to reduce the costs of addiction treatment and to permit addicted people to continue to work while they undergo treatment. The abstinence model programs include the multidisciplinary team of mental health and other medical professionals combined with recovering addiction counselors who work with each patient based on a treatment plan that is individualized to meet each patient's particular needs.

In these specialized addiction treatment programs, patients learn the disease concept of addiction. They learn that they suffer from a progressive and potentially fatal disease. They learn that this disease of addiction to alcohol and other drugs can be understood and that recovery is possible. Addicted people and their families learn that addiction is a family disease, often with a strong genetic component. They learn that getting well means that the family must change, not only the addicted person. Often for the first time, addicted people in intensive treatment meet impressive and believable people who have gotten well from addiction and are living healthy, honest lives free of the use of alcohol and other addictive drugs.

Patients in treatment learn that there are many drugs that produce a high and that all of these drugs are addictive for them. They learn that getting well for alcoholics requires that they not only stop using alcohol but that they must also stop using all other addicting drugs, including marijuana and cocaine. Similarly, cocaine and heroin addicts learn that to have manageable and satisfying lives requires not only that they stop the use of cocaine and heroin but also that they stop smoking marijuana and drinking alcohol. As we saw in Section II of this book, all of these addicting chemicals produce their effects on the brain by way of the single common pathway to the brain's vulnerable pleasure centers, especially the nucleus accumbens and the ventral tegmental areas, the dopamine-triggered reward centers in the brain's control room. Addiction results in the loss of control of the addict's life as the experience of drug-caused highs takes over. Recovery requires a brain free of all use of addicting chemicals.

Patients in addiction treatment learn the predictable course of addictive disease from the early stages to the end stages. They relate their own personal experiences with addictive drugs to this natural history of addiction. They learn the relationship of character defects to the process of addiction, and they learn the role of the family in perpetuating addiction. The most common character defects seen in addicted people are self-centeredness, excessive sensitivity to criticism and rejection, and dishonesty. A major part of recovery involves accepting responsibility for others who have been harmed by their behaviors and making direct amends to these people.

Addicts in addiction treatment learn the triggers for relapse and new ways to handle these triggers to avoid return to the use of alcohol and other drugs. They learn specific strategies for relapse prevention. They learn about the 12-step programs and how these programs promote and sustain recovery. Addicted people in modern treatment programs begin to go to mutual-aid meetings and to develop personal approaches to the first 3 of the 12 steps, admitting that they are powerless over alcohol and drugs and that their lives have become unmanageable. They learn that doing it their way, that is, "running their own programs," was what got them sick and kept them sick. They learn that they have to use the 12-step programs if their lives are to work. In modern addiction treatment, they learn these vital facts from dozens of videos and scores of lectures, as well as from their own 12-step meetings in the program.

From their first days in their treatment programs, patients and their families begin to go to 12-step meetings outside the treatment programs themselves. They begin to appreciate how portable their recovery is and that it is not dependent on any particular addiction treatment program. They discover that recovery through the 12-step programs is accessible to them forever, throughout the world, whenever they need it. Recovery knows no geographic boundaries. Patients are busy every waking minute while they are in good addiction treatment programs.

People who successfully complete addiction treatment commonly say that their time in treatment was the most important and busy time of their lives. They report to whoever will listen that they learned more about themselves and their families, and about how life and addiction works, than at any other time of their lives. The time in an addiction treatment program is a happy and productive time for addicted people, as they develop strong relationships with the program staff and with other patients and families going through treatment with them.

In their treatment programs, addicted people and their family members meet people who have suffered from the same illness for many years and who are working toward recovery. They learn to have hope for a better and more honest life because they can observe people who were "worse than I am" who have gotten well. They learn to express their deep, personal doubts and fears. They begin by feeling that they are different from all the other addicts they have met in meetings and in the treatment program. Once they have gotten more deeply into their own treatment, addicted people usually share their inability to imagine their lives without using alcohol and other drugs: "Sure, I know I cannot use alcohol or other drugs for now, and that I will never be able to use the way I did just before I came in here. But someday I want to use again, in a controlled fashion, the way I once used and the way I know many other people are able to use." Or they say,

"Sure, I know I cannot use cocaine or heroin again, but I have never had a problem with alcohol (or marijuana). There is nothing wrong with my returning to social drinking (or marijuana smoking)."

These feelings are common and understandable early in addiction treatment. The staff at the treatment center explains that patients do not have to think about never using alcohol or other drugs again. They only need to think about today, about taking care of recovery one day at a time. Patients in addiction treatment learn to feel grateful that, for this one day, they have been able to live without the use of alcohol or other drugs.

Family members come to addiction treatment with their own deep hurts and towering angers. Most of all, family members come with their fears. They are angry at their addicted family members and frightened that they will be blamed for the addicts' problems. They think that all will be well in their families if only their addicted family members become clean and sober. They are reluctant to "work their own programs" and "deal with their own issues" because they have spent so much time and energy living their lives in the shadow of their addicted family members. They have all but forgotten that they also have their own lives—lives that have nothing to do with the lives of their addicted family members. These attitudes reflect their codependence. These attitudes of family members early in treatment are as common and understandable as are the attitudes of addicted people early in treatment.

Many addicted people and many family members grew up in families dominated by the addiction of parents and siblings, so they have their own painful feelings as adult children of alcoholics and drug addicts. These issues also are opened up in addiction treatment, and the healing process begins for old wounds. The entire family in addiction treatment begins to be honest with each other and with themselves for the first time in a long time and sometimes for the first time ever. Families undergo this process with other families going through similar experiences in their addiction treatment programs. They deal with their hurts, fears, and hopes. They begin to find better ways of talking with each other and directly expressing to each other the love that they share.

Family members go to their own meetings and work their own programs as part of addiction treatment.

Honesty, the one-word antidote for addiction, is the simplest summary of what good addiction treatment is about. Honesty in personal life, in family life, and in community life—that is central to getting well from addictive disease. In treatment, addicted people and their families begin to think about and discover, or rediscover, the spiritual foundations of their lives. They often keep journals of their feelings and memories. Their lives are shared with more openness and candor. This may sound easy. It is not. Layers upon layers of dishonesty, grievances, hurts, and secrets must be overcome, and personal fears and insecurities must be faced. Not every addiction treatment program has these goals, and not every addicted person or family member in addiction treatment reaches these goals. I describe these characteristics of treatment because, in my experience, this is how good treatment works and how addicted people and their families experience addiction treatment when they are using it effectively to begin their own personal programs of recovery.

The forms of addiction treatment that are not based on the 12-step programs, including methadone maintenance and outpatient drug-free treatment in the public sector, do not have many of the features of the abstinence model. They are more traditional in their approaches to their use of medicines and in their reliance on psychological counseling to deal with addiction to alcohol and other drugs. They often focus on the negative behavior patterns of addicts and teach new, more positive ways of thinking and acting.

These programs that do not rely on the 12-step approach may or may not be committed to the disease concept of addiction, meaning that they may encourage or permit controlled use of one or more addicting drugs, as long as the addicts show evidence that particular drugs have not been "a serious problem" for them in the past. Thus, some addiction treatment programs that are not based on the abstinence model, explicitly or implicitly by ignoring the issue, permit continued "social drinking" and "recreational marijuana use" on the assumption that the continuing use of these drugs is not a serious drug problem for their clients. Within both the public and private sectors, addiction treatment some-times still relies on medical detoxification followed by traditional psychological counseling or psychotherapy.

Increasingly, the strategies, philosophies, and techniques used in the abstinence model, including cognitive-behavior ther-apy relapse prevention, are being incorporated in all forms of ad-diction treatment, including in public sector programs. I strongly support this trend because I am convinced that this is the best way for most addicted people to get well and to stay well. Addiction treatment has a medical, health care dimension. Good addiction treatment also has an educational element and a deep spiritual foundation. The treatment for addiction requires that addicts re-frain from the use of the drugs to which they were addicted, but successful treatment is clearly more than that.

Once an addicted person is free of the use of alcohol and other drugs, that person is in a position to begin to take advantage of other important, positive aspects of life, including vocational, educational, and counseling opportunities. While the addictive disease is still active, all such efforts, however well meaning, avail-able, and attractive they may be, are worthless for addicted peo-ple because the addicted person's brain is preempted by the secret, shameful love of the chemical high.

Treatment for many addicts is the place where they finally get clean and sober. It is the place in which they cannot continue to use drugs without that use being discovered and leading to pain-ful encounters, and it is the place where they learn about the dis-ease concept of addiction and what they need to do to get well. Addiction treatment is a relatively brief interlude in their addic-tion-dominated lives and a unique opportunity to change courses in their increasingly desperate and dysfunctional lives. Is formal addiction treatment necessary to getting well from addiction? No more so than are drug tests and 12-step programs. It is possible to get well without any one of these three elements and even with-out all of them. However, these three components can work to-gether in a synergistic fashion to encourage and support recovery. It is still hard to get well even when all three of these elements are involved. Doing it without one or the other of them is even harder and more unlikely.

Good addiction treatment promotes recovery, but it is not necessary for recovery. As the world begins to face up to the high costs of health care, it will become increasingly important to find more cost-effective ways to help addicted people get well and stay well. There is no better place to begin that search for better, less expensive ways to help sick people than with addiction treatment. However, it is important that addiction treatment not be held to a standard higher than the standard used for other health care. Today even poor addiction treatment is a better buy than many other forms of medical and psychiatric treatment in terms of effectively reducing human suffering and improving economic performance at a reasonable cost.

Addiction treatment is often criticized as ineffective because half or more of discharged patients relapse to drug use within a year or two. This criticism is unfair and unrealistic and reflects a lack of understanding of the disease of addiction. The remarkable fact is that roughly half of treated patients remain clean and sober for a year or two. Many treated patients have stable recoveries that last a lifetime. How many other forms of hospital treatment can meet that standard? Would anyone criticize the treatment of cancer, heart disease, or stroke as ineffective if half of the discharged patients had recurrences of their illness in a year or two after discharge? This comparison brings into perspective the various double standards commonly applied to addiction treatment compared with other medical and surgical treatments.

There are two general observations that can be made with confidence about the growing research into the long-term effectiveness of addiction treatment. First, the longer an addicted person stays in treatment, the better that person does over the long term. Second, the more often and the longer a person stays active with the 12-step fellowships, the better the long-term outcome from any form of addiction.

These two observations are really two parts of one reality. The greatest danger for addicted people and their families is not that they might fail to find the best addiction treatment, it is that they are all too likely to stop treatment and to stop participation in 12-step programs too soon. Once they are not in treatment and/or not going to meetings, many addicted people relapse to their old addictive behavior patterns. This painful reality does not mean that addiction treatment and 12-step programs do not work, it means that the disease of addiction is powerful and lifelong. Only a lifelong program of recovery is likely to succeed, in the long run, for most addicts and their families.

My simple advice to addicted people and their family members is to stick with your treatment program and to keep going to 12-step meetings—the longer the better. Find people who are in solid, successful recoveries and work with them. Stick with the winners. Do what they have done to get well. That way, you and your family will prosper as they have prospered. If you strike out on your own and work your own program in your own way, you are all but doomed to continue active addiction. This dismal process of quitting addiction treatment and 12-step programs means that the addicted person is continuing his or her own personal research on addiction. It is a painful experiment and one that has been conducted many times before. The end is not pretty. The best outcome from this experiment occurs when the new pain it produces leads the addict and the addict's family back into treatment and 12-step meetings.

As a general statement, the 12-step programs always work. The problem with them is not that they do not work, but that too many addicts leave these successful programs and return to their addictive lifestyles. When you feel that you have made a mess of your life and there is no way out for you, go to meetings. When you feel depressed and angry and that you might go back to the familiar rewards of chemical highs, go to meetings. When you see no hope for yourself, go to meetings. When you feel so good that you are confident that you will never even think of using alcohol or other drugs again, go to meetings.

After years of successful work in the 12-step programs, you may not need a lot of meetings—perhaps only one or two a week—but addicted people, no matter how long they have been clean and sober, need to keep going to meetings and work with their sponsor to keep focused and grounded in a new and better way to live. To think otherwise is to become once again the victim of denial, the hallmark of the disease of addiction. Prematurely quitting 12-step meetings reflects a failure to appreciate the seriousness of the problem of addiction and a failure to appreciate that this is a disease from which recovery, with hard and persistent work, is possible.

Can You Get Well Without the 12-Step Programs?

Some readers of this book, especially those who are involved with publicly funded addiction treatment that is not rooted in the abstinence model, will find my heavy reliance on the 12-step programs hard to accept. My experience in the addiction field began in publicly funded treatment that was not based on 12-step fellowships, both when I worked in the District of Columbia government and when I was the director of the National Institute on Drug Abuse. Sometimes these addiction treatments involve cognitive-behavior therapies. Sometimes these programs have a rehabilitation focus, with great emphasis on helping addicts get and hold paying jobs. In most such programs, participation in 12-step fellowships is permitted and even halfheartedly encouraged, even though the 12-step approach is not built into these addiction treatment programs themselves as it is in the abstinence model treatment.

I know that many addicts refuse to go to 12-step fellowship meetings, often telling their counselors that they attended meetings and found them to be both repugnant and unhelpful. Some addicts say that they do not go because the people at the meetings "are not like me." Others do not go because the meetings are "religious," because they have difficulty in groups and therefore they cannot use these meetings, and because meetings are full of phonies and failures.

I have learned that there are many roads to recovery from addiction. Whatever addiction treatment works for anyone is right for that person. I have come to my support for 12-step fellowships as a central part of addiction treatment not from any ideology, accident of exposure, or personal experience as a member of one of these programs. I have come to this belief from finding so many addicts who got well and stayed well through these

12-step programs and from finding so few alcoholics and addicts who got and stayed well in any other way.

Facing Failure

Most of this book about addiction is optimistic. Addiction often can be prevented, and it often can be overcome successfully. The greatest enemy of both prevention and treatment is denial, a complex, deeply ingrained set of attitudes and behaviors that link up with enabling to foster addiction. Two of the factors that underlie both denial and enabling are fatalism and pessimism. This is commonly seen in the view that addiction is a hopeless problem or that it is someone else's problem. Addiction is a hopeful problem, and it is everyone's problem.

Although this is an important perspective on addiction, I am mindful of the many readers of this book who have confronted addiction in themselves—and even more often in a loved one—and who have made use of all the best available techniques for prevention and treatment. Some of these people have paid enormously high prices in terms of personal suffering, in financial burdens, and in the efforts they have made over many years to overcome the problems of addiction only to fail, over and over again.

I know from many personal experiences that such people feel both guilty and angry. They feel guilty because they believe, down deep, that somehow they could have and should have done something different or something more to save the addicted person about whom they care. They feel angry because they have tried so hard for so long and have devoted themselves so thoroughly to the efforts to help, and still they have failed. They are angry because they know that most other people, whether they say so or not, believe that they should have been able to solve this problem of addiction. They hold themselves responsible for their lack of success, and they know that at some level others hold them responsible also. I am concerned that these good people will read this book and think that I, too, am blaming them for their manifest failures to achieve their goals.

Addiction is a serious, potentially fatal disease. My heart goes out to the victims of this desperate disease, both those who use addictive substances and those who love them. I share their feelings of pain daily, as I see in my practice addicts and their families who do not get well and who continue to suffer from this disease in its active and virulent forms. This suffering falls into one of two distinct patterns. The first and most malignant pattern is continuous active addiction or continuing episodes of relapse into awful addiction alternating with often fairly brief periods of abstinence. This pattern of active addiction may go on until the addicted person dies, often of an overdose, an accident, an infectious disease such as AIDS, or violence related to the addiction. My cousin died this way in a drug-caused automobile accident during one of his many relapses.

The second pattern of long-term addiction is, in my experience, more common. These people learn from their painful experiences, from treatment, and even from attendance at 12-step meetings that they suffer from an incurable disease. They either stop their use of alcohol and other drugs by sheer willpower or they moderate and control their alcohol and drug use, more or less successfully. They seem to have a milder form of the addictive disease because the worst alcoholics and addicts cannot even give the appearance of controlling their use of alcohol and other drugs.

The control of these addicts is more appearance than reality. They are not involved in a program of recovery, and they have changed nothing in their lives except their pattern of use of alcohol and other drugs. They may not get arrested for drunk driving, lose their jobs, or have failed marriages. Nevertheless, the losses in their lives pile ever higher as time goes by. Abstaining or continuing to use alcohol and other drugs, but moderating their use with great effort, they are miserable to be around, especially in the evenings when they are most likely to want to drink and use drugs. They miss out on opportunities for relationships with their friends and families. They feel resentful day after day. They eke out an existence in a sort of half-life. It is these addicts and their families for whom I feel especially badly. This is slow-motion suicide, called in Alcoholics Anonymous a "dry drunk" because the character remains that of an alcoholic.

I never see this pattern in people who go to 12-step meetings regularly. In fact, seeing this pattern is one of the reasons I am enthusiastic about the 12-step programs because it seems to be the only way for such people not only to get clean and sober, but to begin living their lives with real joy. This second pattern of long-term addiction is more subtle and more likely to be chronic than the first pattern. The first pattern is so chaotic and destructive that it is likely to lead to some form of definitive bottom, either to an end of the addiction or to death, in fairly short order. This second pattern can go on for decades—decades of suffering for all involved.

For those who experience either of these two common patterns of failure, I can only say that I have seen and shared your suffering. I know that it is awful. I ask family members to go to Al-Anon and to find their own recovery, regardless of what their addict does or does not do, through working that mutual-aid program for family members. This is the way to overcome codependence. I urge addicts to go to more meetings of Narcotics Anonymous and Alcoholics Anonymous. They work, if they will just go regularly to the meetings, find and use a sponsor, and work the program. Remember that today's failure is often the springboard to tomorrow's success. Life is a learning experience and addiction is a tough, persistent teacher.

Case Histories

These are two tales of personal research on addiction. Mitchell hit low bottoms many times and found his own way to get well, educating (or "sponsoring," as it is called in the 12-step programs) his physician along the way. Stephanie, on the other hand, has found gratitude and a sense of peace in her life in recovery from addiction that she has not known for a long time.

Mitchell

Mitchell was about 30 when I first met him in 1980. I didn't know much about AA or NA then, and neither did he. He had been a teenager of the late 1960s, a bright, rebellious kid who, by the 9th grade, had, as he put it, a "great future behind me." He was deeply into drugs, first marijuana and alcohol but later heroin and cocaine. He did everything to extremes, including his drug use. He had severe medical problems, including partial deafness and later diabetes. He dropped out after a year of college.

Mitchell told me that most of his peers from grade school and junior high school were now doctors and lawyers. He was working as a delivery truck driver. He knew the gap between his position in life and theirs was because of his intense drug use. In particular, he knew his marijuana use had led to permanent loss of memory, which limited his academic potential even though he had not smoked pot in many years. I saw him in psychotherapy, about twice a month for 50 minutes a session for several years.

I am not sure how much Mitchell got out of our sessions, but I got a lot out of them because I watched him discover Narcotics Anonymous and begin the long, slow, and ultimately miraculous process of getting well. He started dating, and he worked his way up to manager of all the delivery staff in his company. Ultimately Mitchell got married and bought a house, "almost like it was supposed to be all along." I think I felt worse about the waste of so much of his life than he did. He told me that he felt good about how well he was doing and what a relief it was to him not to be using drugs any more. "The biggest change is that I now save money. Before I not only was always in debt, but I lived in terror every day that my drug dealers would knock on my door demanding payment of my debts to them. Those guys don't take excuses." He went to NA meetings three or four times a week and was one of the leaders in the rapid growth of NA in the Washington metropolitan area. His ability to lead finally showed itself.

I lost track of Mitchell for many years until he called to ask for my help 2 years ago. "I am strung out on heroin, and I don't know what to do. I'm afraid to tell my wife, but our bank account is a mess, and sooner or later she'll figure it out." When he came back to see me for advice, he told me how this cruel fate had befallen him. His best friend from his drug-using days, Jerry, was the son of a rich family. They had remained close. Jerry had not gotten clean, as Mitchell had, or rather he had been clean by fits and starts over the last 10 years. Then a year ago Jerry told Mitchell he had AIDS and was dying. They got much closer. As Mitchell told it to me, he had not gone to NA meetings at all for the previous 3 or 4 years: "I figured I knew it all. I was the wise man to all the newcomers." He developed a pain in his back and went to his doctor. Mitchell did not tell this doctor of his history of addiction. The doctor prescribed Percodan, a synthetic narcotic. It was not long after this that Mitchell returned to using drugs with Jerry, only now it was intravenous heroin.

It is hard to be a psychiatrist when you hear painful life stories. Mitchell's story of going through the final year of Jerry's life was truly sad. Mitchell went down like a stone in a pond when he returned to using drugs. He commented that "for years I told everyone in NA meetings that if you don't use drugs for a long time, your disease of addiction progresses anyway. That means that if you start up using drugs again, you don't go back to where you started with drugs, or even where you were when you stopped using. When you relapse, you start where you would have been if you had never stopped—way down. It seemed nuts to me when I said that, but I found out this past year that it was totally true. I started back on that stuff as a hopeless heroin addict right off the bat."

Mitchell tried to stop heroin on his own. He taught us both what it means to be powerless. He could not stop, no matter how hard he tried. My therapy did nothing to help him stop. He felt he could not go back to NA because "it's just too humiliating." So he joined the local methadone treatment program, starting at a fairly low dose. Methadone allowed him to stabilize his life. He told his wife for the first time what had happened. "I couldn't tell her until I had some control of my life." He almost lost his job, which was tremendously valuable to him. In the methadone program, Mitchell found a wonderful counselor who helped him get back to NA. He gradually reduced his dose until he stopped methadone altogether after about 3 months.

He then came back into therapy with me, "to start to deal with my gambling problem, which is another old addiction that got out of control in the last year." He also needed to talk about his feelings for Jerry, who had died while Mitchell was in the methadone program. "Funny thing about that, he left me some money and it will just about pay off the gambling and drug debts that I ran up in the last year, putting me back where I was before financially. I never could get ahead in life or deal with anything good happening. Even this gift from Jerry I had to screw up with drugs, when it could have been nice for my wife and me to get ahead a bit in our savings."

Stephanie

A few months ago, I received the following letter:

"Dear Dr. DuPont:

"Thank you for sending me to the Betty Ford Center. I'm living in a recovery home in California. Betty Ford sent me here for aftercare (not Betty herself, of course, although she did come to visit while I was there). The only way I can explain what it is like to be a patient at the Betty Ford Center is to tell you how I feel when I think about being there.

"I feel like a child, nurtured, loved, allowed, shown. That's the only way I can describe it. I'm sure you have some idea of what it is like. I'm going to send people there if I am ever able, even if they don't have an addiction. It's just fabulous. I am very grateful for my 94 days of sobriety. (Or was it 10 years!). I wish I lived at B.F.C. I miss it a lot. I'm working my steps, have a sponsor, have a job cooking in a little restaurant, and go to meetings every day. That's really it. Almost seems like too much right now.

"My sister moved back to Philadelphia. I guess I reminded her of Mom. When she left here, she moved to Massachusetts to live with our other sister, but she reminded her too much of Mom too, so she moved in with Mom. Mom is feeling good. I couldn't tell you how she's doing emotionally. I don't know.

"Everyone is really glad I got help. Mom came to family week at Betty Ford. Amazing things happen there. We are all learning from this, somehow. I wish everyone could have come to family week. A lot would have happened. I'm just really grateful that the 'buck is stopping with me.'

"I'm sure you are healthy and content. I hope for that. Thank you again for a gift I could never repay."

These cases show the complexity and difficulty of addictive disease, including the roles of treatment in the process of recovery. Like the other case histories in this book, they are slices of lives in progress, as I share with my patients, often quite briefly, their lives and their struggles with addiction.

Chapter 11

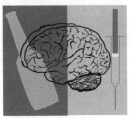

Twelve-Step Programs
A Modern Miracle

In this chapter, we examine the 12-step programs. These programs are not the only path to getting well from addiction, but they are the most widely used and the most secure path. Everyone who is interested in addiction and everyone who cares for the well-being of addicted people needs to understand these unique programs.

ddiction programs based on the Twelve Steps of Alcoholics Anonymous (AA) are the bedrock of lifelong recovery. This chapter is not about group therapy (group meetings of addicts headed by professional mental health specialists such as psychia-

This chapter is based on a book written by Robert L. DuPont and John P. McGovern titled *A Bridge to Recovery: An Introduction to 12-Step Programs.* Also published by the American Psychiatric Press, this book helps people in major social institutions, such as religion, health care, and education, to make better use of 12-step programs in meeting the needs of addicted people and their families.

trists) or about other forms of self-help that are not based on the Twelve Steps of AA. When I see people addicted to alcohol and other drugs who have truly changed their lives and found new and better ways to live (what I recognize as a robust recovery), I usually see people who have made an enduring commitment to one of the 12-step programs. I have never seen anyone who has been harmed by participation in a 12-step fellowship, although there are some risks that are discussed later in this chapter. These programs are the biggest and most secure road to lasting, comprehensive recovery from addiction. They are not, however, the only way to get well from addiction.

Other forms of mutual aid and addiction treatments of many kinds offer hope as well. Whatever works for each addicted person and for his or her family is the best treatment for those people. My focus here on the 12-step programs is not intended to push aside alternatives. It is intended to ensure that you know that this is the largest, most well-traveled, and most accessible road to recovery from addiction in North America and, increasingly, throughout the world today. Everyone interested in addiction needs to know what this road looks like and how to use it, even if another road to recovery is eventually chosen.

The 12-step programs grew out of the experience of addicted people. Their experience, strength, and hope, gained at terrible personal cost, support the view that identifying alcoholism or addiction as a disease helps to overcome the guilt, shame, and isolation of the alcoholic and the addict. Understanding addiction as a disease allows the individual, and the family, to concentrate on conquering destructive behaviors by breaking free of self-defeating denial and futile attempts to solve the problem by willpower. For both the addicted person and the family, admitting loss of control over alcohol and other drug use is the essential first step in overcoming the denial that allows an addiction to maintain control over an addicted person's life.

These are often called self-help or mutual-aid programs to distinguish them from professionally run mental health programs addressing the problems of addiction. All people who want help are welcomed at 12-step meetings, whether they are drug free or not. All that is required is a desire to stop using alcohol and other drugs. Twelve-step programs are not licensed by a government agency or covered by health insurance, nor do they charge fees. Meetings are usually held in public facilities, such as churches and other community locations, as well as in facilities devoted to 12-step meetings. Meetings typically last 1 hour and are held at the same time and place each week.

In most communities there are several groups and, in larger communities, hundreds of 12-step groups that meet each week. The 12-step programs are called *fellowships* because they are made up of members who all contribute actively to the programs. Typical 12-step fellowship members attend from two to seven or more meetings a week for long periods of time, often for their lifetimes. Meetings may have 10 members or less, or more than 1,000 members.

These programs are *mutual aid* as well as *self-help* because one of the great discoveries of AA is that only by banding together and helping others to get well can addicted people get well and stay well themselves. The 12-step programs are spiritually based (but nonreligious) programs run by recovering people. The 12-step programs are not traditional self-help programs, because trying to get well the way the individual addicts chose to do it is how their addictions deepened.

Twelve-step members often reject the designation of their fellowships as either mutual aid or self-help. They do not like mutual aid as a description because they see their strength coming ultimately from the *Higher Power,* not exclusively from other group members. They do not like self-help as a description because addicts have gotten into trouble precisely by doing things their own ways.

The 12-step programs are also not *treatment* because that term is reserved for professionally run programs that charge fees for their services or are paid by taxpayers or some other source. Twelve-step programs are not the result of scientific studies of addiction or its treatment. They have evolved in open and practical ways based on the experience of individual addicted people, with effective techniques continuing and growing, and ineffective ones withering away over time. Members call these programs "fellowships of recovering people," or simply programs of "recovery."

This chapter deals with a wide variety of spiritually based programs modeled on the Twelve Steps and Twelve Traditions of Alcoholics Anonymous.

Twelve-step programs promote a comprehensive lifestyle of recovery. To halt addiction, it is essential that family, friends, and employers recognize addiction and intervene actively. Recovery means living free of the use of alcohol and other drugs, having healthy self-worth, and maintaining sound relationships with family, community, and one's Higher Power. Recovery means being honest.

Group process plays an important role in the success of all mutual-aid programs, including the 12-step programs, which depend on cooperation among members. They are coordinated and led, on a rotating basis, by individuals who are themselves in recovery. The 12-step fellowships provide emotional support to counter the isolation and agony of addiction. Experienced members of 12-step programs, called *oldtimers,* inspire newcomers. Newcomers fresh from active addiction are the most important people at 12-step meetings. Newcomers remind fellowship members of their disease that remains just one drink, or drug use, away. Twelve-step programs help people to control socially unacceptable and self-destructive behaviors, such as addiction, through interaction with others who can identify with them and who have found successful ways to overcome these specific problems so that they can live satisfying and productive lives.

The 12-step programs offer a systematic and carefully planned program for recovery, not just a meeting place or an opportunity to talk about one's problems. Twelve-step fellowships help disaffected individuals achieve successful, healthy social values as well as realistic self-worth. Twelve-step groups offer individuals who share common socially unacceptable behaviors a set of lifesaving guidelines, healthy rituals, and a language to help them understand and overcome their addictions.

Newcomers at 12-step meetings are made to feel welcome and are encouraged to return regularly to fellowship meetings, giving a sense of belonging to addicts who have experienced relentless alienation and rejection. Many 12-step meetings are held in the evening, providing an organized and predictable activity during a time of day when addicts are especially prone to relapse. Use of positive verbal reinforcement and supportive attention by fellow members enhances socialization to prosocial values. Confessing a readiness to accept help is an important part of the 12-step philosophy.

The oldest and largest 12-step program is Alcoholics Anonymous. It helps people overcome problems with alcohol. Narcotics Anonymous (NA) helps people overcome problems with other drugs. Al-Anon is the program for friends and family members of alcoholics. Nar-Anon is the program for friends and family members of drug addicts. Today there are literally dozens of different 12-step programs dealing with many behavioral health problems. This chapter focuses on NA because of its wide reach into the problems of addiction to many drugs of abuse. Many of the characteristics of NA are found in other 12-step programs, including AA from which NA grew.

People new to Narcotics Anonymous and other 12-step fellowships are encouraged to find same-sex members who have been clean and sober for several years or longer and ask them to be their personal guides or *sponsors* to the fellowship and to recovery. The *sponsee* or, as they used to be called, the *pigeon*, is encouraged to learn about the program and to work the 12 steps to recovery "one day at a time." Sponsees typically speak in person or on the telephone with their sponsors every day, at least early in their recovery. Being a sponsor is a major milestone in personal recovery as the more senior addicts "pass on" their experience, strength, and hope to newcomers.

Acceptance leading to forgiveness is a vital component of the 12-step program for getting well. At meetings, discussion of each member's use of alcohol and drugs takes place in a secure, understanding, and accepting environment. The promise of anonymity makes a trusting relationship possible, even with total strangers. A feeling of inclusion is enhanced by the sharing of common experiences. The giving of support is balanced by the expectation of reciprocal encouragement for other members of the group. Stress reduction is another benefit of being involved in a supportive fellowship. Abstinence from using alcohol and other drugs is stressful for addicts, with a tempting remedy for bad feelings of all sorts being the substances that have produced their addictions.

Do I Need a 12-Step Program to Get Well From Addiction?

1. If you use alcohol "alcoholically," or if you use any illicit drug on a continuing basis, you need to stop the use of alcohol and other drugs permanently. If you can do that without anger or resentment, as most cigarette smokers can once they quit, then you do not need a 12-step program to quit and to stay clean and sober.

2. You may still benefit from membership in a 12-step fellowship to improve the quality of your life because some addicts can refrain from the use of alcohol and other drugs nonmedically for many years with what is called *white-knuckle sobriety.* They retain all the dysfunctional character traits of active addicts, even though they no longer use alcohol and other drugs.

3. If you cannot imagine life without alcohol or other drugs, if you have tried several times to stop use and have failed, or if you have had serious problems as a result of your use of alcohol or other drugs, then you probably need a 12-step program, either Alcoholics Anonymous or Narcotics Anonymous.

The Birth of Alcoholics Anonymous

In early May of 1935, just 2 years after the repeal of alcohol prohibition in the United States, Bill Wilson, an unemployed New York stockbroker with a severe history of alcohol abuse, stopped drinking once more and looked for a job. While pursuing an opportunity in Akron, Ohio, he found himself alone, vulnerable, and falling back to old habits in search of a drink. The possibility of reverting to his formerly dissolute and painful lifestyle frightened him. He called a local minister who gave him the name of a member of Akron's Oxford Group.

The Oxford Group at that time was a popular spiritual fellowship seeking to recapture the values of first-century Christianity through a program of personal self-development. Founded in 1921 by Frank N. O. Buchman, a Lutheran minister from Allentown, Pennsylvania, the Oxford Group spread widely throughout the world in the 1920s and 1930s, spawning not only Alcoholics Anonymous but also today's Moral Rearmament (MRA).

The automobile at that time was the central symbol of the American century. Akron, the city that produced most of the tires the nation rode on, was then one of the most successful industrial cities of the American Midwest at the peak of its relative affluence. The Firestone and Seiberling families, in their efforts to assist their community, had brought to Akron the leaders of the Oxford Group and played active roles in the history of AA.

Through this contact, Bill Wilson met a local alcoholic surgeon, Dr. Bob Smith. "Bill W." and "Dr. Bob," as they are called by AA members, met at a Seiberling family home. On June 10, 1935, this friendship culminated in the foundation of what is now Alcoholics Anonymous. On that historic day, Dr. Bob took his last drink—a bottle of beer given to him by Bill W.—on his way to perform surgery at an Akron hospital. Dr. Bob needed the alcohol to steady his hand, which was shaking from his incipient delirium tremens (DTs), the alcohol withdrawal syndrome. That was the last drink of alcohol either man took.

Some of the religious precepts of the Oxford Group had an obvious influence on Bill W.'s development of the AA philosophy, according to the book, *Dr. Bob and the Good Oldtimers,* published by Alcoholics Anonymous World Services in 1980. For instance, the basis of the Oxford Group was the *four absolutes:* absolute honesty, absolute unselfishness, absolute purity, and absolute love. According to Dr. Bob, these absolutes formed "the only yardsticks" that AA had before formulation of the Twelve Steps. The Oxford Group also had five *Cs:* confidence, confession, conviction, conversion, and continuance. The group's five procedures were the following: give in to God, listen to God's direction, check guidance, make restitution, and share.

Bill W. and Dr. Bob soon discovered that alcoholics did not re-

spond well to absolutes or to the formal membership requirements of the Oxford Group. By 1939, Alcoholics Anonymous had
dissolved its connections to the Oxford Group and had begun developing its own completely independent identity. Two additional AA groups were established in Cleveland and New York
City, and *Alcoholics Anonymous*, the "Big Book," which has come to
represent the basic AA authority, was completed by Bill W. and
published.

Alcoholics Anonymous grew slowly for decades. Although
only in the 1980s did it become a major international movement,
the foundations for this quiet global revolution were laid in the
American heartland during the Depression, in the shadow of the
repeal of alcohol prohibition. Ernest Kurtz tells the story of AA,
including the spiritual dimension of the story, in his marvelous
book, *Not-God—A History of Alcoholics Anonymous*, which is available from Hazelden (see Bibliotherapy).

In 1950, AA had 90,000 members in 3,000 groups worldwide.
By 1989, the membership of AA was estimated to consist of 76,000
groups with more than 1,500,000 members in 114 countries.

AA's Singleness of Purpose

As soon as AA developed a track record of success helping alcoholics who had failed at all other efforts to get well from addiction to alcohol, people wanted to apply this remarkable
program to other problems of living, from drug abuse to divorce and from unemployment to depression. In one of its
many early identity-defining exercises, AA articulated the principle of singleness of purpose, committing itself to deal with
one and only one problem: alcoholism. This principle is what
alcoholics mean when they say, "first things first." The first order of business in AA is sobriety.

If that goal is achieved, then alcoholics have genuine hope of
confronting their other serious problems. If that goal is not
achieved, then the alcoholic is not likely to achieve any other important goals. There were many benefits from this focused approach, but one casualty was that many addicts had problems
primarily with drugs other than alcohol. In the early years of the

AA program especially, this meant heroin and cocaine abuse. These other drug problems were officially not welcome in AA unless they were linked to serious alcohol problems. Drug addicts were left in a difficult position in view of the unique effectiveness of the 12-step fellowships once AA defined its singleness of purpose in relationship to alcohol addiction.

Singleness of purpose underlies AA's not being a job program, or a marital therapy program, or a religious or political program. AA recognized early that members had all of these problems, and many more, but that the AA program must limit itself to doing those things that were essential to achieve and maintain sobriety, nothing more and nothing less. Although AA did not deal with primary problems with drugs other than alcohol, from its beginnings AA has included the abstinence from the use of other addicting drugs as well as the abuse of controlled prescription medicines, as clearly within the fellowship's definition of *sobriety*, as a vital part of the organization's singleness of purpose. AA is single-mindedly a program for alcoholics, whether or not they are also abusing other addicting substances.

The valuable lesson here is "less is more." By focusing clearly on the major problem, and doing what must be done to solve that one problem, lives can be reclaimed, and families and even communities can be changed. If this single focus is lost, then the iron grip of addiction to alcohol and other drugs is reasserted and none of these worthy goals is likely to be achieved. If they do not maintain sobriety, then alcoholics are unable to solve their myriad other problems, most of which are made worse by, if not caused by, drinking. In the language of AA, "There is no problem so bad that it cannot be made worse by drinking."

The original 12-step program, Alcoholics Anonymous, uniquely met the needs of alcoholic people. "Singleness of purpose" led AA to ignore officially the needs of people who were addicted exclusively or primarily to drugs other than alcohol, including marijuana, cocaine, and heroin. This same singleness of purpose, the focus on the drinking of people whose lives were made unmanageable by their use of alcohol, meant that AA also was not meeting the urgent needs of members of the alcoholic's family. Thus, Narcotics Anonymous and Al-Anon, respectively, were founded. In more recent years, a seemingly endless range of new 12-step programs have sprung up to address a wide variety of specific needs. Two especially large 12-step programs are Overeaters Anonymous (OA), to help people with eating disorders, and Adult Children of Alcoholics (ACOA), to help adults who grew up in families dominated by the use of alcohol and other drugs.

The Start of Narcotics Anonymous

The first Narcotics Anonymous meeting was held near Los Angeles in 1953. Growth of the fellowship, modeled on AA, was slow at first but accelerated in the early 1980s with the publication of the book, *Narcotics Anonymous*. Like AA's "Big Book," the NA book contained the program guidelines and a series of illustrative personal stories of addiction and recovery. As of January 1988, there were over 12,000 NA meetings in over 43 countries. In recent years, the NA fellowship has grown at a rate of 50% annually. Today there are more than 24,000 Narcotics Anonymous groups throughout the world.

Narcotics Anonymous was started by individuals addicted to drugs other than alcohol who sought recovery but who found that Alcoholics Anonymous did not fully meet their needs. Of the five founding members of NA, three were members of AA. The NA fellowship redefined the rule of "singleness of purpose" to cover all of the many different drugs to which members were addicted. NA developed a somewhat broader program than AA had done, recognizing other compulsive activities and self-destructive mechanisms as contributing factors to addiction and comfortably accepting multiple addictions. Young addicts sometimes are drawn to NA meetings because of the relative lack of slogans, the attention to the extended family, and the NA program's attempts to remain current with drug use trends and treatment innovations. NA meetings often have fewer older, long-term members than do AA meetings. Nevertheless, NA adheres to Twelve Steps and Twelve Traditions nearly identical to those that are the foundation, and the strength, of AA.

The Twelve Steps and Twelve Traditions of Narcotics Anonymous

At the core of NA and the other 12-step fellowships are the Twelve Steps and the Twelve Traditions. The two documents are read aloud at most 12-step meetings to provide a basic orientation to the meeting and to ensure that all fellowship members understand and discuss the basic 12-step program. The repeated reference to the Twelve Steps and the Twelve Traditions also helps maintain the universality and consistency of what are otherwise quite diverse meetings.

The Twelve Steps and the Twelve Traditions were originally formulated by AA between 1935 and 1939 and presented in the "Big Book." Each succeeding 12-step fellowship has adapted them to their specific needs with as few changes as possible. The Twelve Steps form a program of recovery and a blueprint for achieving personal spiritual maturity. The Twelve Traditions are the code of ethics of all the 12-step fellowships. Each point is open to some degree of interpretation—including that of a "Higher Power." The basic AA program has not changed since 1939, and it has been adapted virtually unchanged by NA and all other 12-step fellowships. The experience of over 40 years and in all parts of the world has proved NA to have broad appeal and unique effectiveness in helping addicted people and their families.

Twelve by twelve. Although the Twelve Steps are discussed at meetings, their practice is personal and involves each member and his or her sponsor. The Twelve Traditions are specific, practical guidelines governing the entire fellowship, not a vague accumulation of practices.

The first three of the Twelve Steps provide a foundation for abstinence by acknowledging the problem, coming to believe there is a solution to the problem, and deciding to work to achieve that solution. These steps confront the denial that is the driving force of addiction. The remaining nine steps outline the means of resolving the problem.

Steps Four, Five, Six, and Seven call for a personal moral inventory, revealing the results of that inventory to God and an-

The Twelve Steps of Narcotics Anonymous

1. We admitted we were powerless over our addiction, that our lives had become unmanageable.
2. We came to believe that a Power greater than ourselves could restore us to sanity.
3. We made a decision to turn our will and our lives over to the care of God as we understood Him.
4. We made a searching and fearless moral inventory of ourselves.
5. We admitted to God, to ourselves, and to another human being the exact nature of our wrongs.
6. We were entirely ready to have God remove all these defects of character.
7. We humbly asked Him to remove our shortcomings.
8. We made a list of all persons we had harmed, and became willing to make amends to them all.
9. We made direct amends to such people wherever possible, except when to do so would injure them or others.
10. We continued to take personal inventory and when we were wrong promptly admitted it.
11. We sought through prayer and meditation to improve our conscious contact with God as we understood Him, praying only for knowledge of His will for us and the power to carry that out.
12. Having had a spiritual awakening as the result of these steps, we tried to carry this message to addicts, and to practice these principles in all our affairs.

other human being (usually one's sponsor), having identified one's character defects or shortcomings, being willing to remove these defects, and commencing to exorcise them by asking the

The Twelve Traditions of Narcotics Anonymous

1. Our common welfare should come first; personal recovery depends on NA unity.
2. For our group purpose there is but one ultimate authority—a loving God as He may express Himself in our group conscience. Our leaders are but trusted servants, they do not govern.
3. The only requirement for membership is a desire to stop using.
4. Each group should be autonomous except in matters affecting other groups or NA as a whole.
5. Each group has but one primary purpose—to carry the message to the addict who still suffers.
6. An NA group ought never endorse, finance, or lend the NA name to any related facility or outside enterprise, lest problems of money, property or prestige divert us from our primary purpose.
7. Every NA group ought to be fully self-supporting, declining outside contributions.
8. Narcotics Anonymous should remain forever nonprofessional, but our service centers may employ special workers.
9. NA, as such, ought never be organized, but we may create service boards or committees directly responsible to those they serve.
10. Narcotics Anonymous has no opinion on outside issues; hence the NA name ought never be drawn into public controversy.
11. Our public relations policy is based on attraction rather than promotion; we need always maintain personal anonymity at the level of press, radio, and films.
12. Anonymity is the spiritual foundation of all our Traditions, ever reminding us to place principles before personalities.

The Serenity Prayer

God grant me the serenity
To accept the things I cannot change;
Courage to change the things I can;
And wisdom to know the difference.

Living one day at a time,
Enjoying one moment at a time,
Accepting hardship as a pathway to peace,
Not as I would have it;
Trusting that He will make all things right,
If I surrender to His will;
That I may be reasonably happy in this life,
And supremely happy with Him forever
    in the next.

Note.   Only the first four lines of this remarkable prayer
are used at most 12-step meetings. Those lines are known
as "The Serenity Prayer." The prayer is generally
attributed to Reinhold Niebuhr, who used it in 1934
during a service in the Congregational Church of Heath,
Massachusetts, where he spent many summers. The
prayer was first printed in a monthly bulletin of the
Federal Council of Churches.

Higher Power to remove them. Steps Eight and Nine involve relationships to other people, making amends and restitution to
others. Step Ten is a lifelong maintenance step, bringing together
all of the elements from Steps Four through Nine into a daily process of awareness, self-evaluation, and making amends. Step

Eleven expands the spiritual relationship with God through prayer and meditation, and Step Twelve brings the individual full circle by practicing the principles embodied in the steps and by helping others with alcohol/addiction problems. Only two of the steps (Steps One and Twelve) mention alcohol/addiction, whereas six of the steps mention God or the Higher Power.

The Twelve Traditions of Alcoholics Anonymous were first drawn up in an approximation of their present form in 1946 and later adapted by NA. As the Twelve Steps represent the blueprint for spiritual development of individuals within the fellowships, the Twelve Traditions represent the constitution of the AA and NA fellowships as a group. The traditions can make any interaction with the fellowships difficult for outside programs, institutions, and individuals using more conventional treatment strategies. Professionals and others interested in working cooperatively with 12-step fellowships need an understanding of the Twelve Traditions. The Twelve Traditions define the uniqueness of the 12-step programs and help sustain the smooth functioning of the fellowship. Although these recovery groups are known by their designation of 12-step programs, the Twelve Traditions are no less important. The concepts of anonymity and nonalliance are of special importance. Alcoholics Anonymous will not endorse any nonaffiliated institution. Tradition Ten explicitly forbids expressing an opinion on outside issues; Tradition Six enjoins groups from endorsing, financing, or lending the NA name to any outside enterprise. Traditions Two, Eleven, and Twelve safeguard the fellowship against the development of potentially destructive leaders.

Anonymity is a safeguard for individuals against negative reactions that may result from their exposure as an addict or an alcoholic and a precaution against overzealous, self-serving individuals who may publicly present dubious impressions of the fellowships. Anonymity also encourages individuals in recovery to look beyond themselves to the essential premises of the Twelve Steps.

Broadening the AA principles. In adapting the Twelve Steps to their needs, the only change NA members made was the substitution of "our addiction" for "alcohol" in the First Step and "addicts" for "alcoholics" in the Twelfth Step to show that NA dealt with the disease of addiction rather than with the specific drug alcohol. In answer to the question "Is NA only for narcotics addicts?" the NA answer is, "No. We believe our problem is not the use of any specific drug or group of drugs. Our problem is the disease of addiction, and our program is one of abstinence from all drugs." The book *Narcotics Anonymous* starts with this declaration:

> We cannot change the nature of the addict or addiction. We can help to change the old lie "Once an addict, always an addict," by striving to make recovery more available. God, help us to remember this difference.

Here is how NA introduces itself to members and potential members:

> In NA, we follow a program adapted from Alcoholics Anonymous. More than one million people have recovered in AA, most of them just as hopelessly addicted to alcohol as we were to drugs. We are grateful to the AA. Fellowship for showing us the way to a new life.
>
> The Twelve Steps of Narcotics Anonymous, as adapted from AA, are the basis of our recovery program. We have only broadened their perspective. We follow the same path with a single exception; our identification as addicts is all-inclusive with respect to any mood-changing, mind-altering substance. Alcoholism is too limited a term for us; our problem is not a specific substance, it is a disease called addiction. We believe that as a fellowship, we have been guided by a Greater Consciousness, and are grateful for the direction that has enabled us to build upon a proven program of recovery.
>
> We come to Narcotics Anonymous by various means and believe that our common denominator is that we failed to come to terms with our addiction. Because of the variety of addicts found within our Fellowship, we approach the solution contained within this book in general terms. We pray that we have been searching and thorough, so that every addict who reads this volume will find the hope that we have found.

Based on our experience, we believe that every addict, including the potential addict, suffers from an incurable disease of body, mind, and spirit. We were in the grip of a hopeless dilemma, the solution of which is spiritual in nature.

From the outset, NA defined alcohol as a drug so that members who were abstinent were expected not to use alcohol or other drugs. A cocaine addict cannot continue to use alcohol (or other drugs), claiming that he or she is addicted only to cocaine and uses alcohol "socially." NA sees mood-altering, or what is better called *rewarding*, drugs as the central problem, not the use of the one or two specific drugs on which the addict may have been especially hooked.

This NA attitude toward all addicting drugs is fundamentally not different from that of AA. In AA there is a strong belief that alcoholics cannot use other addicting drugs and maintain their sobriety. The differences between AA and NA are not differences of kind but of emphasis. In AA, emphasis is singularly on alcohol, but there is a broader definition of sobriety, including all addicting drugs. In NA, the primary commitment is to addiction or substance abuse broadly defined, and not to the abuse of any one substance, such as alcohol or cocaine.

In many meetings of both NA and AA, these distinctions are now thoroughly blurred. However, in more traditional AA meetings, especially those with older members who see their problems with alcohol (a single, legal drug) as fundamentally different from those of young drug addicts (who use many illegal drugs and who often have criminal records), the distinction between NA and AA sometimes remains clear-cut, even though many alcoholics have arrest records for driving while impaired (DWI), a serious criminal offense.

Narcotics Anonymous Today

In 1989, Narcotics Anonymous conducted a survey of its membership and received over 5,000 responses. The demographic data based on that survey are shown in the following box.

Demographically, NA meetings tend to reflect the surround-

Age	
Under 20	11%
20–30	37%
30–45	48%
Over 45	4%

Gender	
Male	64%
Female	36%

Duration of uninterrupted clean time	
Less than 1 year	52%
1 to 5 years	41%
More than 5 years	7%

ing community in terms of race, educational level, and occupation. Membership involves honesty and a willingness to work toward recovery, rather than immediate abstinence from all drug use. Only disruptive behavior at meetings is forbidden, but even the disruptive individual, who is asked to leave the meeting, is urged to return to future NA meetings.

Members of Narcotics Anonymous undertake more direct recruitment activities than many other 12-step groups. Individual members volunteer to recruit graduates of formal addiction treatment programs; to contact the criminal justice system release programs; to educate ministers, priests, and rabbis; and to recruit among street addicts. NA is younger, as are many of its members, than AA. It is more flexible but no less dedicated to the Twelve Traditions than is AA.

Narcotics Anonymous and the other 12-step programs have structured techniques for getting better, including the Twelve Steps and Twelve Traditions, a routine of regular attendance at meetings, the reading of books and pamphlets published by the NA organization, and sponsorship by a more experienced member of the fellowship. The written materials on which the NA fellowship is based are authorized and published by the World Service Office, Inc., of NA, located in Van Nuys, California. Each of the 12-step fellowships, including AA and Al-Anon, has a world service headquarters and a wide variety of official published materials. (See Appendix 1 for a listing of the major 12-step fellowships and other mutual-aid groups and Appendix 2 for a listing of other resources for information about the use of alcohol and other drugs.)

Other Fellowships and Groups

In recent years, and usually in urban centers, several subfellowships based on the Twelve Steps of AA and NA have centered on the abuse of individual drugs. Generally, the members of these fellowships also attend AA and/or NA meetings but feel that specific aspects of their particular addictions are not addressed adequately in the general meetings of the larger fellowships. Other organizations based on the Twelve Steps include Drugs Anonymous, Pill Addicts Anonymous (for people addicted to prescription medicines), Marijuana Smokers Anonymous, and Cocaine Anonymous.

In addition to the groups centered on specific drug use, fellowships have been created to meet the individualized needs of women and other groups with special needs such as adolescents and the elderly. Participation in these groups is usually in conjunction with attendance at meetings of AA and NA. Women for Sobriety was formed to address the unique needs of female alcoholics that some women felt were not met by AA. Women who are helped by this alternative organization often initially attend Women for Sobriety meetings and later begin additionally to attend AA meetings. The interplay between the effectiveness of the 12-step fellowships and the special needs felt by women alcoholics has resulted in a dual focus on the traditional and the innovative in Women for Sobriety groups.

Other organizations targeting specific population groups such as Jewish Alcoholics, Chemically Dependent Persons and Significant Others (JACS) and the Calix Society for recovering Catholic alcoholics serve as bridge organizations to the 12-step fellowships. All of these programs use or support the use of the Twelve Steps of AA, adapted to their needs. Many people attend more than one type of 12-step meeting on a regular basis.

Twelve-Step Family Fellowships

Al-Anon

In its literature, Al-Anon describes itself as a 12-step mutual-aid fellowship offering a program of recovery for relatives and friends of alcoholics based on the Twelve Steps and Twelve Traditions of Alcoholics Anonymous. Alateen is a part of Al-Anon for younger family members who have been affected by someone else's drinking.

According to the *1990 Al-Anon/Alateen Membership Survey,* there are over 30,000 Al-Anon groups worldwide. Al-Anon's membership is predominantly white (95%), female (87%), and married (male, 53%; female, 65%), with age distributed throughout adulthood. On the average, Al-Anon members have relationships with at least two alcoholics.

Al-Anon began as a natural outgrowth of Alcoholics Anonymous called the Family Group. Little is known about the first meeting of Al-Anon, but the precedent apparently was set by the wives of the male founders of AA. They realized that families of AA members needed the Twelve Steps as a means of restoring normalcy to their own and to their families' lives.

The alcoholics in AA, most of whom initially were men, went to meetings more or less every evening. They were working the new program, finding new ways to deal with their old problems. What were their spouses to do? They were not welcome at the AA meetings, and they were alone night after night. They did not have a way of understanding what was wrong with their families and with themselves. Family members of addicts needed their own program of recovery from the disease of addiction.

Al-Anon met the important needs of the spouses of alcoholics. Two common characteristics of mental health treatment of addiction were dramatically absent from Al-Anon. First, the Al-Anon groups did not combine the alcoholics and their spouses in the same groups as traditional family therapy does. Throughout the history of AA, the meetings have been separate. One program is for the addicts (e.g., AA, NA), and the other program is for the family members of addicts (e.g., Al-Anon, Alateen, Nar-Anon, ACOA).

Many addicts are themselves married to, or are children of, addicts to alcohol and other drugs, since addiction is both a family and a generational disease. Thus, many addicts also need help in dealing with addicted people in their families of origin and in their current families. When addressing these issues, addicts themselves go to Al-Anon or ACOA meetings. But in keeping with the singleness of purpose concept, addicts are urged to give top priority to their own sobriety, which means their attendance at AA and NA meetings takes precedence.

Second, when family members of alcoholics get together, they often do so to complain about the addicts who run (and ruin) their lives. In contrast, Al-Anon's program, surprisingly to most newcomers, does not build on blaming addicts for the pain in their families. Instead, Al-Anon focuses on ways that family members contribute to the problems in the alcoholic's family. Recovery from addiction to the addict means confronting and overcoming one's own codependence as described in Chapter 8 of this book. Al-Anon is not for complainers and blamers; it is a program that is tough and clear-eyed in its view of the family disease of alcoholism.

Al-Anon, like AA, focuses with singleness of purpose on alcoholism in the family, not on the broader definition of addiction to all nonmedical drug use. Nevertheless, family members of people addicted to drugs other than alcohol are usually welcome at Al-Anon meetings. Al-Anon defines recovery as including abstinence from use of all nonmedical drugs by addicts, not merely abstinence from alcohol use. Although many members of Al-Anon do not drink alcohol, some being themselves recovering alcoholics or addicts, Al-Anon does not require abstinence from alcohol use by its members who are not alcoholic.

The Al-Anon Family Group Headquarters publishes a number of books and pamphlets about recovering from the family disease of alcoholism. The books include *Al-Anon Faces Alcoholism, Al-Anon Family Groups, Alateen—Hope for Children of Alcoholics,* and *. . . In All Our Affairs.*

Alateen

Alateen, a part of Al-Anon, was established specifically for adolescent Al-Anon members to share experiences, learn coping strategies, and offer encouragement to one another. Key issues are the shame of having an alcoholic parent or sibling and learning about their own predisposition to addiction to alcohol and other drugs. Alateen is a fellowship of teenagers whose lives have been affected by the drinking of family members. Alateen is not a teenage AA program. It is a teenage Al-Anon program, devoted to the needs of nonaddicts whose lives have been dominated by the addiction of other family members.

Each Alateen group has an adult sponsor who is a member of Al-Anon. The sponsor is an active participant in the Alateen meeting who provides guidance and knowledge about the disease of alcoholism and about the steps and traditions of AA. These groups, like Al-Anon groups, usually meet at the same time and location as AA meetings to facilitate participation of family members not yet old enough to drive. Members are guided toward awareness that they are not the cause of a loved one's alcoholism or addictive behaviors and that they cannot change or control anyone but themselves. By developing their own spiritual and intellectual resources, based on Al-Anon principles, teenage members of this fellowship can develop a satisfying personal life despite alcohol-related family problems.

Alateen membership in the 4,100 groups worldwide is slightly less demographically homogeneous than Al-Anon. Ethnic representation is 84% white, 5% black, 5% Hispanic, 5% other, and the gender balance is 60% female and 40% male. The school-level composition is 21% elementary, 37% junior high, 36% senior high, 2% college, and 5% not in school. Members of Alateen attend an average of 1.1 meetings per week. The proportion of nonwhite members of Alateen has increased from 9% to 16% since 1987, with minority membership increasing in both urban and rural areas. The number of younger Alateen members is increasing.

Other family mutual-aid groups based on the Twelve Steps include Nar-Anon and Families Anonymous. Although Al-Anon, like AA, officially focuses exclusively on alcohol's effects on the family, these newer groups, like NA, have a broader definition of addiction that includes drugs other than alcohol.

Adult Children of Alcoholics and Co-Dependents Anonymous

Many of today's adults who grew up in households affected by an alcoholic family member did not have access to the burgeoning Al-Anon groups. A child's fear of discovery, shame of a parent's alcoholic behavior, and inability to talk to anyone about addiction in the family frequently result in an adult who has difficulty establishing trusting and appropriate relationships. In the language of the 12-step programs, this denial of addiction in the family is described as the family living with "an elephant in the living room" about which no one speaks. The family does its best to behave normally and to say nothing about the elephant, even though the elephant of addiction, which is often on a rampage, affects every move the family makes.

Children who were confused about and fearful of the dysfunctional family dynamics fostered by alcoholism or addiction commonly become adults without resolving their conflicts or overcoming their shame. Learning that childhood experiences of addiction in the family were shared by others growing up in similar households and understanding the coping mechanisms that were employed to survive in such turmoil are a revelation to many adult children of alcoholics. Even more important is learning the successful techniques to overcome the problems caused by their family experiences with addiction.

Within the past decade, a number of 12-step organizations have emerged to provide education and support to adult children of alcoholics. Books have been written and purchased at an astonishing rate. *Adult Children of Alcoholics,* written by Janet Woititz, has sold 700,000 copies and was on the *New York Times* bestseller list for nearly a year. Through publications such as this, many adults are learning for the first time about the roles that are assumed by children in an alcoholic family. Many are seeking counseling and self-help groups to address long-neglected issues.

Since the early 1980s, over 1,500 Al-Anon ACOA groups have formed in the United States. These groups follow the same Twelve Steps and Twelve Traditions as other Al-Anon groups; however, the focus is on recovery from painful childhood experiences related to parental alcoholism. There is also an ACOA group headquartered in California that has modified the Twelve Steps and Twelve Traditions of AA to address the unique needs of their fellowship. Adult Children of Alcoholics, founded in 1984, currently holds about 1,800 meetings internationally.

A recent and related movement has been the growth of Co-Dependents Anonymous (CoDA), which is not affiliated with Al-Anon. Primary codependence traces its source to early childhood and the influence of being raised by alcoholic, addicted, or otherwise dysfunctional parents. *Codependence,* the subject of Chapter 8 of this book, was defined at the First National Conference on Codependency in Scottsdale, Arizona, as "a pattern of painful dependency upon compulsive behaviors and on approval from others in a search for safety, self-worth, and identity. Recovery is possible." Typically, an individual becomes codependent by adapting to a relationship with an alcoholic or addictive parent or spouse. Although codependence was originally viewed as characterizing family members affected by alcoholism or addiction, it has taken on a broader application to include other dysfunctional behaviors.

Co-Dependents Anonymous was founded in 1986, adapting the Twelve Steps of Alcoholics Anonymous for men and women from dysfunctional families to help them maintain healthy adult relationships. A 12-step organization has also been formed for codependent members of the helping professions. (See Table 11–1 for a guide to the largest 12-step programs.)

Types and Structures of 12-Step Meetings

Twelve-step fellowships have no formal membership or application process and no dues or membership fees. The only money collected is a small voluntary donation, usually $1 or less, made at meetings to cover such expenses as room rental and coffee for the meetings. Most 12-step fellowships do not keep membership records. Individuals become affiliated with a particular fellowship by regularly attending meetings. Although there is a core group of individuals who make up a specific meeting, other participants attend to the extent that the meeting time, place, or availability meets their needs. Meetings of 12-step fellowships are open to everyone who seeks recovery.

Table 11–1.   A guide to major 12-step fellowships

Name	Abbre-viation	Orientation	Number of groups
Alcoholics Anonymous	AA	Personal alcoholism	94,000
Narcotics Anonymous	NA	Personal drug addiction	24,000
Cocaine Anonymous	CA	Personal cocaine addiction	1,500
Al-Anon Family Groups	Al-Anon	Family alcoholism	32,000
Alateen	—	Young Al-Anon members	4,100
Adult Children of Alcoholics	ACOA/ ACA	Adult children from alcoholic families	1,800
Co-Dependents Anonymous	CoDA	People who grew up in dysfunctional families	3,500
Overeaters Anonymous	OA	People with eating disorders	10,000
Gamblers Anonymous	GA	Compulsive gamblers	1,200

The composition of meetings frequently depends on group identity, location, and population density. In rural areas, where there is a smaller and less transient population, memberships of meetings are relatively constant. Urban and high-density suburban areas offer a large number of meetings to a comparatively more mobile fellowship population. In some instances, the membership of a meeting and the focus of the discussion vary dramatically from week to week.

The Meeting

A typical 12-step fellowship group meets once a week at the same time and place. The entire fellowship is made up of all the meetings worldwide of a group, such as AA or NA. Each individual fellowship group has its own identity with a more-or-less consistent format and membership. A specific NA group will meet at a specific time and place throughout the year. Meetings usually last 1 hour, but some are extended to 90 minutes or 2 hours. Twelve-step meetings are held at all times of the day, from early morning to late at night. Because of the large number of individual 12-step fellowship groups, meetings are available for members to attend 365 days a year in many areas. Many new members go to more than one meeting a day, especially when their lives have been disrupted terribly by their addictions. In NA, meetings may have descriptive names such as "Together We Can," "Monday's Miracles," "Talking Heads," or "Out of the Dark."

Twelve-step members usually have what is called a *home meeting.* A home meeting is one that best fulfills the needs of the individual member. The time and place are convenient, and the alcoholic or addict typically finds a particular affinity with other attendees. This is the meeting that a 12-step member attends most consistently, usually varying attendance at several other meetings. Newcomers generally find sponsors at their home meetings and, in time, sponsor other newcomers at their home meetings. Members usually assume volunteer responsibilities in their home meetings, including leading meetings themselves.

Elected or appointed volunteers fill leadership functions at each meeting. A secretary convenes the meetings and takes care of paperwork and recognition of anniversaries of abstinence. The treasurer "passes the hat" for voluntary donations and is responsible for paying any rent or other bills for the meeting. A representative from the local 12-step fellowship committee may attend and report on organizational activities. Another person or persons may be in charge of setting up for the meeting, making coffee, and cleaning up afterward. At larger 12-step meetings, a member may assume responsibility for welcoming newcomers. These leadership functions are usually rotated every 6 months, providing an opportunity for many members to enhance their own recovery by helping others and ensuring that meetings are not dominated over time by particular leaders.

Opening and Closing Meetings

A typical 12-step meeting opens with the secretary introducing himself or herself by first name only as an alcoholic and/or addict, welcoming everyone to the meeting, and inviting visitors and newcomers to introduce themselves by first names only, "so that we can get to know you and talk to you after the meeting." During the first part of the meeting, members may recite the Serenity Prayer. Individual members may read a brief section of the "Twelve Steps of Narcotics Anonymous," "Twelve Traditions of Alcoholics Anonymous," or "How It Works" (from the "Big Book" of Alcoholics Anonymous), depending on the fellowship. (See pages 372–373 for the Twelve Steps and the Twelve Traditions of NA and the Serenity Prayer.) General announcements of interest to group members typically take place either at a break midway through the meeting or at the conclusion of the meeting.

Meetings usually end with everyone standing in a circle, holding hands, observing a moment of silence, then reciting the Lord's Prayer, the Serenity Prayer, or whatever closing the fellowship has decided on. As the meeting disbands, the reminders "Keep coming back!" and "It works!" are often called out. Once a meeting is formed, it usually keeps the same format over long periods of time, even though meetings at other times and locations of the same 12-step fellowship in the same area may have slightly different formats. New meetings are founded when two or three fellowship members decide to start one at a new time or in a new location. Meetings that successfully meet the needs of members flourish and lead to more new meetings, whereas those that do not have declining memberships and often disband.

Types and Formats of Meetings

Twelve-step meetings are divided into two types, *open meetings* and *closed meetings,* each having its own function within the overall fellowship.

Open meetings welcome any interested member of the community. Twelve-step fellowships recognize that visitors may be motivated to attend an open meeting for a number of reasons. Individuals may feel a need to explore a personal drinking or drug problem, may be concerned about a friend or family member, or simply may be interested in educating themselves about the 12-step process. All people are welcome at open meetings. Open meetings are not limited to those people who admit to having an addiction. The only obligation placed on attendance at all 12-step meetings, including open meetings, is that of honoring the anonymity of others by not disclosing names outside of the meeting. Open meetings often conclude with a social time when refreshments are served.

Closed meetings of AA are limited to "people who want to stop drinking," whereas closed meetings of NA are limited to "people who want to stop using drugs." Closed meetings safeguard the anonymity of members and provide a secure and often more stable forum for the discussion of problems best understood by fellow members of a specific fellowship. The meetings are usually informal and encourage participation in the discussion. Newcomers and those who especially may be concerned about their anonymity within the community often find closed meetings particularly helpful. These meetings provide a safe forum for concerns from troubled individuals that may be inappropriate or awkward in an open meeting.

Meetings composed of individuals with similar interests or backgrounds, such as health professionals, may opt for a closed meeting format. By holding a closed meeting, professionals can discuss issues that would not be appropriate in a diverse group and can reduce the likelihood of encountering a problem with doctor-patient or attorney-client relationships that might occur at an open meeting. A number of professional 12-step groups have been established in recent years, such as International Doctors in Alcoholics Anonymous.

Within the two basic types of 12-step meetings are several formats that meetings can take. The following paragraphs briefly describe some of the common 12-step meeting formats.

Discussion meetings are a common type of NA meeting, with other 12-step fellowships following a similar format. The secretary usually presides at a discussion meeting, opening the talk with topics involving recovery and fellowship issues. Recurring themes include relationships, spirituality, and dealing with fear, anger, and anxiety. Attendees are encouraged to participate in turn but discouraged from engaging in *cross-talk*, that is, sustained exchanges between two individuals. Participants are reinforced for their contributions by supportive comments from other members of the fellowship. Emphasis is placed on describing one's own experiences and not on giving advice to others.

At a *speaker* or *speaker/discussion meeting*, one or more members of the fellowship are asked to speak at the meeting. Although the speaker may talk for the entire meeting, more often the speaker's presentation will be limited to a half hour. The secretary usually tries to achieve a balance between regular members and visiting members when scheduling speakers.

The speakers' presentations generally consist of a personal discussion of their life dominated by addiction, their introduction to the 12-step program, and the changes they have experienced through involvement in the fellowship. After the presentation, the speaker may suggest a topic and act as moderator for the discussion portion of the meeting.

The first time a member speaks at a meeting is an important personal occasion marking a passage to a more responsible role within the fellowship. Although new speakers may find the experience difficult, it is nearly always a positive experience and a valuable aid in the process of recovery.

Step meetings incorporating the Twelve Steps provide a blueprint for developing individual spiritual growth within the 12-step fellowship. When a step meeting is initiated, it usually begins by working on Step One at the first session in a discussion format and continues to focus one step at a time through Step Twelve. Then the group returns to Step One. Some meetings elect to work their way sequentially through the Twelve Traditions as well, so the cycle of meetings lasts 24 weeks rather than 12 weeks.

Book meetings are similar to step meetings but involve readings from *Narcotics Anonymous* or other fellowship publications. Passages are read and discussed by those attending the meeting.

Chip, or *birthday, meetings* acknowledge the length of a member's abstinence since his or her entry into the fellowship. Tokens of accomplishment, often in the form of a poker chip or key ring engraved with the fellowship logo and length of abstinence, are ceremoniously given out at the end of an open meeting by the secretary, accompanied by general applause and encouragement. The more commonly acknowledged intervals in the first year of recovery correspond with times that are recognized as those when a newly recovering individual is most vulnerable to relapse, such as 1 day, 1 week, 1 month, or 1 year.

Fellowship members are on the honor system in these self-reports of abstinent behavior. No drug tests are conducted, and no one falsely claiming a chip is confronted, even for obvious lies. The underlying value of the 12-step programs is honesty. Having seen many chip awards, it is hard for me to imagine that more than a few people would want to go to the front of the group and claim a chip dishonestly, simply because of the values of the group. In any event, chips have no force in dealing with employers, courts, or other authorities outside the 12-step fellowships, so there is no incentive for dishonesty in false claims within the fellowships.

Each meeting time and location usually adopts one particular format, which may be reflected in the meeting name, such as "Stepping Free" or "Walking Thru the Pages." Some meetings vary their format by holding 3 weeks of speaker/discussion meetings, then one step study meeting, or a similar combination. There are no established rules on meeting format, and meetings vary among fellowships, regions, and groups. In larger communities, there are 12-step meetings of many different types held at the same time throughout the week, so members have a wide choice of meeting formats throughout every day of the week. Individual members choose the meetings that best meet their needs. Some meetings focus on the needs of newer members of the 12-step fellowships, whereas others are more centered on the needs of long-term members.

Finding a Meeting

Typical 12-step meeting locations include community centers, church halls, schools, and club rooms. Meetings also may be held in institutions such as health centers, hospitals, social service agencies, drug and alcohol treatment centers, and correctional facilities. In urban areas, there are NA and AA clubs that rent space, including general meeting rooms, and hold meetings virtually around the clock, 24 hours a day, 365 days a year. This means that at any time of any day, a person can show up at the club and attend a 12-step fellowship meeting. At such 12-step clubs, meetings are often held for all the larger fellowships and many of the smaller fellowships. For example, there are often simultaneous meetings of AA, NA, and Al-Anon.

An information number can be found in the telephone book of every community with a 12-step fellowship. The white pages of the phone book list the 12-step programs by their individual names (e.g., Al-Anon, Alcoholics Anonymous, Narcotics Anonymous). Specific categories in the yellow pages may vary somewhat by jurisdiction, but they would be similar to "Alcoholism Information and Treatment Centers" or "Drug Abuse and Addiction, Information and Treatment." Volunteers provide meeting times and locations, and "on-call" fellowship members respond to personal requests for help as part of their own Twelve Step commitment. Urban areas with numerous meetings publish a directory with meeting information classified by location, day of the week, time of day, and type of meeting. Directories, often called "Where and When" guides, are available at open meetings or by calling the information number listed in the local telephone directory.

The Role of Literature and Media in the 12-Step Movement

Although the 12-step fellowships do not encourage publicity, an extensive variety of literature is available through the world service headquarters and at local meetings. Narcotics Anonymous offers an extensive array of books and pamphlets. Most of the pamphlets are distributed free of charge, and the books are inexpensive.

The book *Alcoholics Anonymous* was published in 1939 and has been revised twice, the latest revision taking place in 1976. The latest edition is 575 pages long and costs $7.50. *Narcotics Anonymous* is available for $8.25. Both publications are available on audiocassette tapes.

Literature published by the 12-step national organizations is written primarily for the alcoholic or addict entering and continuing in recovery. Many of the pamphlets, however, address programs, professionals, and agencies that refer individuals to the 12-step programs. The pamphlets present information to individuals unfamiliar with the Twelve Steps who interact with and advise those who experience problems with alcoholism and addiction. These titles include, "Am I an Addict?," "For the Newcomer," and "Recovery and Relapse." Similar topics are available from the other 12-step fellowships. (Copies of these materials are available through the General Service Office listed in Appendix 1.)

Alcoholics Anonymous distributes a monthly newsletter, *The AA Grapevine*, that contains articles of interest to the recovering community. The current circulation is 133,000 copies a month to 80 countries around the world. In an effort to make recovery available to as many people as possible, AA also edits a bimonthly newsletter called *Loners: Internationalists Meeting*. This publication is mailed to 2,500 subscribers who are shut-ins or at sea, unable to attend AA meetings in person.

Major publishing houses are now printing books based on the 12-step themes of spirituality, meditation, and recovery. In larger urban areas, there are stores that devote their entire stock to books, tapes, and other inspirational materials related to 12-step recovery. Most libraries and bookstores now have major sections devoted to books dealing with addiction and recovery.

The American Psychiatric Press published *A Bridge to Recovery: An Introduction to 12-Step Programs,* the book on which this chapter is based, to help people in caregiving institutions find new ways to make better use of 12-step programs. Copies can be found at many bookstores or ordered directly from the American Psychiatric Press, Inc., at 1400 K Street, N.W., 11th Floor, Washington, D.C. 20005, (800) 368-5777. Many addicted people and their family members find their way to 12-step meetings through referrals from community organizations, such as schools, hospitals, and churches.

Twelve-step programs have entered the computer age. Some meetings are specifically organized to be accessible via computer modem, allowing people to "attend" meetings from their homes. Computer bulletin boards open up many new possibilities for homebound individuals. Similarly, people who live in rural areas can now participate in more meetings per week via computer link than are available in the immediate vicinity. Some of these meetings are set up on an ad hoc basis among a small group of users. Others are scheduled meetings with a more traditional format where users log in at an appointed time. In addition to being able to interact via computer network, the bulletin boards offer access to 12-step literature, even the "Big Book," that can be read on the screen or downloaded to a printer.

Both Alcoholics Anonymous and Narcotics Anonymous can be reached on the World Wide Web. There are thousands of links, including the "Big Book" online. The official home page for AA is located at http://www.alcoholics-anonymous.org, and the official home page for NA is located at http://www.wsoinc.com.

Twelve-Step Fellowships: The Heart of Stable Recovery

For most people, 12-step fellowships are central to the experience of recovery from addiction. Some people, however, do give up their use of addictive drugs without going to a 12-step meeting. They discover the impossibility of living their lives with the addictive substance, and they find ways to stop using it and to avoid using it in the future. Most cigarette smokers who stop smoking do so without the benefit of any treatment or program, and many of them remain abstinent for years, and often for their lifetimes. Sometimes that same pattern occurs for people addicted to alcohol and other drugs.

My experience, however, leaves me troubled by such apparent recoveries when it comes to alcohol and drugs for people who had a prolonged period of addiction to these substances. I have seen too many of these abstinent people relapse to addiction from this fragile state, called *white-knuckle sobriety* by members of the 12-step fellowships. Similarly, I have seen many people who have entered recovery through regular membership in a 12-step fellowship and who then stop going to meetings, only to relapse again to addiction. Without continuing attendance at 12-step meetings, denial is likely to creep—or spring—back into the abstinent person's life, setting the stage for a painful, dangerous, and prolonged relapse.

Early in recovery, the best course is daily meeting attendance, followed, after several years of abstinence from the use of alcohol

---

Important Features of 12-Step Fellowships

- Based on Alcoholics Anonymous, which started in 1935
- Run by recovering people, not by health care professionals
- Use the Twelve Steps and the Twelve Traditions developed by AA
- Spiritually based, nonresidential, open fellowships
- No charge to join, no dues for membership
- Lifelong participation

and other drugs, by attendance at 12-step meetings two to three times a week. When addicted people are in stable recoveries, meaning that they are certain that they continue to be alcoholics and/or addicts and that this status is lifelong, and when they have been clean and sober for many years, the frequency of attending meetings can sometimes safely be reduced from several times a week to a few meetings a month or even less. Stopping meetings altogether is risky for addicted people in recovery. Most often in successful and stable recovery, reasonably frequent attendance at meetings continues, with the focus shifting over time from sobriety itself to the quality of life that underlies the 12-step fellowships. Dedicated and successful 12-step fellowship members continue to have a clear picture that a relapse is always just "one drink away," and that continued attendance at meetings and working the 12-step programs are essential to maintaining recovery.

Experienced members of the 12-step fellowships also find that more frequent participation in meetings, even years into sobriety, can be helpful in dealing with personal crises of all kinds. For example, a member whose spouse dies or who loses a job may find it helpful to attend meetings once a day for a period of weeks or months to help deal with the feelings unleashed by the crisis, feelings that, if not dealt with, might lead to a relapse to alcohol or other drug use.

When I see a pattern of regular use of 12-step meetings, I am much more secure about the stability of the recovery and the long-term welfare of that person. This pattern is most often associated not only with being free of alcohol and drug use over the long haul, but with a positive and satisfying lifestyle. A good way for an addicted person to join a 12-step fellowship is to go to 90 meetings in 90 days. It is important to establish, early in this process, a home meeting and to get a sponsor who has at least several years of abstinence. The sponsor is the personal guide to the 12-step program for an alcoholic or addict. The 1992 book, *The Recovery Book*, by Al J. Mooney, M.D., Arlene Eisenberg, and Howard Eisenberg, offers clear guidance to anyone new to 12-step programs.

When people first go to 12-step meetings, they are usually

confused, upset, and demoralized. They do not think they can be helped by anyone, least of all a group of nonprofessionals such as the people in the 12-step meetings. They fear making changes in their lives and cling to their old ways of handling their problems, even though their old ways have worked so poorly for them.

Newcomers reluctant to commit themselves to a 12-step program notice that others at the meeting seem different from them in ways that seem to be important. The problems of other members of the 12-step group seem dissimilar and often much worse than the newcomers perceive their own problems to be. The rituals they encounter at the meetings seem alien and even frighteningly cultlike. These rituals appear to be religious as well, confirming their fears that "this is just a disguised form of religion." Most addicted people and their families have not found help in religion, and many are profoundly antireligious by the time they go to their first 12-step meetings. Newcomers find the failures at meetings and conclude that the fellowships do not really work. These perceptions and the tendency to "affiliate out" are part of denial. The disease of addiction is whispering to the addict to flee from the 12-step program.

After a few meetings, many addicted people conclude that they have given the 12-step program a chance and "it didn't work for me." This unfortunate pattern is an expression of the denial that perpetuates the addictive disease in the addict and in the family. My suggestion to newcomers is to keep going to meetings, get a sponsor, and work the program. Find the successful people at the meeting and work with them. Give your fellowship a solid chance to work for you.

One of the major values of modern professional addiction treatment is that it legitimizes the 12-step fellowships, as addicted people and their families meet first-class recovering people who tell their stories of addiction and how they used 12-step programs to get well. Many addicts are simply too confused and afraid to find their way to meetings and to stick with them through their initial fear and unfamiliarity. They fail to derive the benefit of these programs without first going to an addiction treatment program or being literally forced to attend meetings by a judge or other agent of the criminal justice system, or by some other authority in their lives.

When addicted people stick with a 12-step fellowship and learn to use it to help them solve their addiction problems, they also learn to live better, more satisfying lives. They begin to "affiliate into" the program, meaning that they come to see the universality of addiction and just how similar they are to all other addicts. At the start of recovery, many addicts and their family members feel most comfortable in meetings of people similar to themselves in obvious ways, such as gender, age, race, social class, or occupation. Often addicts, especially younger addicts, begin with NA meetings, which have a more open, less structured appearance. Later in their recovery, they often migrate to AA meetings with their greater maturity and sophistication. They also come to realize that their alcoholism or addiction is an important commonality that transcends demographic differences.

Twelve-step meetings not only help to deal with addiction, but to manage feelings of all kinds, including strong feelings and troublesome problems unrelated to the addiction. The 12-step programs are especially adept at dealing with character disorder problems, both the primary character disorder of Type II addicts and the secondary character disorder of Type I addicts as described in Chapter 7.

These fellowship programs are the bedrock for addicts suffering from "dual-diagnosis" problems, meaning that they also suffer from other mental disorders, such as bipolar disorder, anxiety disorders, or schizophrenia. Sometimes such dual-diagnosis people find "double trouble" meetings especially helpful, because most members of these groups suffer both from addictive disease and other mental disorders. The 12-step fellowships are not in conflict with other forms of treatment that deal with other needs of addicted fellowship members. Fellowships generally welcome specific mental health care for members with dual diagnoses of both addiction and other mental disorders. If conflicts do develop between the fellowship and the mental health care, it is helpful for the fellowship members to get together with their sponsors and their professional therapists to work out the conflicts face-to-face.

Critics of the 12-Step Fellowships

Not everyone agrees with this positive view of the 12-step programs for addicted people. There is a vociferous group of professionals, and others, who resist the growing public recognition of the value of the 12-step programs and the principal articles of faith of these groups, including the disease concept of addiction and the importance of the Higher Power in recovery. Stanton Peele, in his book *Diseasing of America* and in other writing, argues, along with other critics, that the disease concept of addiction is simply a glorified excuse for the bad behavior of addicts and alcoholics.

These alternative voices urge that addicts be encouraged to be more rational and to take personal responsibility for their behaviors. The critics of the 12-step programs also argue that the medical treatment of addiction with or without the 12-step programs is less effective than forcing addicts to accept responsibility for their own behaviors. This criticism of the 12-step approach misunderstands the admission of powerlessness in Step One as an abdication of personal responsibility for the addiction and the behavior to which it led. Recall that the two central features of addiction are a life out of control (or unmanageability) and dishonesty (or denial). The admission of powerlessness in Step One is a direct confrontation of both of these problems and is the first, the most difficult, and the most important step on the road to recovery.

Joining a 12-step program is a way to accept responsibility for one's addiction and one's recovery. Nevertheless, disturbing as these assertions are to members of 12-step fellowships, some critics of the disease concept of addiction that underpins the 12-step fellowships go even further by claiming that alcoholics can overcome their problems with drinking and return successfully to controlled or social drinking. A final common criticism of the 12-step approach is that it is a modern cult, a self-serving, shared, and potentially dangerous delusion, or a rogue religion.

Critics of the 12-step fellowships sometimes object to physicians referring patients to 12-step fellowships, the way I do in this book, because they think of these organizations as brainwashing cults or religions. Other people are offended by the requirement that the members of 12-step fellowships admit openly at meetings that they are addicted to alcohol and other drugs, that they have lost control of their lives, and that they can never again drink alcohol socially and moderately. These requirements are all part of the disease concept of addiction held by 12-step fellowships.

When I meet actively addicted people who are skeptical of my advice that they use the 12-step programs, I encourage them to look around for other models of getting well, to find people who have overcome addiction to alcohol and other drugs in other ways, and to learn how they did it. I suggest that they try alternative mutual-aid groups, such as Rational Recovery (RR), which differ from, and are even hostile to, AA and NA. Rational Recovery was founded in about 1986 by Jack Trimpey, a clinical social worker. The RR program is based on the theories of Albert Ellis, who developed the principles of rational-emotive therapy. It is a *cognitive-behavioral* self-help program. RR emphasizes self-reliance, rational thought, and altered behavior during events that trigger relapse.

Programs for Winners

What I have found, and what patients of mine who are willing to do this personal research have found, is that there are many addicted people who have recovered their sanity and have found good ways to live through AA, NA, and Al-Anon. In contrast, it is hard to find addicted people who have gotten and stayed clean and sober in other ways. Similarly, it is easy to find AA, NA, and Al-Anon meetings, but it is harder to find alternative mutual-aid groups. My experience over the last 25 years has convinced me that the reason there are many 12-step meetings, but few alternative meetings, dealing with addiction is because many people find help in the 12-step approach, whereas few people do so in the alternative programs.

What works grows. What does not work withers away. The differences between what works and what does not are easily apparent to anyone willing to go to various meetings and to see for themselves what is happening. This disparity is not because the 12-step fellowships have the support of government agencies, treatment programs, or doctors. Their history is exactly the opposite. Every one of these traditional institutions was initially skeptical of the 12-step fellowships. The 12-step programs have flourished despite the opposition, or more often the neglect, of major social institutions, not because of their support.

You will know the winners of the battle against addiction by the quality of their lives. Go look and see what you find. The most commonly used, the most effective way—but not the only way—to get well from addiction is the 12-step fellowships. It is difficult to go to even one 12-step meeting and not to conclude that the miracle of recovery is at work in the meeting. This easily accessible, direct proof is available to anyone who is open-minded enough to go to a few meetings.

The 12-step groups are not for victims but for survivors. They are not for people who want to blame others for their misfortunes. They are for people who are strong enough and honest enough to shoulder the burdens of responsibility for their own lives, despite the enormous weight of addiction, one of the most powerful and mysterious of human diseases. The 12-step fellowships do not encourage self-pity or withdrawal from life. One of the great discoveries of the founders of Alcoholics Anonymous was that only by helping other sufferers overcome their problems with addiction could members stay sober themselves. The 12-step programs are thus not altruistic in their intent.

Fellowship members have learned through experience that when members begin to think of their goals primarily in altruistic terms rather than in terms of their own continuing needs to stay clean and sober, they are slipping back to denial of their own personal addictions, thereby setting the stage for a relapse. The fellowships are nevertheless profoundly altruistic in their effects (if not in the intentions of individual members) because the only way to achieve the addicts' personal goals is to aid others. This uncompromising and explicit foundation in self-interest is the only one that can support the remarkable achievements that are striking to outside observers of the 12-step revolution. Attendance at these fellowships is the requirement for personal survival, and in this sense they are selfish programs. The good news of recovery requires its being shared with others in need. The 12-step fellowships are voluntary programs that involve the heart as well as the head, the spirit as well as the body.

The 12-step fellowships are not cults. They are open groups of people that welcome addicts from all age, income, and ethnic groups, and from all faiths, as well as those with no religious faith at all. There is no messianic leader of the 12-step communities ready to play the role of pied piper, leading the trusting but misguided followers to their eventual destruction. You cannot join one of these fellowships and give up your wealth and your life to some guru, as happens in cults.

In fact, you cannot give money to these fellowships, no matter how much you may believe in them, except for the very small sums needed to run meetings. There are no salaries paid to the fellowship members who lead the meetings. Twelve-step programs do not use any tax revenues, so they cannot be "downsized" or "eliminated" in budgetary crises. Leadership is rotated on a regular basis so that no one leads on a permanent basis. Term limits are not needed in 12-step fellowships, nor is there danger of salary escalation. When you join a 12-step fellowship, you do not leave your family and community and join a new, alternative community, the way you join a cult.

There are no dues and no membership cards for the 12-step programs. One simply asserts that he or she is a member and that is all there is to it. These are open programs that encourage not uniformity of values, but diversity of values and lifestyles. The 12-step programs do, however, have a highly developed and highly specific belief system about the nature of addiction and about what one must do to get well. This lifesaving belief system has been built over a half century of experience helping over 1 million people get well from addiction. Cults determine and limit beliefs about all aspects of members' lives. The 12-step fellowships focus narrowly on the addictive behavior and that alone. They take no position on anything else, including the political, economic, or religious aspects of their members' lives. Unlike cults, there is no mechanism in the 12-step fellowships for shunning or rejection of heretic members of the group. Diversity of all sorts is welcome in the 12-step fellowships.

How do addicts and their family members get to 12-step meetings? There are many ways, but, as we saw in Chapter 10, one of the most common ways is by going to a formal addiction treatment program. There a person can learn the disease concept of addiction and become familiar with the 12-step programs of recovery. Other addicts find their way to the 12-step fellowships through the programs of criminal justice agencies, such as parole and probation, or through the DWI programs. Others come from their physicians or from religious or educational organizations. Many people are brought by family members or friends. One of most constructive roles for nonaddicts to play in the prevention and treatment of addiction is to learn about the 12-step programs, to learn how to help addicted people and their families find these programs, and to support members of these wonderful fellowships.

Although the 12-step programs originated with AA in Akron, Ohio, more than 60 years ago, most of their growth in the United States and throughout the world has come within the last decade. Other movements, including those dedicated to helping alcoholics and addicts, flourished briefly and then disappeared. It is hard to imagine that the 12-step revolution will peak and then wane in a similar fashion. These programs have benefited from experience and have developed strategies to ensure their survival and growth into the future. Twelve-step programs are not like traditional medical treatment programs, and they are not like religions. They are unique human institutions that are open to diverse populations dealing with addiction in a wide variety of settings. They have shown themselves to be remarkably resilient and adaptable.

Changes are continuously made in the 12-step programs around the enduring Twelve Steps and Twelve Traditions. New 12-step programs continue to spring up to address human problems that have similarities to addiction. The key characteristics of all of these problems are an unmanageable life (loss of control) and dishonesty (denial), which are the central features of addiction. All 12-step programs counter shame, isolation, and dishonesty.

How to Find and Use a 12-Step Program

1. Identify your addiction problem (e.g., addiction to alcohol or other drugs, or loss of control over food, debt, or gambling).

2. Find a friend in the fellowship that deals with your particular addiction who can get you started, or look in your telephone directory for the telephone number of your fellowship and call for information. Choose meetings at a convenient time and place for you.

3. Go to three or four different meetings to find your home meeting, the one in which you are most comfortable.

4. Find someone of your own sex who has at least 1 year of successful time in that program. Choose someone you like and respect, and ask that person to be your temporary sponsor.

5. With the guidance of your sponsor, work the Twelve Steps, going to 90 12-step meetings in 90 days. Read and discuss the written material provided by your fellowship. Speak up, or "share," at every meeting you attend.

6. If you fail to make further progress after an initial positive experience, consider changing sponsors because, as you grow in the program, your needs change and different sponsors can give you different sorts of help.

7. Help other people find and use your fellowship, sharing your own experience, strength, and hope with those you know who have similar problems.

Uses of 12-Step Fellowships and Their Integration With Therapy

Going to 12-step meetings is no guarantee of success in dealing with addiction, although I have never known an addict who went to meetings consistently, had a sponsor, and worked the program who did not get well. Going to meetings is not an alternative to mental health or other medical treatment. The 12-step programs of recovery are not addiction treatment or treatment for any other problem, illness, or disease. AA and NA are not treatment for any other personal or psychiatric problems. Many addicted people find their ways to 12-step programs through formal addiction treatment programs as well as through the care of therapists and doctors. Once in 12-step fellowships, many addicted people are better able to make use of mental health care and other forms of treatment. It is common for recovering addicted people who are in active psychotherapy to also attend 12-step fellowship meetings.

Twelve-step fellowships are the most successful and specific approaches to recovery from addiction. No medical or psychiatric treatment is successful specifically in getting people well from addiction. All too often, not only is formal, professional treatment for addiction not successful, it actually proves to be a screen behind which addiction continues and worsens as addicts and their families believe that they are doing something useful—"all that can be done"—to cure the addiction by participating in a publicly or privately funded health care program. A major goal of the medical and psychiatric treatment of addiction is to help the addict find and use lifelong help in the 12-step fellowships.

For example, methadone treatment of heroin addicts can help desperately ill addicts stabilize their lives, stop nonmedical drug use, and prepare for living drug free. However, in the long run, heroin addicts do best in NA and off methadone, although it may take months or even years of methadone treatment for heroin addicts to get to that stage of recovery. Similarly, Antabuse can be helpful as a bridge to recovery from addiction for some alcoholics. A few heroin addicts find narcotic antagonist therapy helpful in the early stages of recovery.

Formal inpatient or outpatient addiction treatment lasting 4 weeks or longer is a commonly used bridge to lifelong recovery and 12-step programs for addicted people and their families. The criminal justice programs, such as DWI programs, parole, and probation, can also be lead-ins to 12-step fellowships. Urine testing for drugs of abuse and employee assistance programs at work play similar roles for many addicted people today—they provide the incentive and the road map to addicts to help them find recovery in 12-step fellowships.

Sometimes, once alcoholics and addicts are clean and sober in recovery, they and their families want to use formal health care treatments including psychotherapy, the "talking cure." Many times I have seen addicted people who did not benefit from years of psychotherapy join and use a 12-step program, get clean and sober, and then benefit from psychotherapy for the first time in their lives. Many addicted people, once in stable recovery, also are able to make religion a positive part of their new lives.

When addicts are actively using alcohol and other drugs, they are in no position to benefit from counseling or therapy, to say nothing of religion or education. Their minds are so obsessed with and impaired by their use of alcohol and other drugs that they can think of nothing else, certainly nothing that might come between them and their chemical lovers. Once addicts are abstinent, they have a chance of benefiting from diverse forms of therapy. Sometimes, as part of their medical and psychiatric care, addicted people in recovery need, and benefit from, the use of psychiatric medicines.

Risks at 12-Step Meetings

Twelve-step meetings are filled with addicted people in various states of their disease. Some people at meetings are stable in their recoveries and doing well in their lives. They are honest and responsible people. These people are the winners. Other people in the same meetings are right off the streets and are still active in their addictive disease. They are dishonest, and some are actively criminal. A few people attend 12-step meetings while they continue to use alcohol and other drugs. Many of these people will get clean and sober if they continue to attend meetings, get sponsors, and work the program. Some of the successful fellowship members will relapse for longer and shorter periods of time as they struggle with this difficult disease over their lifetimes.

When newcomers go to their first 12-step meetings, it can be hard for them to sort out the winners from the losers. Because the newcomers are often continuing in their own addictive illnesses, some are attracted not to the winners (who may strike them as similar to straight people and thus boring and timid) but to the losers. I had a patient a few years ago who went to 12-step meetings for years, choosing meetings made up almost exclusively of losers. He explained that he did not want to get well because that meant he would have to give up alcohol and other drugs. He went to meetings only because his parole officer required him to go, so he chose meetings where he was most comfortable. "There was no one with a job at those meetings, and not many who were not actively using drugs," he said. "We just complained about our lives from the start of the meeting until the end."

Even more serious than this sort of risk is that of sending a very young adolescent, such as a 13- or 14-year-old, to general 12-step meetings. They are likely to be attracted to the wildest and most irresponsible losers in the meetings. If the adolescent is a girl, the dangers are compounded because of the likelihood that some men in the group will become predatory in their sexual advances toward her. In fact, female newcomers of any age need to be aware of one of the most notorious risks of the 12-step meetings, "the Thirteenth Step." This is the sexual exploitation of newcomer women by sophisticated men in the program, who take advantage of the atmosphere of intimacy and trust that develops.

This is not meant to scare you about 12-step meetings but to alert you to the realities of the serious and challenging process of recovery. Meetings occasionally can be dangerous in the sense that a few people at the meetings may have exploitative sexual, economic, and other interests in others. Some people at meetings may seek to encourage continued alcohol and drug use.

The most risky 12-step meeting, however, is vastly safer than the everyday experiences of addicts of either sex or any age. When addicted people pursue their addictive careers, there are fewer controls over whom they meet and what is to become of them than there are at any 12-step meetings. At least at meetings there is a culture of recovery, and at most meetings there are some, often many, good people who can help the newcomer get and stay well. I have never felt physically endangered or observed any violence at a meeting of a 12-step fellowship. The tamest suburban bar is, in my experience, a more risky place than the scariest 12-step meeting.

To handle the small but real risks at 12-step meetings, it is desirable for adolescents and young women to go to meetings limited to other young people, or to go to regular 12-step meetings with trusted and sober friends, or even to go to meetings, especially early in the program, with a parent or other adult. If it is possible to find a trusted adult, usually of the same sex, who is in the program, to accompany the young person to meetings, so much the better. Once the newcomer starts going to meetings, it is important for him or her to find a sponsor of the same sex who can help sort out the important issues, including risks such as "Thirteenth Stepping."

Not all 12-step meetings are equal. They are all different in important ways. I encourage you to "meeting shop," to go to many meetings and find the ones that best meet your particular needs. Good meetings for one person can be bad meetings for someone else. Good meetings at one time in the lifelong process of recovery can be bad meetings at other times for the same person. All meetings of a 12-step fellowship have foundations that they share, so they are instantly familiar to anyone who is accustomed to the fellowship. On the other hand, each meeting is unique from all others, and meetings change in subtle and important ways over time. The rich diversity of meetings within a single fellowship such as Narcotics Anonymous is one of the many valuable features of these programs. Meetings that meet the real needs of members flourish and those that do not, disappear.

Two Tough Hurdles

The two most difficult aspects of the 12-step approach to addiction for most addicted people are the admission of powerlessness and the Higher Power. These are not minor or expendable program elements, so it is important to understand them and not to let them get in the way of using the fellowships. Addicts all seek to control their use of addicting drugs and believe that they can do so, even if they have repeatedly failed to exercise reasonable control over their use of alcohol and other drugs in the past.

This virtually universal belief is part of the denial that underpins the addiction itself. Using denial, the active addict holds open the hope that the selfish brain can once again use these substances. People addicted to a particular drug may harbor hopes of returning to the controlled use of that substance, or they may hope that they can continue to use another addictive substance in a controlled way. For example, a cocaine addict may bargain with fate by continuing to drink alcohol, justifying this by saying, "I have a cocaine problem. I've never had a problem with alcohol." An alcoholic who loved Scotch whiskey may dream of "having a beer now and then, since beer never was my problem." To believe otherwise is to abandon the hope of the continuing the love affair the addict has with getting high, with the chemical stimulation of the ventral tegmental area of his or her brain. That loss seems intolerable for all active addicts.

Active addicts seek to use techniques that they have developed themselves, or to find advisers who tell them they can successfully use alcohol and other drugs in a controlled fashion so that they can hold onto this highly valued dream of controlled, continuing use of alcohol and other drugs. Sadly, many physicians and other experts reinforce this view that the controlled use of alcohol and other drugs may work for the sick addict. To get well, addicts must start by admitting that they are powerless over their use of addicting drugs. They must admit that their pet techniques for holding on to their chemical lovers will not work in the future, as they have never worked for long in the past. They must face the need to try a new approach, one rooted in the disease concept of the 12-step fellowships and practiced in these programs, one day at a time.

I had a glimpse of just how powerful and persistent the dream of continued use is for addicts when I was invited to the head table with President and Mrs. Ford at the 10th anniversary of the Betty Ford Center. The large and happy crowd celebrating this milestone was entertained by a famous singer who was himself recovering from addiction to alcohol and cocaine. He sang about an alcoholic and his dreams of heaven. One of the guests at the head table, a recovering person himself, laughed and shared with those at our table a recurrent dream of his own: "I figure that my abstaining from drinking as part of my program of recovery applies only to my life on this earth. When I die and go to heaven, I will be able to go beyond my commitment not to drink. In heaven I will have all the alcohol I want, any time I want it." One thing is for sure, nonalcoholic social drinkers do not have that vision of heaven.

Because the obsession with getting high is so intense, persistent, and dangerous, people who speak at 12-step meetings begin speaking by using their first names and admitting that they are alcoholics or addicts, no matter how long it has been since they last used alcohol or other drugs. That repeated, public admission within the program is essential to overcoming the persistent pull of denial, a pull to the dangerous belief that controlled drinking and drug use is possible. Because of the power of this pull, and, to addicted people, the impossibility of imagining that they will never again drink or use drugs, the 12-step programs teach addicts to stay clean and sober "one day at a time" rather than "forever."

The Higher Power is essential to recovery because another central feature of addiction is self-centeredness. Relying on a Higher Power or turning one's life over to one's Higher Power is a way of getting outside the desperate prison of self-centeredness. Anything outside of yourself can be your Higher Power. It can be your family, humankind, nature, or even, as it was for one of my recovering patients, your bed. Many people in recovery are atheists, and even more are agnostics. All religions in the world are represented in the 12-step fellowships. The program reaches out and works for people of any faith and those with no faith at all. Nevertheless, many recovering people, once they have gone beyond their own self-centeredness, find great strength in religion, sometimes the neglected religion of their youths. Many people have lost their religious lives, partly because of their addictions. Twelve-step fellowships can be a road not only to recovery but to a newly fulfilling relationship with religion as well.

This is true for the same reason that 12-step fellowships can be a road into therapy of many kinds and into new relationships with work and family. Once addicts have recovered sanity in their lives, they are more like other people in the world with similar needs, and they respond to similar diverse opportunities for personal and spiritual growth. As long as the active addictions rage, addicts simply have no access to these growth opportunities, as their brains and their lives are preempted by their addictions, by their chemical love affairs. On the other hand, many dedicated members of the 12-step fellowships remain agnostics and atheists without that being any barrier whatsoever to their full participation in the fellowships.

Being Addicted to 12-Step Meetings

One of the common criticisms of the 12-step programs is that addicts who get well through these programs seem to trade in their addictions to alcohol and other drugs in return for an addiction to 12-step meetings. There is an important point here. It is true that recovering people often spend much of their waking time, when they are not working, at meetings. They may have relatively little time for people who are not in their 12-step programs. This is what it takes to get well, especially early in the process of recovery.

Friends and family become frustrated in their attempts to spend more time with the addicts, once they are no longer using alcohol and other drugs. This is an inescapable reality for many people in recovery. As time goes on in recovery, most addicted people spend somewhat less time at meetings and more time with people who are not in the program, but even long into recovery they often spend much time in meetings and with their Twelfth Step work, maintaining their abstinence by helping other addicted people.

Readers of this book will quickly see that no matter how much time recovering people spend in their 12-step programs, this does not qualify as an addiction. An addiction is defined as having two central characteristics: loss of control over one's life (having an unmanageable life because of the use of alcohol and other drugs), and denial (or dishonesty). People who are active in 12-step meetings have lives that are in good control (even though they are often busy), and they are perfectly honest about what they are doing, even with those who do not approve of their going to meetings so often.

If you are concerned about the amount of time an addicted person in recovery spends at 12-step meetings, discuss your concern with that person. Be prepared for this response:

> I am sorry I do not have more time for you than I do, but I have to go to meetings this often to stay clean and sober. When you miss me, remember what my life was like when I was drinking (and using drugs). Remember how little time I had for you then. Recognize that, for me, relapse to active addiction is the alternative to my going to all of these meetings.

There has been a criticism that the 12-step programs are being applied too broadly and that self-help groups of virtually every description have pirated the 12-step approach for use with their own particular concerns. Gamblers Anonymous, Al-Anon, and Overeaters Anonymous have been around for a long time, but now we have Cocaine Anonymous, Marijuana Smokers Anonymous, Pills Anonymous, Debtors Anonymous, Sexaholics Anonymous, Co-Dependents Anonymous, and many more. My answer to that criticism is, "Why worry?" The Twelve Steps and the Twelve Traditions are the basis for programs that prosper when they work and die when they do not work. The jury is still out on many of these new 12-step organizations, but if people find that they meet important needs, the new fellowships will grow. If not, the new fellowships will not be the first apparently good idea to die for lack of results.

Many of the newer and more specific 12-step programs respond to the commonly perceived needs of addicts early in their recoveries to find 12-step programs that meet highly specific, individual requirements. Later in their recoveries, these unique aspects of their needs drop away as fellowship members discover that their needs are the same as those of other alcoholics and addicts. When that transformation takes place, recovering alcoholics and addicts are likely to gravitate to more established 12-step programs. The ultimate end of this journey is often Alcoholics Anonymous, the most sophisticated and the oldest of the 12-step programs.

In the future, an important need is to study the ways of making referrals to 12-step programs and of integrating the 12-step programs more fully into the everyday operations of all social institutions, including the criminal justice system, health care, education, and religion. The 12-step programs have rightly resisted research into their workings, or any implication that professionals or researchers have a valuable contribution to make to these programs. Nevertheless, the referral process to 12-step programs is an appropriate topic for new scientific research. Through such studies it should become possible to make better referrals and to identify those people who are less likely to succeed on their own in 12-step programs in order to provide them with the assistance they need to make better use of these programs.

Controversies are likely to persist about the 12-step programs, especially among those who know little about them. I hope that all readers of this book will go to at least six 12-step meetings to judge the process of recovery for themselves. Pick a meeting near where you live or work. You will find people who look and act like you. Pick a meeting in a different part of your community, and you will find people who look different from you. Spend a little time at meetings and you will see the common threads that create the fabric of addiction in all people. You will also be touched by the miracle of recovery, a miracle you cannot fail to see and feel at those meetings.

Case Histories

Here are three stories involving the 12-step programs. Cynthia found a place where she could talk about a shame she knew she could never escape. Adam found a way to stabilize his out-of-control life and a new forum for his extroverted personality. Mark's successful recovery was a long but eventually triumphant struggle.

Cynthia

Several years ago I attended a 12-step meeting, as I often do. The discussion at the meeting was about the importance of making amends to people whom one has harmed, Step Nine. One group member, whom I will call Cynthia, said she was deeply troubled by this step because, as a dispatcher for the local police department, she routinely and secretly gave information to drug dealers about police activities in return for her drugs. This story brought an unusual hush, even to a meeting used to re-markable confessions. Cynthia said she was never tested for drug use while working for the police force.

Cynthia's question was how she could make amends, "because people have been killed on those raids, some of them po-lice officers." Many opinions were offered, but the dominant view was that she should not reveal such privileged and confi-dential information again at a meeting and also that she should tell no one about it at work because to do so would harm people, most especially herself. She should work on this with her spon-sor, come to meetings, and work the NA program faithfully. I was impressed by the trust Cynthia had in her group and by the support and advice she was able to come up with from peo-ple who could understand her behavior. They could also under-stand that now, as she was clean and sober, she would carry a terrible pain from her life as an addict every day for the remain-der of her life.

Adam

Adam is the oldest of four children of a devoutly religious family. Both of the older boys had terrible drug problems as teenagers, and they were both put into intensive drug treatment programs by their distraught parents. Adam was the smarter one, the one with the outgoing personality, the one with limitless self-confi-dence.

When I knew him he was devoted to AA, had been clean and sober for over 2 years, and was working part-time as a bartender while he pursued his real interest as a commodities trader, "the best way to gamble ever invented because you can get rich risking other people's money." He loved his work as a bartender. I asked him how he could stand to be around alcohol all the time as a vulnerable recovering alcoholic, and what he thought about his drinking customers. "It's not possible for me to be away from alcohol. I know that I cannot drink, that I need to take it one day at a time, and that I need to go to meetings every day if I am to stay sober. It took me 10 terrible years to learn those basic lessons. I am not going to forget them now! When I look across the bar at my customers I see nothing but alcoholics. I figure that I am well paid to give them as much booze as I can so that they can hit their own personal bottoms just as soon as possible. Only when they hit bottom can they begin to pull their lives together. I figure, the faster and harder they hit their own bottoms, the better off they will be. It is my job to speed up the process of recovery, by encouraging their drinking."

I asked Adam if he felt badly thinking about the terrible things that befall his customers as they hit bottom and the fact that some of them will, literally, not survive the experience. He laughed at my naiveté: "No one can stop alcoholics or drug addicts from having all the alcohol and other drugs that they need to have, so why even try? I just tell them that I am saving a seat at AA for them when they are ready for it. Then we laugh together. I figure they are more nervous in their laughter than I am in mine!"

Mark

When our younger daughter Caroline was a college freshman, she dressed up as a cat for a Halloween party in her coed dorm. She was herself scared to death when Mark, a tall, thin freshman, who was one of her best friends, mistook her for "the devil" and said he was going to have to kill her. She called me when she and her friends found out that Mark was high on Ecstasy and marijuana and that he had been spending more time using drugs than he had been studying. Mark was well liked and well respected in this college class. He was considered to be the brightest kid in their dormitory. As a scholarship student and the first one in his family to ever go to college, a lot was riding on his education.

Caroline wondered what to do to help Mark. I suggested that she take him to NA meetings every day for a week and then see what happened. When she indicated that she did not know how to find an NA meeting, I told her to look up "Narcotics Anonymous" in the phone book and then to call and ask for the NA meeting list with information about where and when meetings were held. She and Mark could pick the location and time of meetings that were most convenient for them. They did just that. Caroline said they both got quite an education over that week. Caroline stopped going to meetings, but Mark did not. He kept right on going, the way a drowning person holds on to a lifeline.

Mark finished his freshman year in college with good, but not great, grades. He stayed clean and sober, thanks to regular attendance at NA meetings. Then that first summer, he went home and promptly relapsed to drug use. He called Caroline, upset by his failure. She reminded him that he could go to meetings in his hometown, that his recovery was portable. He found some local meetings and regained his sobriety.

When that college class graduated, Mark was a guest at the dinner we had for Caroline and a few of her friends at a local Mexican restaurant. He chose to sit next to me. He told me how he had found a new life for himself in those meetings and how excited he was about his future. He had come to college thinking he wanted to be a doctor, but he found he had a gift for creative writing, which he linked to his father's talent for jazz music. His father had died of a heroin overdose when Mark was 4 years old, so he barely knew him, but Mark liked what he had heard about him. Mark wanted to write fiction and had won a prestigious national competition for a short story the previous semester. He had a full scholarship to another university to study for a master's degree and to teach while he continued to do his own writing. He was a happy young man. He left no doubt in my mind or in anyone else's that NA had been responsible for his ability to avoid the fate that had claimed his father.

Caroline regretted that Mark had not had much time for her

and their other friends since he had joined NA. Most of his friends were other people in the NA program. Mark explained that only by going to meetings every day had he been able to stay clean and sober. "I am sorry to have disappointed some of my friends, but this is the only way my life works, at least for now." I congratulated him on his accomplishments in college and said I thought he had made a lot of wise choices in his young life. I also told him he had a lot to give to others, and I was glad it looked like he would be able to fulfill his dreams.

More recently, Mark came across the country to attend Caroline's wedding. He told us that he was applying to medical school so he could put his knowledge and his compassion to work to help other people, especially people who suffer from addiction. He told me, "If it had not been for Caroline taking me to those NA meetings day after day and holding my hand when I got scared, I not only would not be going to medical school, I would almost certainly be dead."

The 12-step programs worked for both Cynthia and Adam, in part because they are good programs and in part because these people were dedicated to using these fellowships. The 12-step programs, good as they are, cannot help people who drop out. They are successful only for people who stick with the programs. When people work the 12-step programs, then the programs work for the members.

Mark's scary story has a happy ending. Mark not only found a new life for himself with 5 years of hard work—a life that both fulfilled his identification with his father and went beyond his father's tragically short life—but his recovery also taught powerful lessons to his many friends about addiction and recovery. Whatever else Mark's friends got out of their college educations, they all got good educations about addiction as they went through this experience with Mark.

Although not all the people in the 12-step programs are thoroughly wonderful, many of them are, which is all the more surprising because of the suffering and the character defects many of them experienced earlier in their lives as active addicts. Success in the 12-step programs means living life without alcohol and other drugs. It means living an honest life. After achieving those two goals, successful members of the fellowships simply suffer from all of life's ordinary and extraordinary vicissitudes from which nonaddicts suffer. That may not sound like much of an achievement to people who do not know addiction, but to those who do, that is an immense and, absent active membership in one of the 12-step fellowships, a rare achievement.

Chapter 12

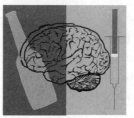

Tough Policy Choices
to Prevent Addiction

*In this chapter, we take a broader look at how both local and
global communities can become more resistant to addiction.*

*T*his chapter is controversial. Although many knowledge-

able experts hold views different from mine on prevention, I do

not consider any of the ideas in this chapter to be political in an

ideological or partisan sense. These ideas are extensions of a public health vision and part of an environmental approach to addiction.

Readers will not be surprised that I support both the wider use of drug testing linked to tough sanctions and the maintenance of strong prohibitions against the sale and use of all illicit drugs. These positions are expressions of the social contract for drug use, which is woven into every section of this book.

Review of the Social Contract for Drug Use

Look again at the social contract for drug use, which has enjoyed wide, bipartisan support in North America for more than half a century: **Self-controlled use, as well as sale, of addictive drugs is prohibited.** The "contract" is between the people of the nation and the government as well as other important social institutions, including work, health, education, and religion. The contract, ratified in laws, regulations, and social customs, contains consequences for failure to abide by it, such as in workplace addiction prevention programs, which provide treatment and rehabilitation for those willing and able to use these options but which also enforce termination of employment for those who continue use of addicting drugs.

The drugs that are included under this contract are spelled out clearly in national laws and international treaties involving virtually every nation in the world. Marijuana, cocaine, heroin, and the hallucinogens, including LSD, are covered under this contract, as is the nonmedical use of such synthetic substances as the barbiturates and the stimulants. The contract also deals with prescribed medicines that have an addiction potential.

These treaties are managed by agencies of the United Nations. Not covered under this basic contract are alcohol and tobacco, two addictive substances that are treated differently under law and in social custom. In North America, the use of alcohol and tobacco is prohibited for youth as a part of an effort to prevent addiction. The extension of the social contract to youthful use of alcohol and tobacco is likely to be adopted by other countries in the next decade as they grapple with the problems of increasing consumption of alcohol and tobacco by highly vulnerable youth.

This social contract was developed in roughly its current form in the first two decades of the 20th century in response to an alarming increase in the problems of addiction that was the direct result of the open access to a rapidly expanding menu of addicting drugs. The social contract captured the values of many nations and cultures over thousands of years in hard-won efforts to protect people from the dangers of addicting drugs. The contract is the heart of the antiaddiction software needed to protect the human brain from addiction.

Assessing Changes in the Social Contract

In assessing any proposal for changes in community responses to alcohol and other drugs, apply this question: "Does the new program or policy support the social contract for drug use?" When the answer is "yes," the proposal is usually sound. When the answer is "no," the proposal is usually hazardous. Prevention questions, however, are not always simple because the general good of supporting the prohibition against nonmedical use of addicting drugs needs to be balanced against competing values that are also important. For example, the values of privacy need to be weighed against the benefits that may be derived from prevention policies that support the social contract. The economic cost of prevention must also be weighed. Ideas that produce little benefit at great cost may be unreasonable even if they support the social contract for drug use.

People disagree about the benefits and the costs of various proposals in this area of life, as in others. When I encounter proposals that will increase the use of addicting drugs in any community, even when the proposals seem to hold out economic or other benefits, I not only am skeptical, but I am generally unsympathetic. After 25 years of working with addicted people and their families, I am convinced that communities benefit from policies that reduce, rather than increase, the nonmedical use of addictive drugs.

In this chapter, we first look at the fundamental critique of the social contract, the proposals to legalize currently illicit drugs. Second, we look at less radical proposals for softening the edges of prohibition against the illicit drugs, which is now labeled "harm reduction." Third, we explore new ideas to intensify the prohibition contained in the social contract. Fourth, we specifically look at drug testing for teenagers. Fifth, we look at new options to deal with alcohol and tobacco. Finally, we consider the issue of medicines that are addictive and how they are treated in the community and in the 12-step programs.

Legalization of Drugs: A False Hope

The idea of drug legalization is appealing to many well-meaning and intelligent people as a way of solving the frustrating drug problem and of winning the war against drugs by surrendering. I am going to spend time on this idea, despite its political impracticality, because drug legalization is winning the support of some thoughtful people today who are seeking new ideas. My assumption is that most of them have not thought much about the idea and what it would entail if it were implemented.

In recent years in North America, there has been yet another revival of interest in solving drug problems by legalizing marijuana and cocaine, the two most widely used illicit drugs. Some people in Europe have rallied to this idea. Dedicated enthusiasts extend this proposal for drug legalization to heroin, LSD, crack cocaine, and all other currently illegal drugs, taking the attitude, "Let the buyer beware." Most proposals to legalize drugs focus on marijuana and sometimes on cocaine, at least for use by adults. Although I am opposed to the legalization of any currently illegal drugs on humanitarian grounds, because I know that it would lead to a serious increase in drug use and drug problems, I am respectful of many of the points made by those who seek to legalize currently illegal drugs.

First, as they correctly point out, the key to prevention and treatment for addiction is in the hearts and minds of the individual drug users or prospective users. Addictive substances, as a realistic matter, are available at some price to almost anyone who wants to pay enough for them. Legalization of all drugs makes clear that the users are themselves responsible for the decision to use drugs or not to use drugs. Legalization of currently illegal drugs might reduce some of the costs of prohibition that are borne by the criminal justice system, such as prosecution and incarceration of people for drug crimes. Legalization might reduce the incentive of criminal drug suppliers, and it might generate tax revenues, assuming the government taxed currently illegal drugs the way it now taxes alcohol and tobacco. These are attractive features of drug legalization. These possible benefits, however, would be bought at a certain high cost in terms of increased health and safety problems because of the increase in the use of addicting drugs if drugs were more easily available. This fact is seldom mentioned by those who propose legalization.

I agree strongly with President Clinton's stance on drug legalization, which he reaffirmed during his first year as president when Jocelyn Elders, M.D., his surgeon general, spoke in support of considering drug legalization as a way to reduce crime. He un equivocally rejected any move toward drug legalization, as have all American presidents of both parties over the past 50 years.

Proposals for drug legalization start from the belief that the current policy of drug prohibition does not work. Legalization advocates point out that alcohol prohibition failed in the United States two generations ago. They argue that the widespread use of illicit drugs, despite prohibition, and the high costs and negative consequences of prohibition, ranging from the police and prison costs to the loss of privacy caused by drug testing in many settings, especially in the workplace, are unreasonably high prices to pay for a failing policy of prohibition.

During the last few years, the drug legalization movement has gained modest public support from some antiauthority political activists and libertarians. It has become fashionable to favor *harm reduction* as an alternative to either legalization or the strict prohibition of illicit drugs. *Harm reduction* is a new term used to describe techniques that seek to reduce the harm caused by illicit drug use, and the prohibition of that use, without reducing the amount of nonmedical drug use. An example of harm reduction is to give heroin addicts clean needles so they are less likely to acquire or pass on HIV infection, even though they continue to use heroin intravenously. Advocates for legalization have blamed virtually all the ills of addiction on the prohibition of drugs. The laws prohibiting drug use have been seen by those who favor legalization to be unwarranted violations of privacy and civil rights.

Drug legalization, like its opposite, drug prohibition, is not a simple alternative. For example, in today's context drug legalization can, in its most radical form, mean a return to open access to all drugs for all people, including limitless medical prescription of addicting drugs to drug addicts to sustain their habits. *Legalization*, the term that is sometimes used, also can mean such modest changes in current drug policies as making marijuana available to certain medical patients (such as AIDS patients and those suffering from vomiting after cancer chemotherapy). Legalization today can mean merely exchanging dirty needles for clean ones in the hope of reducing the spread of HIV among intravenous drug users and eventually attracting them into treatment.

Even outright drug legalizers range from those on the most modest end of the continuum, who propose decriminalizing the possession of marijuana, to those further along the legalization continuum who would create a legal supply of marijuana for all adults who do not have criminal records ("If they can buy handguns, why can't they buy marijuana?"). *Decriminalization* means that the law against using a drug is not enforced or, if it is enforced, the penalty is trivial, such as a $25 fine. Under decriminalization, the availability of drugs remains illegal. For example, decriminalizing marijuana means that users of the drug are not punished legally but there is still no legal supply of marijuana. In contrast, legalization means not only that the users are not punished, but that they can buy the drug from a legal supplier, the way alcohol and tobacco are now treated in most of the world. A more limited relaxation of current drug prohibition, a quasi-legalization, advocates granting licenses for some individuals to purchase and to use specific drugs that are now illegal, such as marijuana and the hallucinogens. The more modest harm-reduction ideas are dealt with in the second section of this chapter.

By the same token, the prohibition of illicit drugs contains a wide range of diverse options. Some who support the continuation of prohibition of currently illegal drugs favor universal drug tests to detect and to deter all users of illicit drugs, whereas others favor reducing the current harsh criminal penalties for drug sales in the hopes of stemming the ever-rising, and ever-more-expensive, number of drug-related offenders in prisons.

Although there are a limitless range of options within the general definitions of both drug legalization and drug prohibition, it is useful to look at the big picture of drug policy options today. In general, is prohibition working, and is it cost-effective? Does legalization offer a reasonable alternative to drug prohibition? There are two models for legalization that can help to sketch an answer to these fundamental questions. The first is a look back at life in the United States 100 years ago when addicting drugs were sold like toothpaste and candy. The second model comes from the comparison of the costs generated by the drugs that now are legal for adults and the drugs that are not. That means looking at alcohol and tobacco on the one hand compared with marijuana, cocaine, heroin, and other illegal drugs on the other hand. The recent trends in the rates of the use of both the legal and the illegal drugs in the United States give valuable perspective when considering lifting prohibition and replacing it with one of the many options for drug legalization.

The American experience with drugs at the end of the 19th century demonstrated serious problems caused by the use of a wide range of drugs when drugs were legally available. These problems were judged by Americans at the time to be unacceptable. In the context of today's debate about prohibition, recall that prohibition was the result of a nonpartisan public outcry over the negative effects of unrestricted drug use. In other words, the legal prohibition of heroin and cocaine did not cause widespread drug use in the United States; widespread drug use caused prohibition. Furthermore, drug prohibition, except for the prohibition of alcohol, has been almost universally supported politically in the United States and throughout the world for more than half a century.

Because the proper goal of a drug policy is to reduce harm, note that alcohol and tobacco produce far more harm than all of the illegal drugs combined. The deaths in the United States from alcohol are estimated at about 125,000 per year, whereas tobacco use causes about 420,000 deaths a year. The deaths resulting from all of the illicit drugs combined are less than 10,000 a year. Similarly, the social costs from alcohol use in the United States in 1990 were estimated at $98.6 billion a year, and the costs of all of the illicit drugs—including all of the costs of prohibition, such as the costs of incarcerating drug offenders in prison—were $66.9 billion. The social costs of smoking tobacco in 1990 were estimated to be $72 billion. In other words, whether the standard is drug-caused deaths or drug-caused economic costs, the drugs that are legal for adults (alcohol and tobacco) cause far more harm than all of the currently illegal drugs combined (see Table 12–1).

Look at the number of users of the legal and illegal drugs in the United States and the trends in the rates of use of these substances from 1985 to 1993 in Table 12–2. These numbers show that prohibition reduces the levels of use compared with legal availability. Compare the totals of alcohol and cigarettes to the totals for marijuana and cocaine, the two most commonly used illegal drugs. Equally important, note that in recent years the rates of use of illicit drugs have fallen much faster than the rates of the drugs whose use is legal for adults.

Would more legal drugs reduce crime, even if it increased

Table 12–1. Economic costs of addiction in the United States, 1990

	Illicit drugs, billions of dollars (%)	Alcohol, billions of dollars (%)	Tobacco, billions of dollars (%)
Medical care	3.2 (4.8)	10.5 (10.7)	20.2 (28.0)
Lost productivity	8.0 (11.9)	36.6 (37.1)	6.8 (9.0)
Death	3.4 (5.1)	33.6 (34.1)	45.0 (63.0)
Crime	46.0 (68.8)	15.8 (16.0)	0
AIDS	6.3 (9.4)	2.1 (2.1)	0
Total cost	66.9	98.6	72.0

Source.   Institute for Health Policy, Brandeis University: *Substance Abuse: The Nation's Number One Health Problem: Key Indicators for Policy.* Princeton, NJ, Robert Wood Johnson Foundation, 1993.

other problems? Take a look at the role that cheap, legal alcohol plays in crimes from highway deaths to murder and from rape to robbery, and you will see that the biggest factor in drug-caused crime is not the high costs of the drugs but the harmful effects of drug use on the brains of drug users. In Table 12–1, note that the costs of illicit drugs are primarily the costs of crime: 68.8% of the $66.9 billion in costs of illicit drugs in 1990 were the costs of crime. Crime produced only 16% of the social costs of alcohol and 0% of the costs generated by tobacco use. In dramatic contrast to these crime costs, the costs of medical care, lost productivity, and death were $14.6 billion for all illegal drugs, $80.7 billion for alcohol, and $72 billion for tobacco. In other words, when drugs are legalized, they are more widely used, and the total costs go up compared with prohibition. The costs of legal drugs are paid for in medical care, lost productivity, and death.

Look again at Table 12–1 and notice that the costs of medical care, lost productivity, death, and AIDS for all illicit drugs are $20.9 billion, whereas the equivalent costs for alcohol are $82.8 billion, and for tobacco they are $72 billion. Recognizing that there are about 12 million current users of illicit drugs, 103 million cur-

Table 12–2. American drug use in the prior 30 days (in millions)

	1985	1993	Decline from 1985–1993
Drugs legal for adults			
Alcohol	113	103	9%
Cigarettes	60	50	17%
The most widely used drugs that are illegal for all			
Marijuana	18	9	50%
Cocaine	6	1.3	78%

Source.   Substance Abuse and Mental Health Services Administration, Office of Applied Studies: *Preliminary Estimates from the 1993 National Household Survey on Drug Abuse,* Advance Report Number 7. Rockville, MD, U.S. Department of Health and Human Services, Public Health Service, 1994.

rent users of alcohol, and 50 million current users of tobacco, the health-related costs (the social burden each year, exclusive of crime costs) per user are the following: illicit drug users, $1,742; alcohol, $798; and tobacco, $1,440. Although some advocates for the legalization of illicit drugs claim that these drugs do not produce health costs on the scale of the costs produced by alcohol and tobacco, these data show that illicit drugs produce higher levels of health and productivity costs per user than are produced by the drugs that are legal for adults.

Under prohibition the overall costs to society are lower, and the costs that are paid show up primarily in police and corrections budgets. It does not require an economic genius to recognize that prohibition is now working effectively to reduce the total costs generated by such drugs as marijuana, cocaine, and heroin. Furthermore, the human suffering reflected in the health care costs would rise dramatically if those drugs were legally available, as alcohol and tobacco are now, because the number of users would increase from the current 12 million to a number similar to the 50 million tobacco users or even the 103 million users of alcohol.

Some supporters of the legalization of currently illegal drugs hold out the hope of large tax revenues from making marijuana, cocaine, hallucinogens, and other drugs legally available, similar to the current taxes on alcohol and tobacco. The 1992 revenue from tobacco taxes at all levels of government from national, state, and local taxes was approximately $12.6 billion. The equivalent figures for alcohol taxes in that same year were about $13 billion. These revenue figures are small in relation to the health burden imposed by the use of tobacco and alcohol in the United States. Trading tax revenue for sickness and death is neither morally nor economically sensible. The health costs now produced by illicit drugs are lower than the tax revenues from either tobacco or alcohol. The tax revenues from tobacco and alcohol are surely larger than the probable tax revenues to be generated from the legalization of marijuana, cocaine, or any other currently illegal drug. If the taxes on these drugs were raised higher than the current taxes on tobacco and alcohol to increase government revenue, one of the principal justifications for legalization would vanish as the incentives for the illicit (untaxed) drug market would persist because of the inflated prices produced by exorbitant taxes.

Supporters of legalization cannot have it both ways. Either the tax revenues from legalization are so low that they do not offset the added health costs, or they are so high that they encourage continuation of the illicit drug traffic. Once more, alcohol and tobacco are useful models for those who would legalize other drugs. These models show that legalization is terribly expensive both in human and in dollar terms.

These uncontested facts show that drug prohibition in the United States works reasonably well to control the costs of addictive drug use and the amount of drug use that occurs. Legalization would result in more use of currently illegal drugs and more harm expressed in greater social costs. Those who would reform drug laws, and who support harm-reduction objectives, should focus their efforts on alcohol and tobacco, where the major drug-caused harm is now taking place in the United States and throughout the world. These two drugs are causing the most harm not because they are more dangerous or more attractive to users than marijuana, cocaine, and heroin. In fact, alcohol and tobacco are both less attractive to many experienced drug users, and they are also much less dangerous. Alcohol and tobacco produce more harm than all of the illegal drugs combined (including the costs of prohibition) because they are so much more widely used. Alcohol and tobacco are more widely used by adults and by children because their use is legal for adults.

If marijuana were legalized, would levels of marijuana use reach, or even exceed, the levels of use of alcohol and tobacco? Many proponents of legalization say that marijuana use would not increase even if the drug were legally available. For a time in the United States, marijuana use was as tolerated for youth as was alcohol use. In 1978 nearly twice as many American high school seniors used marijuana every day (11%) as used alcohol every day (6%). This experience showed that there is a potential for marijuana (and other illegal drugs if their use were more widely tolerated) to be used in modern societies at levels equal to or even exceeding the current levels of the use of alcohol and cigarettes.

If all drugs were completely legal, many people would continue to choose not to use drugs, just as many adults choose not

Drug Legalization

Advantages

- May reduce police and prison costs of prohibition
- May reduce incentives for illegal drug sales
- May raise tax revenue
- Emphasizes the individual responsibility to decide to use or not to use drugs (as is now the case for adults with alcohol and tobacco use)

Disadvantages

- Undermines efforts to discourage drug use
- Increases dramatically the level of drug use in society
- Increases level of drug-caused problems
- Raises total costs to society of drug use, especially costs on the highway, at work, in school, and in family life

to use alcohol and tobacco even though such use is legal. It is equally true that even under the most severe prohibition, some people choose to use prohibited drugs. The relevant question is less black and white. Would legalization increase both the number of drug users and the social harm produced by the use of the drugs compared with the prohibition of these substances? The answer to the question is yes.

Those who support legalization correctly point out that prohibition is an expensive strategy. In other words, making it illegal to consume marijuana, cocaine, heroin, and other drugs costs society large sums of money. These costs are paid in many ways, from the costs of police and prisons to the incentives that prohibition-inflated drug prices provide to the illicit drug traffickers. The costs are also paid in some loss of privacy as, for example, drug tests are more widely used in the criminal justice system, in the workplace, and elsewhere. Those who support prohibition do not help their case by denying the magnitude of these costs. Are these costs of prohibition justified in terms of reduced harm and improved quality of life for most citizens? The evidence is clear that prohibition is worth its high costs.

Legalization is an old siren call that promises to reduce the high societal cost burdens of drug use. Abundant evidence shows that legalization would raise the total costs society pays for drug use, not reduce them. We do not need new experiments to make this point. Those experiments have already been conducted at the cost of great human suffering.

Arguments for the radical dismantling of drug prohibition find increasingly common expression in the media because of the appeal of this shocking and apparently new idea. Despite incessant media attention to the concept of drug legalization, the possibility that anyone could buy any drug on the open market the way people now buy Coca-Cola is so hard for most people to accept that outright legalization has almost no political appeal. I have found that those who would legalize drugs are stumped by obvious questions such as these:

- Will there be any limits on who may buy LSD, crack cocaine, and heroin, or will anyone with a little money be able to walk into a store and buy whatever drugs he or she wants?
- What forms of drugs will be available and at what potencies? Will everyone be able to buy cheap, clean syringes and sterile heroin, for example?
- Will children of any age be able to buy any drugs they want? If not, how will children be kept from buying the immensely more available supply of drugs after legalization, given the dismal record of North America with alcohol and tobacco use by youth?

Whenever would-be legalizers start to put barriers between potential consumers and the drugs they want to purchase, they are repeating the problems of prohibition which they seek to solve by drug legalization. For example, if they say, "Drugs will only be available to registered addicts, not to anyone who wants them," then the incentives for illegal suppliers remain in place. In addition, there would be a great financial incentive for the registered addicts to sell their drugs to people who are not registered, as now happens with methadone.

When legalizers propose high taxes to discourage drug use and to provide public revenue, they have created incentives for illegal distribution, as occurs now with high cigarette taxes. Only if all drugs were legalized in all dosages and in all forms (e.g., suitable for intravenous injection and smoking) for anyone who wanted to buy them, and only if taxes on drugs were kept low (as they are now on alcohol), would the hoped-for economic and criminal benefits of legalization be realized.

Most often those who support drug legalization back away from these fundamental questions, saying that they want to try new ideas, or, as many politicians put it, "I am merely proposing that we study alternatives to the current prohibition policies." This is an irresponsible position that allows the politician to gain media attention for the seemingly daring idea of drug legalization without bearing the political responsibility for supporting that idea.

My answer to politicians who hide behind such manipulations is this:

> The proposal that people should have legal access to whatever drugs they want is not new. That was the situation in the United States before we had drug prohibition. If you do not know that history, or if you have not learned from the world's experience with drugs during the 20th century, I suggest that you do a bit of homework before you grab the bully pulpit of your public position to mislead people.

One curious aspect of the contemporary legalization argument is that people who are involved in drug treatment almost all oppose drug legalization. If they were operating on their own self-interest, they would welcome drug legalization because it would substantially increase the need for the treatment of addiction. Treatment professionals generally oppose drug legalization because their dedication to the welfare of drug users is more powerful than their own economic interests. Talk, as I have, to drug abusers in treatment or to those who have successfully developed solid, personal recovery programs. Few of them support legalization because they know that such an approach would make life harder for them and for all other recovering people.

More than 20 years ago, Stewart Alsop, a distinguished journalist, wrote a column for *Newsweek* magazine proposing that the heroin addiction problem would be solved by legal access to heroin. As the head of the Narcotics Treatment Administration for the District of Columbia government, I called Mr. Alsop, who lived in Washington, and asked him to come with me to talk with a group of heroin addicts about his ideas. He took me up on the offer. The reaction of these recovering men and women to his ideas left a lasting impression on both me and Mr. Alsop. They laughed, telling him that they were having a hard time staying off heroin when heroin was illegal, but that if it were as available as alcohol, they would surely relapse to heroin use. "But would you then commit crimes?" Mr. Alsop asked. They answered that they would if they did not die of an overdose. To his credit, Stewart Alsop published a follow-up article in *Newsweek* reversing his position. I wish more of today's would-be legalizers would listen to both addicted people and professionals in the field of addiction treatment.

The politics of drug legalization has interested me over the years. Some political liberals are attracted to drug legalization, but so are some politically conservative libertarians. I have found a simple way to separate the two groups: ask what they think about gun control and limits on advertising cigarettes. Almost all the liberals who support drug legalization are staunch supporters of gun control and tough limits on cigarette advertising, whereas the libertarians generally oppose not only drug prohibition, but also gun control and limits on cigarette advertising. The libertarian position is clear and consistent, if scary in terms of the public health. The liberal positions favoring drug legalization puzzle me. Are drugs considered safe but guns and cigarettes considered dangerous? Is there a role for the government in gun control and cigarette advertising but not in drug prohibition?

This political analysis of drug legalization should not obscure the fact that most liberals and most conservatives strongly favor continued prohibition of all illicit drugs, including marijuana. Only a small minority of each group have been won over to the camp of the drug legalizers. For the record, I support drug prohibition and strict limits on alcohol and cigarette advertising. I also support not only gun registration but strict limits on the access to guns. I consider that each of these positions reflects a consistent concern for the public health. I also know that although such tough and desirable government policies will reduce problems with the prohibited behaviors, these prohibitions—no matter how tough they are—will not end our serious problems with alcohol, tobacco, illicit drugs, or guns. For some people the decisions to use any of these products is determined by personal choices and not by government policies. On the other hand, prohibiting gun ownership and stopping all cigarette advertising will reduce, but not end, gun-related violence and cigarette use, just as the prohibition of illicit drugs has not stopped the use of those drugs.

When they look at the fact that the currently legal drugs produce far higher costs for health and productivity than the currently illegal drugs, many supporters of drug legalization conclude that legal availability would not lead to increased use of the currently illegal drugs. They deny that the currently illegal drugs cause, or would cause if legal, serious health problems. They accept that alcohol and nicotine cause huge health and productivity problems, but they believe that such costs would not occur if marijuana, cocaine, LSD, and heroin were legally available.

One physician who supported drug legalization told me she did not believe that cocaine, heroin, and other illegal drugs caused serious health problems other than the problems caused by their prohibition: "It is gunshot wounds and AIDS that kill illicit drug users, not their drugs." She believed that if addicts could get "cheap, pure drugs," they would have few health- or work-related problems and would cause others in the society few problems. Such ignorance of the devastating negative impact of currently illegal intoxicating drugs shocked me, but it is not uncommon. This doctor was simply wrong on the facts: the currently illegal drugs do cause serious harm even when they are available cheaply in pure forms.

Some supporters of legalization want to let "good adults" who use marijuana in the privacy of their homes live free of harassment from legal authorities and employers. This is an interesting point of view, but it is unrelated to the argument for drug legalization because such a small part of the overall societal drug problem is involved with such marijuana use. Decriminalizing marijuana would not make streets safer or reduce the incentives for drug dealers to continue their work.

Many supporters of legalization are personally opposed to the use of illicit drugs. They support legalization the way I supported marijuana decriminalization in the mid-1970s, in order to promote humane values against what they perceive to be harsh and counterproductive uses of the government's power. If they stay with the drug legalization issue long enough, and if they are honest with themselves, they will find, as I did to my shame, that many of the most active supporters of legalization actively encourage the nonmedical use of drugs. Even worse, they will discover that most of the public who listen to views that are sympathetic to drug legalization and/or decriminalization perceive these views to be prodrug, no matter how often the speakers disavow this interpretation of their views.

Support for the legalization of currently illegal drugs strengthens those forces in the society that want to see the use of illicit drugs go up, including those who benefit from the lucrative but deadly illicit drug traffic. Drug traffickers know that the supply of drugs such as marijuana, cocaine, and heroin will never become legal in any major nation of the world, so they need not fear competition from big companies that now sell tobacco and alcohol. They are smart enough to know that support for the drug legalization lobby blunts the will of the modern world to curb both the supply and the use of currently illegal drugs. They know that support for legalization builds their criminal business of drug trafficking.

Because many thoughtful people have proposed the legalization of drugs as a solution to the war we are waging against the financial, social, medical, and political ravages of drug abuse, I want to share my projection of such a decision. Here is my fantasy when it comes to drug legalization: some community or nation will try it. I would say, "Go right ahead and put heroin, cocaine, LSD, and all the rest of the modern menu of addicting drugs for sale in your local food markets." The results of the experiment would not be long in coming, and they are not hard to predict. The good news as a result of drug legalization would be that crime costs (prisons, courts, and police) might fall, tax revenues would rise, and the illegal market for these drugs would be reduced. The bad news would be that health and productivity costs would increase dramatically so that the net costs to society would rise substantially. Worse, the human costs from drug use would rise over time as more people used these drugs and became addicted. The highest costs of drug legalization would be paid in those groups that are the most vulnerable to addiction: youth and the disadvantaged. If any community in the world would be so foolish as to try outright legalization for drugs including marijuana, cocaine, heroin, and LSD, we might have less discussion of this thoroughly unworkable and dangerous (but endlessly seductive) idea.

It is often said that although democracy is a messy, expensive, and flawed system of government, it is better than the alternatives. The prohibition of currently illegal drugs is also a messy, expensive, and flawed system but, like democracy, it is better than the alternatives. This is not to say that either democracy or drug prohibition cannot be improved, but abundant evidence from many societies and over many years has shown that, in general, prohibition of drugs such as marijuana, cocaine, and heroin is a reasonable and generally effective way to deal with a difficult human problem.

Harm Reduction: Incremental Legalization

Although the people who would dismantle drug prohibition use the language and the media attention of full-blown legalization, there are few of them with the courage of their own rhetoric. Instead of proposing outright legalization, more moderate voices offer a set of reasonable-seeming modifications in the current drug prohibition policy, designed, as they claim, to reduce harm.

They do not want to reduce drug use. They want to reduce drug prohibition bit by bit rather than in one grand stroke. They say they want to reduce the harm caused by drug prohibition. That may sound like a minor distinction, but in the world of addiction it is vitally important. The prohibitionists, in contrast, want to reduce drug use as a way to reduce the harm caused by drug use. *Harm reduction* is a new term that accepts the use of illicit drugs but seeks to reduce the pain that drug prohibition causes to individuals and to communities at large. Here are some current harm-reduction proposals:

- Provide addicts with clean needles to reduce the spread of HIV (the AIDS virus) that results from intravenous drug use with shared needles.
- Reduce the penalties for drug sale and eliminate the penalties for drug possession and drug use to reduce the costs of police and prisons resulting from drug prohibition.
- Use marijuana (and heroin, LSD, and other illegal drugs) in the treatment of many illnesses, including AIDS, multiple sclerosis, alcoholism, cancer pain, and the nausea and vomiting from chemotherapy.
- Make marijuana special. Make it the one allegedly safe, socially acceptable currently illegal drug. This is a variant of the overall drug legalization proposal—do not legalize all drugs, just legalize marijuana. Some add LSD and the hallucinogens to their short list of drugs for special treatment.
- Register addicts and give them drugs in medically supervised clinics—whatever drugs they want—as some people now perceive is done for heroin addicts receiving methadone.
- Stop drug tests at work and elsewhere because they are expensive and unreliable, as well as an invasion of privacy.

Although each of these ideas has some appeal, they all represent incremental abandonments of drug prohibition. They would all encourage wider use of illicit drugs. Harm reduction today is the reincarnation of the "responsible use" movement of the 1970s. Let us examine these ideas one at a time.

Clean Needles

Providing addicts with clean needles accepts their criminal and deadly drug habits. Intravenous drug users have at least four potentially fatal problems as a result of their IV drug use: HIV infection from shared needles, death from overdose, death from accidents, and homicide. At best, giving them clean needles reduces only one of those risks, the possibility of HIV infection. Having worked with many IV drug users, I know that most addicts continue to use dirty and contaminated needles no matter how many clean needles they have. More important, why not cure the underlying problem—the drug addiction itself—so that all four lethal risks are reduced? Involuntary treatment of IV drug addicts makes more sense, and is more humane, than giving them clean needles. Giving IV drug addicts clean needles to save their lives is about as sensible as making sure that all drunk drivers have air bags in their cars and then turning them loose on the highways.

Reduced Penalties for Drug Possession and Sale

Reducing penalties for drug possession and sale reduces the pressure on addicts to stop using drugs. As such, it is an enabling step. As will be seen in the final section of this chapter, which deals with new ideas to make drug prohibition work better, what is needed is not lesser or eliminated penalties, but strategies to make the penalties for possession and sale of illicit drugs more effective and less costly in society. Removing penalties for drug sale and possession is surrendering to the illicit drug epidemic.

Medical Use of Illicit Drugs

The social contract for drug use contains a clear exemption for the medical use of substances with high abuse potential, as is now done for morphine. The problem with marijuana and other currently illegal drugs as medicines is that they have not met the routine medical standards as effective treatments. If and when any of the currently illegal drugs does meet those medical standards, I will be eager to support them as medical treatments. It is inconceivable that marijuana would ever be approved as a medical treatment, since marijuana smoke contains more than 2,000 chemicals in an unstable and unpredictable mix. Modern medicine uses purified chemicals in controlled doses to treat specific illnesses.

At some future time a chemical found in marijuana, most likely synthetically produced, may prove useful for one or another medical treatments. Today Marinol (dronabinol), synthetic delta-9-tetrahydrocannabinol (THC), is approved in the United States for the treatment of the nausea and vomiting sometimes resulting from cancer chemotherapy. There are other medicines that are better and more easily tolerated by chemotherapy patients for this problem, but Marinol is available to physicians today. If other currently illicit drugs meet the routine standards for safe and effective medical treatments, and if there are not other agents at least as good that have lower abuse potentials, then they (like morphine) should be approved. This approach does not satisfy many harm-reduction advocates because these advocates want to have sick medical patients using exactly the substances that are widely abused. This insistence reveals that their fundamental motivation is the encouragement of the use of currently illegal drugs. When modern scientifically trained doctors prescribe medicines, they prescribe specific chemicals in known doses. Smoked marijuana simply does not meet this everyday medical standard since the smoke contains thousands of different chemicals in unstable and unpredictable dosages. Doctors do not prescribe crude smoking drugs, they prescribe specific medicines.

Making Marijuana Legal

Carving out marijuana as the one safe currently illegal drug would add marijuana to alcohol and tobacco as legal drugs for adults. That would increase the use of marijuana, a dangerous drug. We had some experience in the United States with almost-legal marijuana in the mid-1970s, and the results were bad. Marijuana use increased rapidly, especially among youth, as did the problems associated with marijuana use, from school failures and family disruptions to auto accidents and decreased productivity at work. Adding the hallucinogens, including Ecstasy and LSD, to the list of newly legal drugs is an even more frightening thought.

Registering Addicts to Give Them Drugs

Registering addicts and providing them with drugs, like giving IV drug users clean needles, encourages and supports nonmedical drug use. It is the wrong way to go. It is also impractical. Which drugs would the doctors in such clinics give to their "patients" and in what dose? Would they charge for these drugs or give them away? What if a "patient" asked for more drugs than the doctor thought wise? If the doctor said "no," the "patient" could respond, "If you don't give me the drugs I want right now, I will buy them on the illicit market!" How could the doctor resist this blackmail? If the doctors were stingy with their "patients," then the incentive for the illicit drug trade would persist. If the doctors were generous, there would be an irresistible temptation for "patients" to give away or sell the drugs they got from these clinics.

There is no medical precedent for doctors giving drugs to patients in this way. It is not a sort of medical practice that any ethical physician would be part of. How could doctors think they were helping such "patients" when the drugs they were giving out were killing them and spreading to other people in the community?

Methadone treatment appears to be a notable exception to the social contract. It is a reasonable exception because methadone is a unique medicine. When taken orally, methadone needs to be taken only once a day to provide long-lasting relief from both craving for heroin and withdrawal symptoms. Because tolerance develops rapidly and completely to the behavioral ill effects of the methadone after regular doses over a few weeks or longer, methadone-maintained patients function normally at work and in family life.

Methadone is a unique temporary treatment that permits heroin addicts to stabilize their lives. Methadone itself does nothing to discourage the use of drugs other than opiates. Methadone treatment, however, gives the program staff powerful leverage to promote prosocial behaviors, from gainful employment to cessation of the use of other addicting drugs such as alcohol, marijuana, and cocaine and other stimulants.

There is no equivalent for methadone that would substitute for LSD, marijuana, cocaine, or other illicit drugs. All of these drugs are taken many times a day, and tolerance for their negative behavioral effects is incomplete. Because tolerance to the negative effects is incomplete for these drugs, people who used clinic-supplied cocaine or heroin would continue to be impaired and unable to function in society whether driving a car or going to work. They would be dysfunctional as friends and family members. Take-home drugs would have to be dispersed in large amounts (in contrast to once-a-day methadone), and the "patients" taking these drugs would not be able to work or to function in family life.

Giving away currently illegal drugs in so-called "clinics" would be like setting up clinics to give alcohol to alcoholics and calling it medical treatment. The alcoholic "patients" at such clinics would be drunk and dysfunctional, as well as being grossly impaired and dangerous to themselves and to others. Giving away drugs such as cocaine, LSD, and heroin at "clinics," if the practice were widespread so that anyone who wanted the drugs could get them at no cost, would eliminate the incentive for the illegal drug market. It would do this, however, at the cost of flooding the community with these drugs, leading to far worse problems overall than are now seen when the drugs are prohibited.

Eliminate or Reduce Drug Tests

The final harm-reduction idea to be considered is to abandon drug tests at work. Drug tests in the workplace and elsewhere are now widely conducted in ways that are fair and accurate. When linked to sanctions, drug tests pull back the curtain of denial and expose the secret of nonmedical drug use to the antidrug forces in families and in communities. Drug tests are a major element of effective prohibition of illicit drug use. Drug tests reduce drug use and reduce the overall social burden imposed by drugs in the community. Drug tests at work powerfully reinforce the social contract for drug use, making clear that use of illicit drugs on or off the job is incompatible with gainful employment. Stopping drug tests at work and elsewhere is a step backward to greater permissiveness toward illicit drug use.

Harm-reduction proposals are promoted as alternatives to either strict prohibition or legalization. They are usually supported by pointing out the failings of the current policies of prohibition. Each step in the harm-reduction agenda is small and, in itself, unlikely to produce either much benefit or much risk to the drug problems of the country. The major costs of these proposals, and the reason I oppose them, is that they undermine the country's will to reject nonmedical drug use. Harm reduction is incremental appeasement in the work of preventing addiction. Harm reduction is dangerous for the same reasons that it attracts supporters, because of its symbolism. In my view, the symbolism of harm reduction is dangerous because it accepts and tolerates illicit drug use. When drug use is tolerated, it increases, producing not less harm, but more harm.

Strengthening Prohibition and Supporting the Social Contract

Having looked at proposals to eliminate or relax the prohibition against nonmedical drug use, we now turn to proposals that would strengthen the social contract for drug use. With respect to local, national, and even global efforts to reduce both the availability and the nonmedical use of drugs, there is a great prevention opportunity. Think of the "drug abuse chain" as being U-shaped. The drug producer and the drug user are at each high end, with the production process dangling in between. The chain is most vulnerable at each high end, where the personnel and the product are more visible (see Figure 12–1). The manufacturing process is much more easily concealed. Let me explain.

When drug crops are grown, they must be exposed to the sunlight. Both marijuana plants and opium poppies from which heroin is produced are visible for several months prior to harvest, and coca bushes from which cocaine is produced must be exposed to the sun for 3 or 4 years before their initial harvest. Countries with the will to destroy drug crops can destroy most of them fairly easily. International efforts can help developing countries destroy drug crops by providing them with the means to apply biodegradable herbicides from airplanes. Today, many countries lack the political will to destroy their highly visible and lucrative drug crops.

Not all drug crops are grown in developing countries. North America now has a large domestic marijuana crop to supply much of its own market. Synthetic drugs are mostly produced locally in all parts of North America. LSD, Ecstasy, and other hallucinogens, phencyclidine (PCP), and methamphetamine are produced in large quantities within the borders of the United States, Canada, and other economically developed countries.

The site of initial cultivation or production of drugs is one vulnerable end of the drug chain. The other vulnerable end of the drug chain is the drug addict, the ultimate consumer of the drugs. Countries with the will to stop illicit drug use can identify nonmedical drug users fairly easily and can apply strong sanctions to deter nonmedical use. However, once the drug crop is harvested and enters the international drug traffic, the drug becomes small, valuable, and easily concealed. Interdiction between the growing

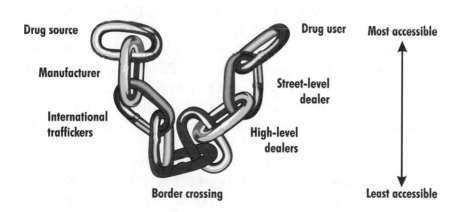

Figure 12–1.   The Drug Abuse Chain.

plant and the ultimate drug user is fraught with difficulty.

The supply of drugs is more easily stopped close to either the plant or the laboratory source, or within the ultimate drug user. The farther the drug moves from either end of the drug chain, the more difficult it is to detect and to eliminate. This is the U-shaped chain because the higher and more vulnerable parts are the two ends of the drug supply chain, and the lower parts of the chain are the middle, when the drug supply is hidden and most difficult to interrupt. Most countries today try to solve their nonmedical drug problems primarily by dealing with this least visible, least vulnerable part of the drug chain, where the nonmedical drugs are close neither to their plant or laboratory origins nor to the drug users.

More concerted national and international efforts are needed to detect and destroy drug crops and drug laboratories and to identify and deter nonmedical drug use by individual drug users. By destroying drug crops while they are still in the ground, prevention efforts make drugs physically unavailable. By identifying nonmedical drug users and applying strong sanctions against continued drug use, drug abuse prevention efforts make drugs psychologically unavailable. More needs to be done throughout the world to destroy both drug crops and illegal laboratories where synthetic drugs are manufactured. Modern satellite technology could be used to swiftly and reliably identify most drug crops. Aerial crop destruction techniques could eliminate most of these crops.

Surely traffickers would respond to such measures by using smaller and more disguised means of cultivation of drug crops and by switching to synthetically produced drugs. Illicit drugs constitute an industry that has more than $100 billion a year in revenue. The illegal drug industry will not simply accept defeat. But smaller, more dispersed cultivation is less efficient than the current wholesale approach to drug crop cultivation. This switch to more dispersed, less efficient production would raise the cost of drugs and make them less accessible to people all over the world. There are many relatively effective techniques for dealing with synthetically produced drugs, especially the control of chemicals needed to produce synthetic drugs.

Similarly, although universal drug testing with tough sanctions applied to drug users will not end drug use, it can powerfully discourage nonmedical drug use. Widespread drug testing linked to sanctions for nonmedical drug use will reduce the demand for drugs by reducing the size of the user population. By shrinking the demand for drugs, wider use of drug testing will reduce the financial incentives to drug suppliers.

Nations of the world, through international agencies and other mechanisms, can band together to promote these understandable, achievable goals of drug abuse prevention. A good start has already been made by the United Nations. The United Nations holds an annual meeting to deal with addicting, illegal drugs and has a staff headquartered in Vienna, Austria, that helps the nations of the world deal more effectively with both the supply of and the demand for addicting drugs. International prevention efforts need more support, both politically and financially. They need to get far tougher than they have been in the past. The same controversies that frustrate antidrug action in North America are played out every day on a global scale. Coming to understand addiction and what to do about it will be no easier in other nations than it has been in North America. But the goal of real, lasting prevention can be reached. The time is ripe for action as the pain generated by addiction becomes more severe, year by year, in all parts of the world.

I make these suggestions for the future with humility. They are controversial. Many well-meaning and experienced experts tell us that these are impossible and even undesirable goals. They encourage us to focus our efforts on the drug traffickers who are handling highly purified drugs. They ask us to educate and persuade people not to use drugs nonmedically or to provide drug users with services and assistance so that they will not want to use drugs nonmedically. They want to offer drug growers alternative crops. I wholeheartedly support those humane efforts. I know they work. But they do not work well enough.

The stronger approaches I suggest will add significantly to the current success in preventing tragedies caused by addiction. These new ideas are not meant to undermine current efforts, including law enforcement, education, and treatment efforts. In the final analysis, making drugs unavailable either physically or psy-chologically will always be an unfinished task. *Physical availability* refers to whether the drugs are available in a person's environ-ment as a practical matter. *Psychological availability* refers to whether the person considers drug use to be an option. Some people who live in environments with high physical availability nevertheless choose not to use them, making them psychologi-cally unavailable. Cigarettes, for example, are widely physically available, but their availability is irrelevant to many people who choose not to use them. Prevention seeks to make drugs such as marijuana, cocaine, LSD, and heroin both physically and psycho-logically unavailable.

All efforts are successful or unsuccessful in relative, not abso-lute, terms. Being realistic, we must recognize and accept that no efforts, however effective, will stop all nonmedical drug use. Con-versely, no efforts, however ineffective (including outright drug legalization), will cause everyone to abuse drugs. Good policies are aimed at reducing the use of addicting drugs, not eliminating all nonmedical drug use.

When it comes to preventing drug use, the central goal is to give users and would-be users many good reasons not to use drugs. Primarily that means discouraging drug use by making drugs expensive and hard to get and by using drug tests with tough sanctions for positive tests. Educating people not to use drugs is pleasant and generally not controversial, although it is expensive. It is both unpleasant and controversial to conduct drug tests and to impose serious consequences on those who use illicit drugs. Given the powerful brain mechanisms at work to encour-age and perpetuate drug use, only tough love approaches are likely to work for many people of all ages and all social classes.

The workplace has been a site of the application of a drug test-ing approach in the last decade in the United States. Many other institutions would benefit from the same general approach. The highest priority is the criminal justice system, where many of the most serious drug addicts are to be found, many of whom gener-ate high social costs as a result of their drug use. It needs to be clearly stated and actively enforced that any person who is re-leased to the community on parole or probation is subject to frequent drug tests, with incarceration being a swift and certain consequence of illicit drug use. Such incarceration need not be prolonged, just long enough to convince the probationer or parolee that the policy is inescapable.

Repeated infractions of the no-use policy should be met by graduated sanctions, with more prolonged reincarceration for each subsequent offense until the point is made. People arrested for any offense need to understand the risks and the consequences of violating the no-use policy right from the start. Progressive sanctions linked to regular drug tests need to become the standard of care in the criminal justice system.

This antiaddiction approach contrasts starkly with the widely supported view that long, mandatory prison sentences are the best way to deter crime and to protect the community from criminals. The best way to stop crime and protect law-abiding citizens is to impose zero-tolerance standards for nonmedical drug use on everyone who is released conditionally from any criminal justice agency. Only when offenders fail repeatedly to adhere to this standard should they be incarcerated for long periods of time. What is needed most at this time to reduce crime and relieve overcrowded prisons is mandatory, universal drug testing with graduated sanctions for failure to meet the drug-free standard.

Similar approaches are needed for all entitlement programs including public assistance and public housing and for both public and private disability programs. Programs to aid the homeless and the unemployed also need a zero-tolerance standard for illicit drug use. All too often today, humanitarian assistance programs are turned into perverse systems promoting addiction to alcohol and other drugs. Money is toxic for active addicts. In many cases today, the result of income transfer programs is tax-supported addiction to alcohol and other drugs.

This process is similar to the sad state of affairs in families dealing with an addicted member. The more the family gives to the addict, the deeper the addiction becomes as the disease turns the family love into a cruel caricature. Everyone loses when enabling is the response, regardless of the good intentions that are behind it. Only a tough love approach offers hope for real help to addicted people caught in these all-too-common traps. Remember that the word *love* is part of the term *tough love.* Tough love is not rejecting or hostile; it simply enforces the concept that with rights come responsibilities.

Drug Testing for Teenagers

Given the reality that most nonmedical drug use begins in child-hood, especially between the ages of 12 and 20, there has been a gratifying rise in school-based prevention programs discouraging the use of alcohol and other drugs. Not only are more youth exposed in schools to antidrug information programs, they increasingly are exposed also to programs that teach specific and effective refusal skills especially to high-risk youth. Nevertheless, high-risk youth and high-risk environments continue to produce tragically high levels of new nonmedical drug use among vulnerable teenagers. Schools can do a better job than they have so far in educating parents to the dangers of drug use by children and to what parents can do to stop teenage alcohol and drug use before it begins.

There is a need today for routine drug tests for schoolchildren. If we can require children to get a vaccination or to have an eye or hearing test as a condition of being in school, a modern nation can surely require a drug test as a condition of school attendance. Who is harmed by making school attendance conditional on not using illicit drugs? Surely not the schoolchildren themselves, whether they use drugs or not. Today, even children who do not use drugs are harmed by the nonmedical use of drugs in their schools because drug use causes not only poor academic performance but also disruptive behavior, drug sales, and violence in schools. Why is it disturbing to conduct drug tests of teenagers in school using either urine or hair samples? How many children would be helped by giving teachers and parents access to routine drug tests for children who show signs of possible nonmedical drug use, such as falling grades, socially disruptive behavior, or truancy?

What is to be done with youths who fail drug tests at school? Putting drug-using youth out of school is a bad answer for them, for their families, and for their communities. Instead of expulsion, drug-using students need to have their families and their schools work together so that they become and remain drug free. They need to be taken out of their routine classrooms and assigned to "in-school suspension" until they are drug free. This means that such youth should not have the freedom of movement of other students in school so that they can be more closely supervised. They should spend their school time in a quarantine/detention status where they can get intensive counseling and education based on the disease concept of addiction. This is what is done today to automobile drivers who have been arrested for alcohol and drug offenses in driving while impaired (DWI) programs. Parents of drug-using children need education and support to help their children resist the lure of continued drug and alcohol use. Once these drug-using youth are drug free, they need regular follow-up drug tests to ensure that they remain drug free.

Drug testing in the schools is not only controversial, but when it has been proposed it has been widely opposed, and when it has been tried it has suffered legally at the hands of judges in all parts of the country. Few educators have talked about drug testing students, not because large numbers of children do not use drugs but simply out of a practical decision that this is not a politically workable idea. I have focused extensively on the idea of routine drug testing in the schools because it is such a good idea if a community is serious about stopping drug abuse before it begins.

The fact that the idea of drug testing in the schools has fared so poorly tells more about the political state of drug abuse prevention than it does about the merits of the idea itself. Too many people are frightened by or hostile to drug testing. Too many people deny the deadly impact of teenage drug use. Too many people believe that some level of illicit drug use is normal and reasonably safe for kids and that tough sanctions against drug use by kids is unfair or even cruel. Too many people believe that educational efforts can prevent drug use. No matter how innovative and clever, drug education is only weakly effective in reducing the use of alcohol, tobacco, or other drugs among teenagers. In the United States we have two decades of expensive experience to prove that point.

Unfortunately, drug testing schoolchildren, as they are now tested for other health problems, is not likely to be tried beyond a few private schools, and even there the interest in drug testing is limited. That means that parents and others who are concerned about the possible drug use of children will have to negotiate the troubled waters of teenage vulnerability to drug abuse on their own without the guidance and support of the school and the community when it comes to drug tests. For more active, responsible parents with low-risk children, this is not a great problem. For parents with high-risk children, and for parents who are not active in protecting their children from drug abuse, the passivity and tolerance of the society are the major problems that fuel the continuing drug abuse epidemic.

The same argument for universal drug testing coupled with tough sanctions for illicit drug use could have been made here with equal force, and equal futility, about many other areas of contemporary life in North America. Why not make drug testing a requirement for getting a driver's license or a license to practice medicine? Denial of the serious problems caused by drug abuse and the misunderstanding of drug tests have coupled with concerns for the costs of such programs and their legal vulnerability to take these options out of consideration today. I write in the hope that tomorrow we will be better able to think about these options and to find practical, affordable ways to use them to save lives.

This concern about the failure of adults to help kids stop using drugs by getting tough about youthful illegal drug use (including the routine use of drug tests for kids) is not limited to the abuse of illicit drugs, such as marijuana, cocaine, and heroin. It extends also to the prevention of the use of alcohol and tobacco, which is illegal for children. The minimum drinking age today in the United States is 21, and the minimum smoking age is 18.

Who is enforcing the criminal laws against drinking and smoking by youth? Far more needs to be done to enforce the laws against the sale of alcohol and tobacco to youth. Every seller of these substances needs to be held accountable for each sale to be sure that alcohol and tobacco are not sold to youth. Similarly, youth need to be strongly punished for attempting to buy alcohol and tobacco and for using fake identification cards that falsify their ages. The same forces of denial and inertia that handicap potential strong efforts to curb the use of illicit drugs also handicap efforts to combat the underage use of alcohol and tobacco. For now, teachers, parents, and public health officials concerned with youth must be content to focus on education and creative "jawboning" approaches to these vital health problems. On the other hand, drug testing can now be made available to parents on a case-by-case basis by knowledgeable physicians.

Although conflicts remain about drug testing in schools, including questions about the costs and the most appropriate responses to positive tests, in 1995 the U.S. Supreme Court ruled decisively that drug tests were constitutionally permitted in public schools. I was the expert in the original case that formed the basis for the Supreme Court ruling. The testing program in Vernonia, Oregon, involved student athletes who were tested at the start of the school year and then subsequently during the year on a random basis. In that program, positive urine tests indicating illicit drug use led to parental notification and evaluation for treatment as well as suspension from athletic competition until the student was drug free. This was a nonpunitive, community-based intervention with the goal of preventing drug problems before they started by giving student athletes another good reason not to use drugs.

Educational approaches to drug abuse prevention do work, as shown by the long-term drops in the rates of drug use documented in Chapter 3. Those statistics also show that the use of these addicting substances by youth not only remains high, despite the best efforts for two decades to talk youth out of these unhealthy habits, but that use of some drugs is now increasing. A central point of this book is that the use of rewarding chemicals is supported by powerful biological forces that affect people unevenly, with some people biologically at higher risk than others. Furthermore, the environment in which youth decide to use or not to use addicting substances plays a powerful role in establishing the rate at which these chemicals are used in any population. The more tolerant the environment, the greater the use of addicting substances.

Admittedly, drug testing coupled with sanctions is strong medicine, but after nearly a quarter of a century working with the problems of addiction, I believe it is the best way to prevent drug use for many people who are highly vulnerable to the lure of addicting drugs. Tests and sanctions will not end the problem of addiction. They need to be coupled with treatment and the use of 12-step programs. But routine drug tests and sanctions make clear, in practical and real ways, that the community is serious about combating addiction and helping young people. Drug testing teenagers is a good way to use the environmental approach to addiction in order to prevent initial drug use, to raise bottoms for addicted people, and to save lives.

Although I do not find privacy arguments persuasive against drug tests in many settings, including in the public schools, I am sensitive to concern for the potential costs of routine drug tests. Drug testing in any setting needs to be balanced by careful cost-benefit calculations. Even in these low-risk settings, cost considerations justify relatively infrequent drug tests. In these settings, drug tests are needed to act as a deterrent to nonmedical drug use, even if the tests are conducted relatively infrequently.

Customs officers at national borders cannot search every incoming passenger's baggage for contraband materials, including drugs being smuggled into the country. Inspections cannot be conducted on every piece of luggage because of the costs and the delays such universal scrutiny would create. The reason to use discretion in selecting only some bags for inspection is not a matter of civil rights or privacy, it is a matter of practicality. The same is true for urine tests in low-risk environments. Tests can be infrequent, but everyone needs to know that they could be tested at any time, just as all travelers know they may have their luggage checked when they enter the country. Without that potential for testing, however infrequently it is done, the deterrent value is lost. Similarly, the fact that customs officers could choose to search any person or piece of baggage is a powerful deterrent to all would-be drug smugglers. The desirable social goal for drug smuggling and for illicit drug use is to pull back the denial that permits criminal behaviors to continue. That is a big step in raising the bottoms for drug users. Wider use of drug testing is the cornerstone of effective environmental prevention programs.

Some readers will think that this vision of the future is shocking and even repugnant, comparing it to George Orwell's *1984,* a totalitarian nightmare. I understand these opinions because they were my opinions 20 years ago. The well-meaning approach of opposing wider use of drug tests indirectly supports tolerance for nonmedical drug use. This more tolerant approach assumes that education and information can solve the problems of drug abuse prevention for youth. Education and information about drug-caused problems, and the new drug refusal skills training approach to prevention, do work. The modern parents' education and support programs to help parents team up to keep their children drug free also work. I strongly support these valuable programs.

However, under the best of circumstances and with the best available educational approaches, too many high-risk youth will continue to fall victim to nonmedical drug use. Attempting to solve the drug problem by education alone is similar to solving the problem of airline hijacking by relying only on education and information. Such an approach has value, but it is not good enough to protect the public interests without searches and strict sanctions. Educating people to wear seat belts and not to speed is a good idea, but many people will not wear seat belts or avoid speeding on the highways without the strong arm of the law. So it is with drug abuse prevention in the modern world.

In the early 1970s the central controversy in drug abuse prevention was the use of methadone treatment. Ten years later the central controversy was the decriminalization of marijuana. In the late 1980s the central controversy was the use of drug tests in the workplace. In the 1990s the issue will be the wider application of drug tests, linked to serious consequences, in all aspects of modern life, from going to school, to driving a car, to getting a license to practice medicine. The criminal justice system is especially in need of universal drug testing linked to tough consequences for positive test results.

Although I advocate an early intervention approach that includes drug tests and sanctions, this approach is not absolutely necessary given that addiction is a progressive, incurable, and potentially fatal disease. Such early interventions are not required because addiction just keeps getting worse so that, sooner or later, interventions cannot be avoided. A more tolerant and permissive approach will work, although it will produce lower bottoms and ultimately higher costs. Addicted people then will have to get worse before they confront their addictions. They and those who care about them will have to suffer more before interventions take place and recovery begins. Arguments for raising bottoms are expressions of humane concern. They are efforts to confront addiction earlier, before the prices paid become unnecessarily high.

I have come to these views slowly and reluctantly, during more than two decades of painful dealings with addiction. I no longer think it helps drug users to allow them to continue nonmedical drug use, because I have seen the awful consequences of letting the drug dependence syndrome play itself out. Addiction is modern chemical slavery. Uncompromising antiaddiction actions are the first step in modern emancipation.

This long discussion of drug testing of teenagers is not meant to imply that drug testing linked to sanctions is the only thing young people need to avoid drug use. There is a wide range of good new prevention ideas being used in schools in all parts of the world. One of the most constructive new approaches is the Student Assistance Program (SAP) modeled on the Employee Assistance Program (EAP) in the workplace. SAPs are small organizations within schools that bring together counselors, teachers, parents, and community experts to help students and their families cope better with a wide range of problems, including addiction. SAPs help families sort out many problems and find appropriate and affordable community resources to deal with them. SAPs also help students and families use 12-step programs when that is appropriate. SAPs provide an expertise about addiction and other problems that is beyond the capability of most teachers and counselors.

New Ideas to Deal With Alcohol and Tobacco

It is not only when it comes to the illicit drugs that new ideas are needed to make our families and communities more resistant to addiction. Outright prohibition throughout society is impractical for either alcohol or tobacco, so new ideas need to be found that fall short of total prohibition but that, nevertheless, reduce the use of alcohol and tobacco and thereby reduce the high social costs created by these substances. It is unwise to treat either alcohol or tobacco as routine items of commerce. Instead, additional taxes and restrictions of their sale and use need to be applied.

When it comes to tobacco, there has been a major, positive change in social attitude in North America over the past two decades as the acceptability of smoking tobacco has diminished in many public and private places. It is widely recognized that there is no safe dose of cigarettes, so the modern public health goal is a smokeless society. How that goal can be achieved without total legal prohibition of tobacco use is hard to imagine. The most recent increase in the levels of use of tobacco by high school students makes clear that efforts at education and persuasion are insufficient. Especially when it comes to youth, prohibition is exactly what is needed. The legal age for smoking cigarettes needs to be raised from 18 to 21. We need family, school, and community policies that enforce the zero-tolerance standard when it comes to smoking by youth under the age of 21. The zero-tolerance standard for tobacco use, including smokeless tobacco, needs to be enforced with drug tests and tough sanctions, including the denial of drivers' licenses and participation in extracurricular activities for youth who use tobacco.

Alcohol also needs to be the target of new efforts to curtail use, especially drinking by youth under 21 and heavy drinking by adults. The guidelines contained in Chapter 9 of this book provide a standard against which alcohol use can be judged. In the workplace and on the highway, the zero-tolerance standard needs to be enforced when it comes to alcohol use by adults and youth.

The major institutions in society need to continue trends to restrict the use of both alcohol and tobacco, limiting the use by adults to private homes. Public education about the harmful effects of both alcohol and tobacco use needs to become more common and more graphic.

Of all the new ideas for dealing with alcohol and tobacco, the most urgent is to help youth grow up free of the use of either substance. Alcohol and tobacco are the leading gateway drugs into the drug dependence syndrome in all parts of the world. By simply delaying the age at which people choose to use either alcohol or tobacco, the rates of use will fall sharply. Once people reach the age of 21, they are far less likely to initiate the use of either alcohol or tobacco, or of any other drug. It is unrealistic to think that curtailing tobacco or alcohol advertising would have a large effect on the rates of use by young people. It is equally unrealistic to think that education and peer refusal teaching can have more than a marginal effect on the rates of use by youth. This is shown by the continuing high levels of the use of drugs by North American youth and the most recent rise in the rates of use of some illicit drugs.

The only way that youth are going to stop using alcohol and tobacco is for families, schools, physicians, and others who deal with youth to get serious about the prohibition against their use that now exists in law in North America, but which is almost never enforced. The first line of defense against alcohol and tobacco use, as well as against the use of other illegal drugs, is the family. Families need to be empowered and encouraged to take whatever actions are necessary to ensure that their children do not use alcohol or tobacco. To leave such decisions to children is to leave the large majority of youth to the untender mercies of the selfish brain.

Medicines Versus Drugs: Safer Use of Potentially Addicting Substances in Medical Practice

The final area of public policy to be dealt with in this chapter is use of medicines that have addictive potentials. The basic social contract for drug use makes clear that physicians need to be able to prescribe, and patients need to be able to use, medicines that have addictive potentials as part of responsible medical care.

For such an approach to work, doctors, patients, and families need to have guidelines for the recognition of addiction and to be honest with each other about these treatments. The Controlled Substances Act (CSA) and related international treaties establish which medicines are potentially addicting. Patients need to recognize this distinction and to be open with their families and their doctors about their use of potentially addicting medicines. For patients who do not have a preexisting history of addiction to alcohol and other drugs, the use of these medicines poses little risk, although the risk is not zero. If the patient escalates the dose beyond the usual therapeutic level, and especially if the patient obtains these medicines from more than one physician or from physicians who are not fully informed about the patient's use of these substances, then serious addiction can occur.

Distinctions must be made between the appropriate medical use of controlled substances and the illegal, nonmedical use of these substances. These distinctions can be clouded by misunderstanding the role of physical dependence. Any substance taken repeatedly can produce a simple cellular adaptation so that the body reacts to abrupt discontinuation by experiencing "withdrawal symptoms." Most addicted people do not experience withdrawal on abrupt discontinuation, meaning that they are not physically dependent. Some medical patients do show withdrawal symptoms on abrupt discontinuation of their medicines.

Addiction is a malignant lifelong disease of the entire self. Physical dependence is a benign cellular adaptation to the presence of a substance, which can occur after prolonged use of medicines other than controlled substances, such as antidepressant and antihypertensive medicines. The following boxes distinguish between medical use and nonmedical use and between physical dependence and addiction. These concepts are useful to physicians, patients, and family members, as well as to regulatory and legal authorities.

The universal antidote to addiction is honesty. If the patient remains honest with the family and the doctor, the risks of addiction are low and easily managed. It is important that patients who use controlled substances not be subject to harassment or made to feel guilty about their appropriate, medical use of these medicines in the name of tough-minded addiction prevention. It is especially important that law enforcement and regulatory agencies

Distinguishing Medical From Nonmedical Use

	Medical Use	Nonmedical Use
Intent	To treat a diagnosed illness	To party
Effect	Improves the user's life	Harms the user's life
Pattern	Sensible, low dose	Chaotic, high dose
Control	Shared with physician	Self-controlled
Legality	Legal	Illegal (except alcohol use by adults)

not intervene in medical practice in ways that have a chilling effect on proper medical care. It is also important that patients themselves and their families do not avoid the use of effective medical treatments because of misplaced fear of addiction.

The Twelve-Step Solution

Whether dealing with addiction in the workplace, in the criminal justice system, in families, or in schools, the most effective way to help people overcome the problems of addiction is to help them find their ways to the 12-step programs of Alcoholics Anonymous and the myriad programs modeled on it as discussed in Chapter 11. It is important, when thinking of new ideas to combat addiction, to encourage everyone to learn more about addiction and

Physical Dependence Versus Addiction

Physical Dependence

- Reversal of substance's effects on abrupt discontinuation
- Not a disease but a simple cellular adaptation to the presence of substance
- Treatment is gradual dose reduction

Addiction

- Loss of control (unmanageability of life)
- Denial (dishonesty)
- Incurable disease of the entire self
- Treatment is lifelong recovery

to reach out a helping hand to addicted people and their families. A cold, rejecting, moralistic rejection of addicted people is never the right answer either in personal life or in institutions that deal with people. No addict is hopeless. Genuine concern and caring can make a difference, once that caring is protected from becoming enabling by a recognition of the potentially fatal disease of addiction.

In this chapter, we have explored only a few of the new proposals for modification of contemporary drug and alcohol policies. You now have the tools to think about all of the proposals you will meet in the future. Many readers will reach conclusions about the best way to proceed that are different from those I have reached. I respect that diversity of views. I am mindful that the problem of addiction—as is stated in AA's "Big Book," *Alcoholics Anonymous*—is truly "cunning, baffling, and powerful," and that no ideas, old or new, will solve or end the problem of addiction to alcohol and other drugs. Addiction is with us, both individually and collectively, forever. The questions we all face are not how to rid ourselves of addiction but how to learn from addiction so that we can reduce the burdens addiction imposes to the lowest feasible levels in ourselves, our families, and our communities.

The major conclusion that I have reached after many false starts looking for new ideas for community-wide prevention is that the social signals—the values that are expressed in the basic social contract for drug use—are not only widely understood and of great importance but that attempts to soften them are perceived by many people to be signs that illicit drug use is socially acceptable or even "almost legal." Therefore, any proposal that can be seen as being tolerant of illicit drug use is potentially damaging to the will of individuals, families, and communities to resist the seductions of addicting drugs. Given the vulnerability to addiction that is hardwired into the human brain, it is important that antiaddiction software be kept in good working order and updated periodically to ensure that it works as well as it can to reduce the risk of addiction in the modern world.

Case Histories

The following case histories illustrate the different faces of addiction. Jan's story illustrates the power and complexity of the disease of addiction. She was unaware of the brain mechanisms underlying her behavioral problems; she simply reacted to the insistence of her selfish brain ("more, now"), which demanded the stimulation of its pleasure centers. Jan showed the sometimes confusing picture of addiction to medically prescribed controlled substances. Although many people, and even many physicians (both by prescribing addicting drugs to addicted people and by mislabeling nonaddicted medical patients as addicts), confuse appropriate medical treatment with addiction, it is my hope that no reader of this book will make that mistake.

Mary lost her fiancé to his prosocial and powerful addiction to competitive athletics. Mary's case shows some of the extensive range of human experiences that are affected by the loss of control over pleasurable activities and the value and the generalizability of the understanding of addiction.

Sally's story illustrates the frightening potential consequences that can result from the absence of policies and procedures for the use of alcohol and other drugs in the workplace.

Jan

A psychiatrist called asking for my help with a difficult case. He had been treating a nurse, Jan, who had a painful back as well as chronic depression and anxiety. He thought that she needed to use an antianxiety medicine, such as Valium, but other doctors had raised questions about this treatment. The psychiatrist asked my help, saying, "You are not hostile to the use of these medicines when they are needed." I agreed to see the patient, feeling confident that there had been a misunderstanding and that I could simply support the psychiatrist in his judgment. I looked forward to helping both Jan and her obviously well-meaning therapist.

Jan told me that she had seen her psychiatrist during the previous 4 years, more or less once a week. She had never asked for medicines from him, including Valium, and he had not prescribed any. She had been "caught" at her work as an intensive care nurse stealing controlled substances from her patients for her own use. She assured me that in the particular instance for which she was being investigated she was innocent, but she added that "plenty of other times, which they know nothing about, I did take narcotics, stimulants, and antianxiety medicines to inject into myself." Jan also said she had been sent to an addiction treatment program a year ago but had signed herself out within a few days because the treatment seemed inappropriate to her. "I don't consider myself to be a drug addict because I don't use the drugs every day," she said.

I told Jan that I considered her to be a drug addict and that she should go to an addiction program immediately. I also suggested that she regularly attend Narcotics Anonymous meetings and that right now she should turn herself in voluntarily to her hospital's impaired health care workers program. She was shocked by these recommendations and rejected them. I called her psychiatrist and said it would be unwise to prescribe Valium or any other controlled substance to Jan and that he should do whatever he could to see that she got treatment for her addiction. I pointed out to him that she was not an anxious patient in need of an antianxiety medicine or a pain patient in need of narcotics but that she was a run-of-the-mill desperate drug addict who happened to be a nurse. Jan had lied to him for 4 years in confidential psychotherapy about her drug use. She had never told him of her pattern of stealing drugs from her patients, until she almost got caught and wanted his help, not to get well but to get more drugs.

A month later I got a call from another psychiatrist to whom Jan's psychiatrist had referred her after he, too, rejected my advice. The new doctor took a different approach from the one I took. He referred Jan to a physician, an expert in chronic pain, who prescribed methadone for her chronic back pain on the condition that she go to an expert in addiction treatment for urine monitoring to ensure that she did not continue to use drugs other than methadone. This treatment is in clear violation of the rules governing the treatment of addiction, which prohibit physicians from prescribing methadone or other narcotics to drug addicts in the treatment of their addiction, except as part of a licensed narcotics treatment program. The doctors justified their unorthodox actions by saying that Jan did have chronic back pain (which they felt justified her use of methadone as an analgesic) and that the drug testing would ensure that she did not abuse other medicines.

The doctors agreed with her that she could stop drug use if they gave her the methadone and that she did not need addiction treatment. They also agreed that her career was in jeopardy if she turned herself in at her hospital as a drug addict. Based on my experience I strongly disagreed, but I figured they needed to find out for themselves the hard way, as I had over the years, just how tenacious addiction is and how vital it is to be open and honest if one is to recover.

Mary

Mary, a 30-year-old beauty queen, brought her fiancé to me. She was a cheerleader for the Washington Redskins, an impressive and beautiful person. Her fiancé, Rick, was a triathlete who competed at high levels in the combined running, biking, and swimming contests held in various parts of the country. She complained that all Rick did was train. He also went to his job as a senior government worker 5 days a week, but he found little pleasure in it. Rick stayed at work as little as possible. He had little time for Mary or anything else because his training schedule called for him to work out 4 or more hours, 7 days a week.

When we got into the issues of their relationship, Rick was quick to admit that his major love was training and competing. In truth, he did not care much for Mary or anyone else and could not imagine that situation ever changing unless he got injured (read, "hit bottom"). Therapy for this couple became a matter of helping Mary give up on Rick before she married him. She was never going to win that competition because he already had a lover, his training and competing, in his life before he met her.

Sally

I was giving a talk about drug testing in the workplace to a group of lawyers a couple of years ago. A woman I will call Sally came up to me afterward with a sad story she did not want to share with the others at the meeting. She said she was the chief counsel for a large national hospital chain. She had received an emergency call from a nurse at one of their hospitals, who said: "I am calling from a phone booth outside an operating room. The surgeon who is about to do this case is drunk. What should I do?"

It did not take Sally long to answer, "Do what you would ordinarily do, and hope for the best." I was shocked and asked, "Why did you tell her that?" Her answer was simple and direct: "I figured we were less likely to be sued by the patient for malpractice than we were to be sued by the surgeon for harming his career. We have no policy for handling such cases, so there was no procedure for the nurse to follow. Whenever we have tried to institute a policy, our medical staffs object." I asked what happened to the patient in the story. Sally replied, "I don't know. The nurse never called back."

Chapter 13

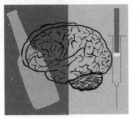

The Future of
Addiction

*Addiction is growing worldwide, but so are understanding
and realistic hopes for both prevention and recovery. These
hopes are the subjects of our final chapter.*

*T*his book is about the terrors of addiction, the wonders of

recovery, and the mysteries of both. In this final chapter we look

back on the territory explored and speculate about where

the new, rapidly growing field of addiction is headed over the remaining years of the 20th century. I am a doctor, not a historian. I am a clinician, not a writer. If my view of the past is limited, my capacity to see the future is even more restricted. What follows is offered with humility but also with awe because I know that addiction is a profoundly important window on the human experience. By learning from addiction we can grow as individuals, as families, and as communities.

A Positive View of the Future

This examination of addiction offers glimpses of a better future for many people. Out of the suffering of addiction have come marvelous responses, the most important of which are the 12-step fellowships. In addition, there have been many valuable community responses to addiction, including Mothers Against Drunk Driving (MADD), the parents movement, and the new efforts to make schools and workplaces drug free. My hope for the future is that MADD will increasingly focus on preventing teenage drug and alcohol use in addition to their focus on preventing impaired driving. Individuals who confront addiction not only regain the control of their lives made unmanageable by nonmedical drug use, but they also develop a new sense of the meaning of life and a new capacity to form caring and healthy relationships.

The same can be said for families and social institutions. Once the slavery of addiction is faced honestly and without fear, there are many options to reduce problems caused by addiction and to enhance the institutions themselves. The Employee Assistance Programs (EAPs) in the workplace are an excellent example of constructive responses to addiction. Originally focused on alcohol problems in the workplace, today's EAPs have been broadened to include other drug problems and a wide range of human difficulties, from mental health disorders to gambling and financial problems. EAPs in the workplace not only help reduce problems with alcohol and other drugs but also provide a good way for the workplace to identify and help solve a broad range of serious human problems.

Many more victims will be claimed throughout the world by

the modern plague of addiction to alcohol and other drugs in the coming decade and well beyond, regardless of the efforts that are made to combat addiction. To be human is to be susceptible to addiction. One does not have to be bad or defective to become addicted. All one has to do is to use drugs, to try them. The selfish brain takes over from there. The more individuals, families, and communities can accept our shared human vulnerability to addiction, including the often cruel diversity of relative risk, the better.

Future Directions of the Drug Abuse Epidemic

The severity of the drug epidemic in the last three decades ensures that the cultural forces favoring tolerance for drug use will be under pressure in all parts of the world for at least the next decade. Although it is unlikely that any nation will promote the use of currently illegal drugs within the foreseeable future, the global rise in modern values and modern lifestyles ensures that the levels of the use of addicting drugs will rise in most of the world in a relentless fashion for a long time to come.

As the growing intolerance for nonmedical drug use begins to shrink the illicit drug market in some subpopulations in developed nations, especially in mature middle-class North America, the illicit drug market will increase in nations and in communities that are less well defended against drug traffickers. Eastern Europe, the former Soviet Union, and especially the developing nations of the world are the primary targets for expansion of the illicit drug markets in the next decade. Today 80% of the world's population lives in developing nations. In the next decade, these nations will experience 95% of the world's population growth. The developing nations are also the most vulnerable places on earth to addiction in the next decade.

Another trend for the future is increased use of drug tests. When an employer institutes drug tests, it forces addicted workers either to stop nonmedical drug use or to move to employers that do not conduct drug tests. As drug tests in the community become more widespread, drug abusers are increasingly concentrated in those organizations that do not do tests.

Decreased social tolerance for nonmedical drug use and increased use of drug tests in all of the developed nations increasingly will pull back the curtain of denial and expose more and more addicts to the dominant antidrug values of their societies. A growing awareness that life, liberty, and the pursuit of happiness do not include the nonmedical use of illicit drugs is essential for survival of individuals, communities, and nations as the 20th century comes to an end. This will mean pulling back some of the protections of privacy now provided to drug abusers by those who are deeply devoted to the principles of individual liberty.

In the 1970s, the threat of terrorism in the air led to worldwide agreement that privacy had to be limited somewhat to protect airline passengers. Airport searches, which used modern technology, were entirely new experiences. Today, air travelers in all parts of the world must be searched for guns and explosives. This search, without individual probable cause, has not raised a cry of violated civil liberties, as about 3 million people are searched each day of the year.

Are drug tests a more threatening search for the citizens of the modern global village? I do not believe that being searched before I get on an airplane violates my rights to privacy and, after 20 years of being drug tested as a routine part of my employment, neither do I believe that drug testing is a violation of my privacy. We need nonmedical drug detectors placed so widely throughout our communities that people would not consider using illicit drugs any more than they would consider getting on an airplane with bombs or guns.

A Tragic but Unavoidable Reality

There is a dark side to my view of the future of addiction in the modern world. There are many individuals, many families, and entire communities that will not accept antiaddiction values. They helplessly will live out the imperatives of the selfish brain's hardware without the benefit of the new and more effective antiaddiction software. Theirs is a terrible journey of self-discovery from which many travelers do not return alive.

Some who take this dangerous path into addiction to alcohol and other drugs, led by the demands of their selfish brains, are handicapped by their own biology, which makes them especially attracted to the siren call of addictive substances. Some are handicapped by family and community environments that are relatively permissive of alcohol and drug use. Some have other mental and physical problems that make them especially vulnerable to addiction. Some people with mental illness, such as bipolar disorder, schizophrenia, and antisocial personality disorder, engage in impulsive behaviors. They are especially vulnerable to addiction, a disease associated with reward now and pain later. Of course, many people with all types of psychiatric diagnoses are not reckless or impulsive. They are no more, and no less, vulnerable to addiction than are any other people in the society. It is impulsiveness and recklessness that lead to addiction.

A person who lacks personal recklessness may develop panic disorder and turn to alcohol for temporary relief, just as a depressed person may turn to amphetamines or cocaine for relief. If that person lacks the unique biological vulnerability for addiction, and if that person lacks the recklessness of character disorder, then the brush with addictive drugs usually will be short-lived because they are not effective treatments for these disorders. Not only do these nonmedical drugs not work in the long run, they produce many problems of their own, including anxiety and depression. If, on the other hand, the person suffering from a psychiatric diagnosis does have a strong pattern of recklessness and a biological vulnerability to addiction, this brush with addicting drugs may be the start of a long-term career as an alcoholic or drug addict.

In addition, there are people who have great success, whose belief that they are above or beyond normal human vulnerability also places them at high risk of addiction. This added risk is seen in sports figures, entertainers, and the winners in financial markets. All of them, like some of the poor and some of those suffering from mental disorders that promote impulsiveness, are at added risk of using, and therefore of falling in love with, addicting drugs. The similarity between society's winners and society's losers in addiction risk underlines the fact that addiction to alcohol and other drugs is an equal opportunity destroyer.

Some people who are at high risk for addiction have inadequate human support networks, which makes them more susceptible to the powerful, immediate reinforcement of alcohol and other drugs. Some people live in communities already overwhelmed by the devastating effects of addiction. In these communities, addiction is a malignant, multigenerational disease. In a vicious cycle, the more these communities deteriorate, the more the people living in them become addicted to alcohol and other drugs. And the more they use alcohol and other drugs, the more their fabric of social supports deteriorates.

The tragic escalation of this destructive cycle is common in many parts of North America today. People in these communities are especially likely to be victimized as their selfish brains are tyrannized by addicting drugs. Many of the people who are most concerned about the welfare of people in these suffering communities are dedicated to resisting the use of drug tests linked to tough sanctions as a way of helping addicted people in these communities. They actively fend off the forces that can act to reduce the use of alcohol and other drugs in the name of protecting the privacy and dignity of the members of these communities.

The risk of addiction is related to both genetics and the environment. In many impoverished communities in North America, there is an increasing concentration of those who are genetically vulnerable to addiction, and of environments that are either tolerant to addiction or ineffective in curbing it. One of the major reasons that people become poor is addiction. One of the ways people escape poverty is by overcoming addiction. Today in North America there is an inescapable but horrifying sorting going on, as those who are addicted to the nonmedical use of alcohol and other drugs tend to move into poverty and, once there, to be increasingly victimized by their own and their neighbors' addiction.

A Silver Lining

This dark cloud has a silver lining. Addiction can provide a valuable wake-up call to individuals, families, and communities. Religions have a long history of finding their most eager and enduring converts in those communities that are the most afflicted by addiction to alcohol and other drugs. It is certain that in the next decade there will be more and better efforts of many religions to reach into the communities hardest hit by addiction to help them overcome this most solvable of the many causes of poverty, violence, and social disorganization.

The path to recovery from addiction is reasonably well recognized. The limiting factor today is the will to follow it. That path is lowered social tolerance for illicit drug use, in families and in community institutions. This lowered tolerance for illicit drug use needs to be imposed through drug testing coupled with strong consequences, especially within the agencies most powerfully influencing the lives of people affected by addiction to alcohol and other drugs. These agencies include the criminal justice system and the welfare and disability systems, as well as public housing and public schools. When social institutions raise the bottoms for nonmedical drug use, more people will seek to overcome addiction and use the ladders around them to climb not only out of addiction but also out of poverty and spiritual degradation.

This same determination to raise the bottoms for illicit drug users needs to be extended in all other areas of community life, including the sports, entertainment, financial, and medical communities. In these areas, the most remarkable development over the past decade has been the use of drug testing in Olympic and professional athletics. This approach, now universally accepted in all parts of the world, is a valuable model to all of us who are not world-class athletes. We can learn about addiction and its consequences through the modern mass media. We can learn from the preventive efforts applied in sports at the highest levels with drug tests and tough sanctions.

More is needed than just raising the bottoms in hard-hit communities, as it is for all addicted people. The way to recovery needs to be identified; usable road maps to overcome addiction need to be widely available. For most addicted people, that way to recovery will be through membership in one of the 12-step fellowships. Many religions help answer the fundamental questions posed by addiction: the questions of what life means and how people can best relate to one another. Religion can rarely solve the problem of addiction without a specific recovery program such as AA or NA but, once recovery is under way, religion is, for some addicted people in recovery, a vital part of living a better life.

With respect to the abuse of alcohol and other drugs, we each face the potential with weighted factors. We are not all equal. Many people who escape the ravages of addiction would like to believe that it is because they have virtue that is not possessed by those who succumb to addiction. Although this sometimes is the case, more often there are forces in our lives over which we have no control, and often little knowledge, that put us at either high risk or low risk of addiction. One should feel no more virtuous for avoiding the problems of addiction than one should feel guilty for catching this modern plague.

Two Truths About Prevention of Addiction

The first and most important truth is that if you do not use addicting substances nonmedically, you cannot get addicted to them. In the final analysis, the drug problem is a one that must be faced by drug users and potential drug users—one person at a time, one day at a time. The focus of all efforts to prevent and treat addiction to alcohol and other drugs comes down to individual people making highly personal choices. The consequences of these choices are often life and death, and they spread out to affect families and communities far beyond the individuals who make the choices.

Nevertheless, the opportunity for preventive action lies within the individual who chooses each day to use or not to use alcohol and other drugs. That is where the rubber meets the road. No community program can change that fact. Sadly, many of the people, families, and institutions that are the most well meaning in our societies are helping addiction to flourish by their unwitting enabling behaviors. This risk is one of the major dangers that each person must face and cannot escape. A seemingly loving community and a seemingly loving family, when in the grip of denial, are part of the problem of addiction and not part of the solution.

The second important truth about prevention is that if you remain honest, you cannot become addicted to alcohol and other drugs because the forces in all communities that reject addiction ultimately will confront you with so much pressure that either you will have to become a liar or you will have to give up your use of alcohol or other drugs before you develop a major problem. Only by using the addicting substances nonmedically in the first place, and then only by lying about your use of them and the consequences of that use, can you become addicted. The road to dishonesty, or as it is more charitably called, denial, is often paved with good community and family intentions and is easily traveled by those who find pleasure in the use of addicting drugs. For people infatuated with the highs of alcohol and other drugs, dishonesty is as natural as eating. A family or a community that condones or excuses nonmedical drug use and dishonesty is a suffering family or community.

There is real and valuable learning down the painful road of addiction. The lessons learned at such high cost by addicts and their families are applicable not only to those who travel that road but to all people. Those lessons point us back to sound values that are available to everyone. Addiction is both endlessly mysterious and utterly understandable.

The world will see big increases in the addiction to alcohol and other drugs in future decades as the world's population of 5.5 billion human beings grows by an additional 1 billion in each of the next few decades. An ever larger percentage of the people in the world will be exposed to addicting substances in environments that are increasingly anonymous and permissive of individual control over behavior. The North American experience with addiction over the past 100 years predicts the future of the world. There will be furious battles for the hearts and minds of people in all parts of the world with respect to the use of alcohol and other drugs, as well as tobacco. The stakes are high. The issues are complex and controversial. Good options are available, but they are not easy for many people to accept and to use.

In all parts of the world, there are strong legal, religious, and cultural counteractions to the increasing threat of addiction, but these are frustrated by the powerful forces of the selfish brain, by the increasingly permissive values in modern life, and by the tremendous economic incentives for wider use of addicting drugs. The global market for these drugs is already large, and it will increase dramatically in the coming years. The global market in illegal drugs is more than $100 billion a year and growing rapidly. Every day more people are joining the lucrative criminal narcotics traffic industry in all parts of the world. These people, for personal economic reasons, will spread the supply of addicting chemicals to every corner of the globe in their search for money.

Narcotics trafficking has a corrosive impact both on law enforcement and on political processes. It is associated closely with the marketing of illegal guns and with the corruption of legal and political authorities. Today more than one-third of the world's illicit drug supply finds its way to, or originates in, North America. It is likely that this percentage will fall in the next decade as the global market for illicit drugs expands far faster than the market in North America.

Developing Nations, Drug Traffic, and Higher Education

Over a decade ago, I saw firsthand the impact of the global narcotics traffic on Culiacán, a midsized town in western Mexico. It was a model of what happens when narcotics trafficking takes hold of a local economy. Opium poppies and marijuana were newly grown in large-scale operations in this lovely area. The drugs were sent into the international market, mostly destined for the voracious appetites of drug addicts in the United States. The local economy in Culiacán then was booming as people had more money than they had ever seen before. I spoke with one middle-class woman who could not find a maid. She told me,

> My maid of the past 10 years quit. She asked for an unpaid vacation last summer. When she came back, she owned a slightly used Chevrolet and announced that she had joined the narcotraffic. She worked for me for a few more weeks and then left, saying she could make a lot more money working for the traffickers.

Every day there were several murders in the small town's streets. Ordinary people walked through town with guns to protect themselves. The wealthier citizens of Culiacán traveled outside only with bodyguards carrying machine guns. People were afraid to send their children to school or to go to a movie because of the random violence. A businessman told me he had lost heart when the Rotary Club was taken over by the narcotraffickers.

As a representative of the United States government, I flew over the opium and marijuana fields in a helicopter, observing small, carefully tended plots growing both marijuana and opium in the arid mountainous terrain. When the leading candidate for president of Mexico visited Culiacán a few weeks later, during the election season, the local people, who had benefited economically beyond their greatest hopes from the sudden boom produced by narcotrafficking, pleaded with the politician to help end the narcotraffic. Although narcotics traffic had made them all rich, their lives had become unlivable, frightening nightmares dominated by criminal violence. Illicit riches had turned this stable and relatively poor town into a sort of modern Dodge City of the Wild West. Home had suddenly become a dangerous place governed by bullets and gangsters.

At about the same time, I visited the opium-growing fields of the Golden Triangle in northwest Thailand and saw remote villagers take the international money given for "crop substitution," which was intended to encourage new crops such as strawberries, corn, and coffee to replace their large-scale opium cultivation. The local communities took this money and grew the new, highly subsidized crops, and then just kept right on growing opium. As a village headman told me,

> Why would we stop growing opium? The money we get for that is far more than for any other crop. We just take the new money and add it to the money we get for opium. New people are coming in here to work all the time since we are doing so well now that we have a new government aid program.

This local leader also said that opium had been grown in that area of Thailand for a long time, but until about 1970 opium was grown in small quantities mostly for the limited local market, to be used by a few addicted sad, old men. But, stimulated by the huge growth in the demand for heroin produced by the flood of American servicemen into nearby Vietnam, their well-established small-scale opium cultivation suddenly became a megabusiness. Opium became the principal source of income in the region. To call opium in the Golden Triangle a "traditional crop" was a misnomer. Opium had been grown there for generations, on a tiny scale. Only in the past 20 years had it become a major crop, a crop that fed the modern global heroin epidemic, not the small and local traditional appetite for opium. Much of that newly grown opium was used in Thailand by addicts in the hill country and by the even larger number of new, young intravenous heroin addicts in Thailand's major cities.

A visit to the coca-growing areas of the Andes gave me the same message. Coca had been grown in those areas for hundreds, if not thousands, of years, but only in the last two decades had coca cultivation become large scale. Ninety-nine percent of the coca was now destined for the illicit global drug traffic. Local, traditional coca leaf use was merely a convenient disguise for denial and neglect of this new and increased cultivation and the illegal cocaine traffic to which it gave rise.

Denial characterized not only local governments in all growing areas but all national governments of both the producing and consuming nations. Sophisticated people used traditional cultivation of coca and local use of coca leaves as a veil to hide from world view the devastating and thoroughly modern tragedy of vast new drug crop cultivation. I saw rain forests on the Amazon side of the Andes being cleared by bulldozers to plant coca bushes. I saw remote Andean villages transformed into dangerous modern crime meccas filled with the most expensive pickup trucks and luxury automobiles as the result of the profits from the explosively growing international drug trade.

After my visits to these and other so-called traditional drug cultivation areas of the world, I realized that drug crop substitution was a losing proposition. What was needed was the eradication, the destruction, of drug crops. The clear message must be given to the growers of illicit drug crops in all parts of the world that their lovingly tended plants will never see a harvest.

Crop substitution on the supply side of the drug abuse equation is the direct analogy of relying on education and treatment on the demand side. These are good ideas, but to depend on them alone without tough sanctions against drug cultivation and drug use is wishful thinking by people who do not understand the power of addiction, a power rooted in the brain and fed by the billions of dollars in the illicit drug market. The generous helping-hand approach of crop substitution, education, and treatment, unless coupled with strong antidrug measures, is no match for the grip of addiction on either the supply side or the demand side of the addiction equation. The same conclusion is always reached, eventually, by the family facing the addiction of one of its members. To think otherwise is not merely to be deluded, it is enabling on a global scale. Wishful thoughts about drugs on the world scene today—despite the good intentions of most of those involved—are an aspect of the disease of addiction, of codependence, reflected in international relations.

Modern societies with long histories of exposure to drugs such as marijuana and opium had developed reasonably effective cultural techniques to contain the damage done by the use of these drugs. Mexico and countries of the Middle East, for example, had long experiences with the use of marijuana or cannabis. Several South American countries had a long exposure to coca leaf chewing. Many Asian countries had long exposure to opium smoking. In general, these societies adapted to the persistence of these drugs by limiting drug use to relatively small percentages of the lower social classes, with the dominant classes showing great contempt for the users of these drugs. Children of more affluent and better educated families in these societies grew up knowing that "people like us do not do things like that." This approach was part of the cultural learning that has taken place over the last hundred years or so in relatively heavily exposed countries.

Within the last two decades, however, this pattern has broken down in an alarming fashion. Widespread alcohol use was carried from North American and European nations to all parts of the world, especially to the cultural elite in other nations where the values of the more economically developed nations have been widely imitated. In particular, the heavy use of alcohol became a marker of sophistication and wealth in developing nations during the last 50 years. Cigarette smoking showed a similar pattern, producing malignant health consequences throughout the world.

During this same period, this already tragic pattern of behavioral contagion, in which some of the worst health practices of the developed nations spread rapidly to developing nations, was compounded in a cruel fashion as highly vulnerable youth from developing countries came to economically developed nations to pursue their educations. Often these students were the best and the brightest youth of the developing nations. Many were the children of the emerging elites in their countries. In North American and European universities, these youth found an unaccustomed freedom of behavior, including a wide exposure to alcohol and other drugs in a value system that glorified the ability to drink excessively and to use illicit drugs freely. These behaviors were seen to be badges of unconventionality and courage in prestigious universities.

The prodrug values had a bad effect on many youth from the economically developed countries. Sad to say, there were many other youth from developed countries to take the places of the youth lost to addiction during their student years. This could not be said for the youth of developing nations who came to these same universities for their educations. They were relatively few in number. Their skills were sorely needed in their home countries. All too many of them dropped out because of addiction to alcohol and other drugs. They returned home, not with valuable new knowledge and experiences, but with drug habits that they exposed to those with whom they had contact at home.

It is ironic that many developing nations that had more or less successfully contained the use of one or two abused drugs by cultural means, limiting that use to a relatively few lower class people, are today finding that their elite youth, in their own universities and in foreign universities, have become the new sources of alcohol and drug abuse contagion, not of the relatively traditional use of single drugs such as marijuana, opium, and coca leaves, but of the modern, high-potency use of the full range of abused drugs.

The Role of Religion in Prevention and Treatment

Religions increasingly will reach into the population groups most affected by addiction to alcohol and other drugs to find converts, as people flee in terror from the consequences, both personal and communal, of addiction. The world, already filled with inequity in many areas including levels of drug use, will become more stratified and unequal as some people will have values and/or brains that are relatively resistant to addiction, and others will be more victimized by addiction.

It is no accident that the modern miracle of recovery, based on the 12-step programs, relies heavily on the spiritual values of honesty and community, replacing the self-centeredness of addiction. Only when recovery has a spiritual foundation does it work, for most addicted people, over a lifetime. In the world beyond North America, in the last decade of the 20th century, it is certain that religion and traditional cultural values will play the dominant role in the efforts to reduce the demand for nonmedical drugs. The North American model of addiction treatment based on medical care and the drug test are unaffordable in much of the rest of the world. Less developed nations to a large extent will be unable to use these approaches in responding to their own addicted populations. They have a compensating advantage, compared with North America. These nations are made up of communities that have more traditional, cohesive, cultural values than do most communities in North America.

Deeply rooted and widely shared values, and the institutions that embody them, will be the major sources of recovery from addiction in developing nations, rather than the medical addiction treatment, which has formed the principal response to the problems of addicted people in North America during the last quarter century. The North American addiction treatment programs' use of 12-step fellowships, with their spiritual foundation, will be a useful bridge to new programs in less developed, more traditional cultures in all parts of the world. Religion will play a major role in both the prevention and treatment of addiction in all parts of the world, especially in developing nations.

For many people, however, faith is not enough either to prevent or to treat addiction to alcohol and other drugs. To be truly effective in preventing addiction, religion needs a clear and effective prohibition against the use of addicting drugs. To help people who are already addicted, religion usually requires the help of the specific recovery programs of Alcoholics Anonymous and Narcotics Anonymous. Without these programs, religions are not accessible, as a realistic matter, to many addicted people as long as they continue to use alcohol and other drugs.

The fact that religion will play a large role in recovery from addiction will be relatively easy for people in more traditional societies to accept. It is unfamiliar and even disturbing to many people in economically developed nations who have grown accustomed to thinking that science and technology can overcome all serious health problems. No matter how rich or sophisticated the individual or the community, the experience of addiction will force a reconsideration of that assumption.

Addiction is a model for modern health problems where behavior—individual choices—is at the root of the disease. As modern medicine becomes increasingly technical and scientific, it is humbled by the realization that individual human choices can produce devastating costs that cannot be prevented by science alone. The spread of AIDS and the role of tobacco in health make this point as clearly as do problems with alcohol and other drugs. To really work, new prevention efforts must be rooted in life-sustaining values, and they must touch everyone, not only those who are easily accessible but the hard-to-reach people I have labeled "high risk," especially impulsive youth and the disadvantaged in society.

Watch what happens in the lives of individuals when they get well from addiction. Watch what happens in the lives of communities when they reduce addiction. You will find that there is a deeply spiritual foundation to the healing process of both successful prevention and successful treatment of addiction. This does not mean that modern science and medicine do not have important, positive roles in both the prevention and the treatment of addiction. It certainly does not mean that sophistication, education, and even technology cannot help people understand and overcome addiction to alcohol and other drugs. But the easily verifiable reality of the spiritual underpinnings of addiction and recovery does mean that addiction is both a biological and a spiritual disease. Getting well and staying well have a great deal to do with personal and community values, which, for most people in all parts of the world, are rooted in religion.

The most fundamental lessons from the North American experience with alcohol and other drugs are applicable and affordable in all of the countries of the world. In particular, the modern North American use of 12-step programs, based on mutual aid from addicted people and their families, is a widely applicable model. Those interested in learning from the recent North American experience with addiction can do nothing more useful than attending 12-step meetings and furthering the worldwide expansion of these specific and successful antiaddiction programs. The global dissemination of the culture of recovery is already occurring in all parts of the world.

The earlier North American flirtation with increased tolerance for nonmedical drug use is an object lesson in how to make drug problems worse. In contrast, the more recent North American experience with decreased social tolerance for nonmedical drug use provides a solid basis for efforts aimed at reducing nonmedical drug use in other countries.

Overcoming Denial and Enabling

This discussion of the future of addiction has focused thus far on developing nations. In developed nations, the large and costly welfare state is all too often twisted into a deadly caricature by addiction to alcohol and other drugs, as people falling into the safety net because of their addictions are rescued from the consequences of their choices to use alcohol and other drugs. In many cases, they are provided with cash subsidies that are used directly to purchase addicting drugs. In the future, the security nets of developed nations need to be equipped with tripwires to identify alcohol and other drug use and to intervene to stop it as a condition of continued access to benefits. This will be a painful process in all parts of the world because of the pervasive process of denial that now grips caring institutions and the dedication to privacy that veils addiction.

The awareness of the devastation caused by addiction within caring social and medical systems, like the problem of addiction in families, just gets worse and worse until, finally, it must be faced honestly and openly. The way that is both easy and quick to get to the place where recovery can begin is to require alcohol and drug tests for all social and health care programs. Such testing will peel back denial and, ultimately, force those responsible for these programs to confront the problems caused by addiction.

Within developed nations, addiction treatment based on the use of mutual aid and self-help, and linked to spiritual values, is a useful model for treatment and intervention in many medical and mental disorders. It is likely that addiction treatment in the future will be the teacher for many other forms of medical and social services, just as workplace addiction programs, including the EAPs and drug tests, are now proving to be valuable models for other social institutions, from education and religion to health care and the criminal justice system. In all these ways, successful treatment of addiction points back to shared, deeply held values and to the importance of the community of caring people and a relationship with a Higher Power (or, in the words of the Twelve Steps of Alcoholics Anonymous, God "as we understood Him").

Some Useful Next Steps

There are good public health reasons to do a better job than is now being done in most countries, both developed and developing, to monitor the extent of the nonmedical use of addicting drugs and the consequences of that use. Research is needed so that sound responses can be developed and so that the results of these efforts can be scientifically measured. International agencies, especially the United Nations and regional international groups, can do more than is now being done to support global epidemiological studies of nonmedical drug use. Technical assistance should be more widely shared globally for epidemiological studies to aid both the prevention and the treatment of addiction.

In this same spirit, all nations of the world can do a better job of recognizing their shared vulnerability to global criminal narcotics trafficking. Countries that produce drugs need to recognize that the highest costs for the production of drug crops are paid within their own borders. It is not possible to grow and manufacture illicit drugs without having the producer country's own population suffer intensely from the use of those drugs. The selfish brain knows no ethnic, national, or economic boundaries. If addicting drugs are widely available, they will be used by high-risk people, first and most intensively by urban young men, in all parts of the world. The risk of addiction is a human risk that cannot be denied or escaped if drugs are available and if their use is tolerated.

Although most drug crops now are grown in developing nations primarily for ultimate consumption in developed nations, additional perspectives need to be added to balance this conventional picture. The developed nations often produce pharmaceutical drugs, limited to prescription use within their own boundaries, which are shipped to developing nations and sold openly without the safeguards of tightly controlled prescription drug distribution systems. In this way, developed nations are producer nations and major contributors to the problems of addiction in developing nations.

In addition, developed nations are becoming increasingly involved in the growing of drug crops for local consumption, a trend that shortens and makes less vulnerable the drug distribution chain. This trend diversifies the sources of agriculturally produced addictive drugs. Every nation in the world is now, or can easily become, both a consumer and a producer nation when it comes to addicting drugs. It is not a matter of "us" versus "them." When it comes to the risk of addiction in the world today, it is only "us"—all of us on this planet.

The responses to the dangers of addiction to alcohol and other drugs, including law enforcement, prevention, and treatment, need to fit the values and experiences of each national culture as well as specific subcultures within individual nations. The social contract for drug use, which has been the foundation of the North American experience with addicting drugs and of all international drug abuse prevention treaties throughout the 20th century, can prove increasingly useful in all parts of the world. This social contract calls for no use of addicting drugs, except for a few that might be kept under tight medical or religious control, and except for restrained alcohol use by adults.

Some well-meaning people are now disguising purely self-controlled addictive use of these substances under the cloak of traditional practices in medicine and religion. It is easy to distinguish dangerous pseudotraditional drug use from truly traditional use of addicting drugs. If the users control the access to the drugs and set their own doses and frequency of use, then this represents modern addiction flying under a false flag. It is not traditional, socially controlled substance use. If the user comes to the "religion" from the drug culture rather than from a long-standing, well-established religious commitment, and if the "religious" drug use is a central part of a drug-using lifestyle rather than a small part of a religious lifestyle, then the use is simply drug abuse. If the user of addicting substances repeatedly and frequently consumes high-potency drugs by highly addictive routes of administration, then this is modern drug addiction, not traditional medicine or religion.

The experience in all parts of the world during the 20th century has shown that traditional, limited, and controlled use of addicting drugs is pushed out by modern addictive use because of the workings of the selfish brain. Modern addictive drug use provides more intense and frequent brain reward than does low-dose infrequent traditional use of substances by less rewarding routes of administration. Modern addictive drug use fits best with values that promote personal control of people's lifestyle. Traditional cultures in all parts of the world have proved to be even more vulnerable to addiction with modern high-potency drugs than are modern societies. Use of low-potency traditional drugs does not reduce the use of high-potency drugs; rather, it sets the stage for and encourages such dangerous use.

Children and youth under 21 are an important special case. Is anyone, even the most ardent advocate of legalizing drugs to take the profit out of drug sales, advocating making alcohol and other drugs available to children and youth? Whatever else we may disagree about, let us team up in the future in all parts of the world on the simple goal of helping children grow to adulthood free of the use of alcohol and other drugs as well as free of the use of tobacco. This goal is partly a responsibility of youth, but it is mostly a responsibility of adults. The explosive, worldwide growth of tobacco, alcohol, and other drug use by youth in the last two decades is devastating evidence of the failure of adult responsibility for the vital welfare of children and youth.

Surely when it comes to youth using tobacco, alcohol, and other drugs, it is not a matter of "choice" to be made by the youth. Such an attitude reflects an ignorance of the vulnerability of the selfish brain to addicting substances, a lack of understanding of the unique vulnerability of young people, and a shocking abdication of adult responsibility for the world's most precious resource, its young people.

Those individuals, families, and communities that have the best ability to resist the lure of chemical highs will prosper, relatively. And those that are less able to resist these biologically inescapable temptations will suffer more intensely, until, like the addict hitting bottom, they reach a point that the only way for them to survive is to admit their powerlessness and to join together to develop new and more effective lifestyles based on shared, powerful values that include a commitment not to use addicting drugs nonmedically.

Learning about addiction is expensive and painful. If learning does not take place, the outcome of addiction for an individual, a family, or a community can be death. Reading books and learning from the experience of others can help some people, but many good people have to learn about addiction to alcohol and other drugs the harder way by experiencing firsthand the inescapable suffering addiction causes. I call this process "doing personal research on addiction." This remains the most common route—and for many people the only practical route—to learn from addiction, in families, in communities, and in entire nations. Trial by fire is the most dangerous and expensive way to learn. Many researchers do not survive. But the fire of active addiction is an excellent teacher for those who do survive. The conclusion of such personal research into addictive disease can be a rebirth of the spirit, a rediscovery of hope and serenity, and the creation of a sense of both personal identity and of community solidarity based on compassion and a shared sense of vulnerability. That is the gift of addiction.

In this book, I have focused on the human brain, which is made up of as many as 1 trillion separate brain cells, or neurons. The most basic feature of the brain, unlike the lungs, kidneys, and heart, is its plasticity. Life changes the brain. Neurons are continually making new connections, or synapses, in response to personal experience. Although it is true that once it is addicted to alcohol and other drugs the brain has changed forever, it is also true that all human experience permanently changes the brain. Not only is the vulnerability to addiction hardwired into the brain, but the human brain has the capacity to acquire new operating instructions from experience, from the environment in which the brain exists. This environment includes the rules for living a good life, which is culture. Human cultures are enduring, shared, but ever-changing responses to human experiences over long periods of time. The addicted brain—the selfish brain—seeks immediate rewards from the chemical stimulation of the pleasure centers. The brain can learn from addiction but with difficulty and at high cost.

Individual people, families, communities, and even nations can learn from addiction and thus add to the cultural guidance for our lives. Two simple tests can be added to any personal decision to pursue a pleasure or not: the honesty test and the long-term test. If an activity that produces pleasure can be completely shared with those who love us, then it meets the honesty test. If a pleasure-producing behavior leads to good feelings that last over time, say for a week or a month, then it is usually reasonable and safe. When pleasure cannot pass the honesty and the long-term tests, as the use of addictive drugs generally cannot, then danger signals need to be heeded.

At a deeper level, learning from addiction means learning what makes a good life, for individuals, families, and communities. Real recovery from addiction, and real prevention of addiction, can only come one person at a time, from the inside out. Recovery and prevention are as much about the heart as the head, which is why addiction is a spiritual disease and not just a problem of chemicals acting in the synapses of the brain.

Seen whole and without distortion, addiction is a mighty teacher.

A Personal Footnote

A friend who read an early draft of this book commented that I made addiction seem so simple and easy to understand that she assumed my readers would think that they could easily prevent, identify, and cure the disease. She and I knew that anyone who reached this conclusion would soon be humbled by the power and mystery of addiction. Addiction to alcohol and other drugs is truly cunning, baffling, and powerful, as well as being a progressive and potentially fatal disease. No book can make it anything less. I hope this book helps you on your own personal journey of discovery. Armed with the ideas in this book—a software program to help you cope with the selfish brain—you are better equipped to confront addiction.

At the very least, I hope the book will help us talk with other people about what we see and what we have learned about addiction so that the suffering of addiction need not be endured in silence, isolation, and shame as it now is. Addiction is a uniquely human disease, one that offers not only many roads to recovery but much benefit from the painful journey.

Some parts of this book are controversial and easily misunderstood. I appreciate your willingness to hear me out and to consider my views. Deep wisdom about addiction is most likely to be found in the community of recovering people, addicted people, and their families who are living their lives, one day at a time, by the sound principles of the Twelve Steps and the Twelve Traditions of Alcoholics Anonymous, Narcotics Anonymous, and the other mutual-aid programs based on the original AA. I have one request that I now repeat at the end of the book. I ask readers who are not familiar with these programs to go to at least six 12-step meetings with an open mind and learn for themselves about the slavery of addiction and the miracle of recovery. I have never been to a

12-step meeting where I could not see the miracle of recovery happening right before my eyes. I have never been to a meeting where I did not learn something valuable for living my own life. Go to meetings. They work.

This book is dedicated to my own teachers about addiction, my patients who have taught me the meaning of a cure for addiction. A cure is knowing what is wrong and what to do about it. If this book helps you know what is wrong and what to do about it when it comes to addiction, if it helps you learn from addiction, then I have succeeded.

Drug Facts

Here is a quick summary of the major drugs of abuse in the modern world, along with their common slang names, the ways they are used, and the effects of their use. This is a review of the more comprehensive material on these drugs found in Chapters 5 and 6, especially the four drugs that are the primary focus of this book: alcohol, marijuana, cocaine, and heroin.

Drugs are the lovers of drug abusers, so they are often given pet names. These intimate names for drugs are chosen so that nonmedical drug users can demonstrate to each other that they are "hip" or "cool." These special words to describe their drugs are intended to be incomprehensible to straight people who do not use drugs. They are a code that addicted people use to define themselves and their passionate attachments to the objects of their love, their addicting drugs.

The specific names that drug abusers use are often limited to geographic areas or even to specific subgroups of people within geographic areas. For example, young users often use different names for the same drug than do older users. Women may use different names than men. Ethnic groups have specific and unique names for particular drugs. Urban addicts use different names than rural addicts, and East Coast addicts sometimes use different names than West Coast addicts. The names used by drug abusers change over time. All of this seems both confusing and complex. The drugs chosen by drug abusers, for the most part, are only a handful. Unlike the pet names used for them, these drugs change little over time. This is all the more remarkable considering that modern science produces a nearly limitless number of potentially abusable substances. For all their complexity of slang, addicted people tend to be highly traditional when it comes to the drugs they most commonly use.

Alcohol and Other Depressants

Alcoholics often show deep attachments to the particular brand names of the alcohol they drink. Because alcohol is the only legal (for adults) nonmedical drug, it is the only one that has extensive, well-advertised commercial affiliations. If other drugs were legally available, they would show a similar pattern of brand name loyalty.

The effects of depressants are in many ways similar to the effects of alcohol. Small amounts can produce calmness, reduced inhibitions, and relaxed muscles, but somewhat larger doses can cause slurred speech, staggering gait, and altered perception. Very large doses of alcohol and other depressants can cause respiratory depression, coma, and death. The combination of depressant drugs and alcohol can multiply the risks of impairment and even overdose or death. The use of depressants, including alcohol, every day can cause physical dependence. Regular use over time results in a tolerance to the depressant, leading the user to increase the quantity consumed in order to get high. When regular users suddenly stop taking large doses of alcohol and other depressants, they develop withdrawal symptoms ranging from restlessness, insomnia, and anxiety to convulsions and death. For alcohol, the withdrawal syndrome is called *delirium tremens*, or DTs.

Babies born to mothers who abuse alcohol and other depressants during pregnancy may be physically dependent on the drugs and show withdrawal symptoms shortly after they are born. Birth defects and behavioral problems also may result. Fetal alcohol syndrome (FAS) is a specific group of congenital defects, usually including mental retardation, which result from maternal alcohol use during pregnancy.

The alcohol and other depressants section of the table at the end of this chapter applies only to the nonmedical use of alcohol and other depressants, all of which is illegal, except for the use of alcohol by adults. Some of these substances are used legitimately and beneficially in medical practice. See the distinction between medical and nonmedical drug use on page 458.

Marijuana (Cannabis)

All forms of cannabis have both short-term and long-term negative physical and mental effects. Several regularly observed physical effects of cannabis are increase in the heart rate, bloodshot eyes, dry mouth and throat, and increased appetite. Use of cannabis impairs short-term memory and comprehension, alters the sense of time and distance, and reduces the ability to perform tasks requiring concentration and coordination, such as studying or driving a car. People do not effectively retain information when they are high on marijuana. Motivation and clear thinking are markedly reduced by marijuana use, making new learning, and even simple tasks, difficult. Marijuana use can also produce paranoia, psychosis, and panic attacks. Driving an automobile and use of other complex equipment are severely affected by marijuana use.

Because marijuana users often inhale the unfiltered smoke deeply and then hold it in their lungs as long as possible, marijuana smoke is damaging to the lungs and pulmonary system. It contains more cancer-causing chemicals than tobacco smoke. Marijuana use also adversely affects the endocrine and immune systems of users. Long-term users of cannabis may develop tolerance and require more of the drug to get the same effect. The drug use becomes the center of their lives. Marijuana use makes users stupid and lazy, encouraging carelessness and discouraging motivation and goal-oriented efforts.

Cocaine and Other Stimulants

Cocaine stimulates the central nervous system. Cocaine's immediate effects include dilated pupils and elevated blood pressure, heart rate, respiratory rate, and body temperature. Cocaine can stimulate the brain and the heart pathologically, causing epileptic seizures and heart abnormalities that can be fatal, even after a single use. Occasional use of cocaine by snorting can cause a stuffy or runny nose, whereas chronic intranasal use of cocaine can ulcerate the mucous membrane of the nose and lead to perforation of the septum between the two sides of the nasal cavity. Injecting cocaine with contaminated needles and syringes can lead to AIDS, hepatitis, and other serious infectious diseases. Preparation of freebase, which involves the use of volatile solvents, can result in death or injury from fire or explosion. Cocaine produces severe dependency, a feeling that the user cannot function without the drug. Tolerance develops rapidly after repeated use of cocaine.

Crack or freebase rock is extremely addictive when smoked. Its effects are felt within 8 seconds. The physical effects of crack smoking include dilated pupils, increased pulse rate, elevated blood pressure, insomnia, loss of appetite, tactile hallucinations, paranoia, irregular heartbeat, and seizures. The use of cocaine by any route of administration can cause sudden death by cardiac arrest or seizures.

All brain stimulant drugs cause increased heart and respiratory rates, elevated blood pressure, dilated pupils, and decreased appetite. In addition, stimulant users may experience sweating, headache, blurred vision, dizziness, sleeplessness, anxiety, and panic attacks. Extremely high doses of stimulants can cause a rapid or irregular heartbeat, tremors, loss of coordination, and even sudden death. An amphetamine injection, or smoking of methamphetamine ("ice"), creates a sudden increase in blood pressure that can result in stroke, very high fever, or sudden heart failure.

In addition to the physical effects, most stimulant users report feeling restless, anxious, and moody after drug use. Higher and repeated doses of stimulants intensify the effects. People who use large amounts of amphetamines over a long period can develop an amphetamine psychosis that includes hallucinations, delusions, and paranoia. These symptoms usually disappear within days of stopping drug use, but they may persist for months or years after stimulant use stops.

Khat is a plant that contains a chemical called cathinone, which is similar to amphetamine. It has been chewed for centuries by people living on the horn of northeast Africa and nearby Arabia. Local use of khat is similar to coffee use in its effects, but heavy use can lead to an amphetamine-like psychosis. Chronic use of khat leads to discolored teeth and gums, constipation, raised blood pressure, and impotence.

Heroin and Other Opiates

Opiates, usually taken by injection or smoked by experienced nonmedical drug users, initially produce a feeling of euphoria that is often followed by drowsiness. Early in the use of these drugs they cause nausea and vomiting, but these symptoms disappear after repeated use. Opiate users also experience constricted pupils, watery eyes, and itching. An opiate overdose produces slow and shallow breathing, clammy skin, convulsions, coma, and death. Tolerance to narcotics and physical dependence develop rapidly after repeated opiate use over days or weeks of everyday use. The use of contaminated needles and syringes may result in contagious diseases such as AIDS, endocarditis, and hepatitis. Opiate addiction in pregnant women can lead to the birth of premature, stillborn, or addicted infants who experience severe withdrawal symptoms.

Other Commonly Abused Drugs

Hallucinogens

Lysergic acid diethylamide (LSD), mescaline, and psilocybin cause illusions and hallucinations. The physical effects may include dilated pupils, elevated body temperature, increased heart rate and blood pressure, loss of appetite, sleeplessness, and tremors. Sensations and feelings may change rapidly. It is common to have an upsetting reaction to LSD, mescaline, and psilocybin, called a *bad trip*. The user of hallucinogens may experience panic, confusion, suspicion, anxiety, and loss of control. Delayed effects, or flashbacks, can occur even weeks or months after hallucinogen use has ceased.

Phencyclidine (PCP) broadly and unpredictably interrupts many of the functions of the brain. Because PCP blocks pain receptors, PCP use may result in self-inflicted injuries. The effects of PCP vary, but users frequently report a feeling of distance and estrangement. Time sense and body movement are slowed down. Muscular coordination worsens and the senses are dulled. Speech may be blocked and incoherent. Users may look wide-eyed and drool uncontrollably. Chronic users of PCP report persistent memory problems and speech difficulties. Some of these effects may last 6 months or longer following prolonged daily use of PCP. Severe mood disorders—depression, anxiety, and violent behavior—also occur after PCP use. In later stages of chronic PCP use, users often exhibit paranoid and uncontrolled behavior and experience hallucinations. Chronic use leads to *burnout*. Large doses of PCP may produce convulsions and coma, as well as heart and lung failure leading to sudden death.

One group of hallucinogens, chemically related to amphetamines, includes MDMA or Ecstasy. These drugs produce a stimulant rush and muscular restlessness (as befits their relationship to the stimulants) and distorted thinking, including frequently a sense of being "connected" to other people. The effects of use last for 3 to 4 hours. These drugs, including Ecstasy, flood the brain's serotonin neurotransmitters and may cause permanent loss of these brain cells. The aftereffects of use typically include lethargy and loss of appetite. These drugs are commonly used at "raves," the all-night dance parties of teenagers.

Inhalants and Abusable Gases

The negative effects of inhalants include nausea, sneezing, coughing, nosebleeds, fatigue, lack of coordination, and loss of appetite. Solvents and aerosol sprays decrease the heart and respiratory rates and impair judgment. Abused gases such as amyl nitrite and butyl nitrite can cause rapid pulse, headaches, and involuntary passing of urine and feces. Long-term use of volatile solvents may result in hepatitis or brain damage. Deeply inhaling the vapors of solvents, or using large amounts over a short time, may result in disorientation, violent behavior, unconsciousness, or death. High concentrations of inhalants can cause suffocation by displacing the oxygen in the lungs, depressing the central nervous system to the point that breathing stops. Long-term inhalant use can cause weight loss, fatigue, disordered blood chemistry, and muscle fatigue. Repeated sniffing of concentrated solvent vapors over time can damage the brain permanently.

Look-Alikes and Act-Alikes

Illicit drugs have no official status in society and therefore no quality control. Drug users do not know what drugs they are taking into their bodies or the potency of the drugs they are using. This creates abundant opportunities for drug sellers to deceive their customers. Drug dealers themselves may not know what they are buying for resale to their customers. *Look-alikes* are pseudodrugs. They contain nonscheduled substances manufactured to look like controlled substances. Many teenagers are sold pills made to look like LSD, MDMA, amphetamines, barbiturates, and other controlled substances. Sometimes these pills contain caffeine to mimic stimulants, or antihistamines to mimic depressants.

Drugs of deception, or *act-alikes*, are controlled or prescription substances sold as other, more attractive addictive drugs. For example, diazepam (Valium) is sometimes sold as illicit Quaalude, and local anesthetics, such as procaine and novocaine, are sold as cocaine. Both look-alikes and act-alikes can cause serious and even fatal reactions.

Drug	Appearance	Route of administration	Popular or slang names
Alcohol and other depressants			
Alcohol	Liquid—color from light and clear to dark and nearly opaque	Oral	Booze, hootch, rot-gut, brew, suds
Barbiturates	Usually capsules, which are often colorful (e.g., red, yellow, and blue)	Oral, injected	Barbs, blue devils, red devils, yellow jacket, yellows, sleeping pills, candy, goofers, blue-birds, reds, beans, Christmas trees, dolls, peanuts, rainbows, Nembutal, Seconal, Amytal, tuinals
Methaqualone	Tablets	Oral	Quaaludes, ludes, sopors, Q
Antianxiety medicines	Tablets, capsules	Oral	Tranqs, mother's little helper, downers
Marijuana (cannabis)			
Marijuana	Looks like dried parsley mixed with stems—may include seeds	Smoked, oral	Pot, grass, weed, reefer, dope, Mary Jane, sinsemilla (also California sinsemilla), Acapulco gold, Thai sticks, Maui wowee, joint, herb, Colombian, Panama red

(continued)

Drug	Appearance	Route of administration	Popular or slang names
Tetrahydrocannabinol	Soft gelatin capsules	Oral	THC
Hashish	Brown or black cakes or balls	Smoked, oral	Hash
Hashish oil	Concentrated syrupy liquid varying in color from clear to black	Smoked— mixed with tobacco	Hash oil
Cocaine and other stimulants			
Cocaine	White crystalline powder, often diluted with other ingredients	Inhaled through nose, injected	Coke, snow, flake, white, blow, nose candy, big C, C, snowbirds, lady, girl, the white lady, toot, happy dust
Crack cocaine (freebase)	Light brown or beige pellets or crystalline rocks that resemble coagulated soap; often packaged in small vials	Smoked	Crack, freebase rocks, rock, eggs, fries, base
Amphetamines	Capsules, pills, tablets	Oral, injected, inhaled through nose	Speed, uppers, ups, black beauties, pep pills, copilots, bumblebees, hearts, footballs, brownies, black Mollies, jelly beans, wakeups, As, bennies, dexies, crossroads, greenies, beans, Benzedrine, Dexedrine, biphetamine

Methamphetamines	White powder, pills, a rock that resembles a block of paraffin (ice)	Oral, injected, inhaled through nose, smoked	Crank, crystal meth, crystal, crystal methedrine, speed, ice
Khat	Leafy twigs	Chewed	Khat, qat
Additional stimulants	Pills, capsules, tablets	Oral, injected	Ritalin, Cylert, Preludin, Tenuate, Ionamin
Heroin and other opiates			
Heroin	Powder, white to dark brown, tarlike substance	Injected, inhaled through nose, smoked	Smack, horse, brown sugar, junk, mud, big H, black tar, dope, skag, hard stuff, boy, H
Methadone	Solution, tablet	Oral, injected	Dolophine, Methadose, Amidone
Codeine	Capsules, tablets, dark liquid varying in thickness	Oral, injected	Empirin compound with codeine, Tylenol with codeine, codeine, codeine in cough medicines
Morphine	White crystals, hypodermic tablets, injectable solutions	Injected, oral, smoked	Pectoral syrup

(continued)

Drug	Appearance	Route of administration	Popular or slang names
Meperidine	White powder, solution, tablets	Oral, injected	Pethidine, Demerol, Mepergan
Opium	Dark brown chunks, powder	Smoked, eaten	Paregoric, Dover's powder, Parepectolin
Fentanyl and related synthetic opiates	White powder resembling heroin	Inhaled through nose, injected	Synthetic heroin, China white
Synthetic drugs related to meperidine	White powder	Inhaled through nose, injected	Synthetic heroin, MPTP (new heroin), MPPP
Other opiates	Tablets, capsules, liquid	Oral, injected	Percocet, Percodan, Tussionex, fentanyl, Darvon, Talwin, Lomotil
Hallucinogens			
Lysergic acid diethylamide	Brightly colored tablets, impregnated blotter paper, thin squares of gelatin, clear liquid	Oral, licked off paper, gelatin and liquid can be put in the eyes	LSD, acid, green or red dragon, white lightning, blue heaven, sugar cubes, microdot, purple or orange haze, California sunshine, pink wedges

Mescaline and peyote	Hard brown discs, tablets, capsules	Discs—chewed, swallowed, or smoked; tablets and capsules—taken orally	Mesc, buttons, cactus, businessman's acid
Psilocybin	Fresh or dried mushrooms	Chewed and swallowed	Mushrooms, magic mushrooms, 'shrooms
Phencyclidine	Liquid, capsules, white crystalline powder, pills	Oral, injected, smoked—can be sprayed on cigarettes, parsley, and marijuana	PCP, angel dust, loveboat, lovely, hog, killer weed, dust, white powder, flakes, superjoint (when laced with marijuana), rocket fuel, embalming fluid, peace pills, busy bee, DOA (dead on arrival), green, elephant tranquilizer
Synthetic drugs related to amphetamines and methamphetamines	White powder, tablets, capsules	Oral, injected, inhaled through nose	MDMA (Ecstasy, XTC, X, Adam, essence), MDM, STP, PMA, 2,5-DMA, TMA, DOM, DOB, Eve

(continued)

Drug	Appearance	Route of administration	Popular or slang names
		Abusable gases	
Nitrous oxide	Propellant for whipped cream in aerosol can, small 8-gram metal cylinder sold with a balloon or pipe	Inhaled	Laughing gas, whippets, buzz bomb
Amyl nitrite	Clear yellowish liquid in ampules	Inhaled	Poppers, snappers, amys, pears
Butyl nitrite	Packaged in small bottles	Inhaled	Rush, bolt, locker room, aroma of men, bullet, climax
		Inhalants	
Chlorohydrocarbons	Aerosol paint cans, containers of cleaning fluid	Inhaled	Aerosol sprays, scrubwoman's kick
Hydrocarbons	Cans of aerosol propellants, gasoline, glue, paint thinner	Inhaled	Solvents
		Look-alikes	
Look-alikes	Capsules, tablets, often similar to stimulants and depressants	Oral	The same names used for stimulants and depressants and other drugs of abuse

Act-alikes		
Act-alikes	Capsules, tablets, powder, pills; often similar to the major drugs of abuse	Oral, smoked, inhaled through nose, injected	The same names as the major drugs of abuse

Bibliotherapy

Healing through reading books is called *bibliotherapy*. Books tell good stories, they contain useful ideas, and they offer workable plans for living better lives. A group of 18 newly recovering alcoholics met in Akron, Ohio, in 1937 to consider how they could best spread the word to others about the new program they had used based on the Twelve Steps that were pioneered by Bill W. They considered establishing a national chain of hospitals or taking their message on the road to explain it. Then they hit on their most powerful idea: they wrote a book so that people everywhere in the world could learn about the new program. Only after the book was finished did the group choose a name for itself. They choose the name *Alcoholics Anonymous* for their organization. Their book, popularly known as the "Big Book," is also titled *Alcoholics Anonymous*. Over 11 million copies are now in print. With this remarkable book, all can see the power of the written word to change the world, one person at a time.

Because addiction is such a huge problem that affects so many people, and because the good news about recovery is just beginning to be understood, there is a rapidly rising tide of good written and other material available to help people who are seeking ways to understand and to overcome problems of addiction. Today, many books are available from Alcoholics Anonymous and from the other 12-step programs and mutual-aid groups; these are listed in Appendix 1. Several major organizations and publishers have devoted substantial efforts to the issues of addiction; these are listed in the resources in Appendix 2. Many libraries and bookstores also have extensive collections of useful books on addiction. In recent years, bookstores that specialize in material on addiction and recovery have become more widespread as interest in these issues grows. These specialty bookstores may be listed under "Book Dealers, Retail" in the Yellow Pages of your telephone directory. I have listed below some books that you can consider, but I urge you to follow your own instincts to the books that best meet your personal needs.

Beattie M: Codependent No More—How to Stop Controlling Others and Start Caring for Yourself. New York, HarperCollins, 1987

Bradshaw J: Bradshaw On: The Family—A Revolutionary Way of Self-Discovery. Deerfield Beach, FL, Health Communications, 1988

Cermak TL: A Primer on Adult Children of Alcoholics, 2nd Edition. Deerfield Beach, FL, Health Communications, 1989

DuPont RL: Getting Tough on Gateway Drugs: A Guide for the Family. Washington, DC, American Psychiatric Press, 1984

DuPont RL (ed): Stopping Alcohol and Other Drug Use Before it Starts: The Future of Prevention, OSAP Prevention Monograph-1 (DHHS Publ No ADM-89-1645). Rockville, MD, U.S. Department of Health and Human Services, Office for Substance Abuse Prevention, 1989.

DuPont RL, McGovern JP: A Bridge to Recovery: An Introduction to 12-Step Programs. Washington, DC, American Psychiatric Press, 1994

Falco M: The Making of a Drug-Free America—Programs That Work. New York, Times Books, 1992

Ford B, Chase C: Betty: A Glad Awakening. Garden City, NY, Doubleday, 1987

Fox CL, Forbing SE: Creating Drug-Free Schools and Communities: A Comprehensive Approach. New York, NY, HarperCollins, 1992

Gold MS: The Facts About Drugs and Alcohol, 3rd Edition. New York, Bantam Books, 1988

Gold MS: The Good News About Drugs and Alcohol: Curing, Treating and Preventing Substance Abuse in the New Age of Biopsychiatry. New York, Villard Books, 1991

Gold MS: Tobacco. New York, Plenum, 1995

Goldstein A: Addiction: From Biology to Drug Policy. New York, WH Freeman, 1994

Hamilton T, Samples P: The Twelve Steps and Dual Disorders: A Framework of Recovery for Those of Us With Addiction and an Emotional or Psychiatric Illness. Center City, MN, Hazelden Educational Materials, 1994

Help for Helpers: Meditations for Counselors. Park Ridge, IL, Parkside Publishing, 1987

Johnson VE: I'll Quit Tomorrow: A Practical Guide to Alcoholism Treatment, Revised Edition. San Francisco, CA, HarperSanFrancisco, 1980

Kirkpatrick J: Turnabout: New Help for the Woman Alcoholic. New York, Bantam Books, 1986

Kurtz E: Not-God: A History of Alcoholics Anonymous, Expanded Edition. Center City, MN, Hazelden, 1991

Kurtz E, Ketcham K: The Spirituality of Imperfection. New York, Bantam, 1992

May GG: Addiction and Grace: Love and Spirituality in the Healing of Addictions. San Francisco, CA, HarperSanFrancisco, 1988

Milam JR, Ketcham K: Under the Influence: A Guide to the Myths and Realities of Alcoholism. New York, Bantam Books, 1981

Mooney AJ, Eisenberg A, Eisenberg H: The Recovery Book. New York, Workman Publishing, 1992

Nowinski J, Baker S: The Twelve-Step Facilitation Handbook: A Systematic Approach to Early Recovery from Alcoholism and Addiction. New York, Lexington Books, 1992

Rivinus TM (ed): Children of Chemically Dependent Parents: Multiperspectives from the Cutting Edge. New York, Brunner/Mazel, 1991

Robertson N: Getting Better: Inside Alcoholics Anonymous. New York, William Morrow, 1988

Rogers RL, McMillin CS: Don't Help: A Positive Guide to Working With the Alcoholic. New York, Bantam Books, 1988

Serendipity Support Group Series: 12 Steps: The Path to Wholeness. Littleton, CO, Serendipity House, 1990

Seymour RB, Smith DE: Drug Free: A Unique, Positive Approach to Staying Off Alcohol and Other Drugs. New York, Facts on File Publications, 1987

Sher K: Children of Alcoholics: A Critical Appraisal of Theory and Research. Chicago, IL, University of Chicago Press, 1991

Starck PL, McGovern JP (eds): The Hidden Dimension of Illness: Human Suffering. New York, National League for Nursing Press, 1992

Sturz EL: Dealing With Disruptive Adolescents and Drugs. New York, Argus Community, 1992

Tobias JM: Kids and Drugs: A Handbook for Parents and Professionals, 2nd Edition. Annandale, VA, Pandaa Press, 1989

U.S. Department of Health and Human Services, Public Health Service: Catalog of Publications 1990-92 (DHHS Publ No PHS-93-1301). Hyattsville, MD: Centers for Disease Control and Prevention, National Center for Health Statistics, September 1993

Washton A, Boundy D: Willpower's Not Enough—Recovering From Addictions of Every Kind. New York, HarperPerennial, 1989

Washton A, Stone-Washton N: Step Zero: What to Do When You Can't Take It Anymore, A Hazelden Book. New York, HarperCollins, 1991

Wasserman H, Danforth HE: The Human Bond: Support Groups and Mutual Aid. New York, Spring Publishing, 1988

Wegscheider-Cruse S, Cruse JR: Understanding Co-Dependency. Deerfield Beach, FL, Health Communications, 1990

Whitfield CL: Healing the Child Within: Discovery and Recovery for Adult Children of Dysfunctional Families. Deerfield Beach, FL, Health Communications, 1987

Wing N: Grateful to Have Been There: My 42 Years With Bill and Lois and the Evolution of Alcoholics Anonymous. Park Ridge, IL, Parkside Publishing, 1992

Woititz JG: Adult Children of Alcoholics. Deerfield Beach, FL, Health Communications, 1990

Wolin SJ, Wolin S: The Resilient Self: How Survivors of Troubled Families Rise Above Adversity. New York, Villard Books, 1993

Appendix 1

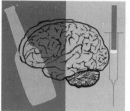

Twelve-Step Fellowship and Other Mutual-Aid Group Descriptions

Many of the 12-step fellowships and other mutual-aid groups listed below offer published materials as well as guidance about referrals, group development, retreats, and speakers bureaus. Call or write for further information.

Adult Children of Alcoholics. International organization founded in 1976 and based on the Twelve Steps of Alcoholics Anonymous (AA). Mutual-aid group for adults who grew up with alcoholic parents. More than 1,800 groups.

Adult Children of Alcoholics World Service Organization
P.O. Box 3216
Torrance, CA 90510
(310) 534-1815

Al-Anon Family Groups. International organization based on Twelve Steps and Twelve Traditions adapted from AA. Founded in 1951 as mutual-aid program of recovery for family and friends of alcoholics. More than 32,000 groups.

> Al-Anon Family Group Headquarters
> P.O. Box 862
> Midtown Station
> New York, NY 10018-6106
> (212) 302-7240
> (800) 344-2666 (meeting information)
> (800) 356-9996 (general)

Alateen. An international fellowship that is part of Al-Anon Family Groups. Founded in 1957 for teenagers and young adults affected by someone else's drinking. Adult member of Al-Anon serves as group sponsor. More than 4,100 groups.

> Alateen
> Al-Anon Family Group Headquarters
> P.O. Box 862
> Midtown Station
> New York, NY 10018-0862
> (212) 302-7240
> (800) 344-2666 (meeting information)
> (800) 356-9996 (general)

Alcoholics Anonymous. International organization of men and women devoted to helping themselves and others overcome alcoholism by following 12-step program to recovery. Founded in 1935. More than 94,000 groups.

> Alcoholics Anonymous World Services, Inc.
> General Service Office
> Box 459
> Grand Central Station
> New York, NY 10163
> (212) 870-3400

Calix Society.   National organization for Catholic alcoholics in Alcoholics Anonymous fellowships. Founded in 1947. About 45 chapters.

> Calix Society
> 7601 Wayzata Boulevard
> Minneapolis, MN 55426
> (612) 546-0544

Cocaine Anonymous.   International mutual-aid organization of men and women helping themselves and others achieve recovery from cocaine addiction. Founded in 1982. More than 1,500 groups.

> Cocaine Anonymous World Services, Inc.
> 3740 Overland Avenue, Suite H
> Los Angeles, CA 90034
> (310) 559-5833 (business office)
> (800) 347-8998 (meeting information)

Co-Dependents Anonymous.   National organization of men and women who grew up in dysfunctional families. Founded in 1986. About 3,500 groups.

> Co-Dependents Anonymous
> P.O. Box 33577
> Phoenix, AZ 85067-3577
> (602) 277-7991

Drugs Anonymous (formerly Pills Anonymous).   National organization for those recovering from chemical addiction. About 10 groups.

> Drugs Anonymous
> P.O. Box 473, Ansonia Station
> New York, NY 10023
> (212) 874-0700

Dual Disorders Anonymous. Illinois model program for men and women suffering from both mental disorder and addiction to alcohol or other drugs. Founded in 1982. About 25 chapters.

> Dual Disorders Anonymous
> P.O. Box 4045
> Des Plaines, IL 60016
> (708) 462-3380

Families Anonymous. International organization of family and friends of individuals with substance abuse or behavioral problems. Based on Twelve Steps of Alcoholics Anonymous. Founded in 1971. About 500 groups.

> Families Anonymous
> P.O. Box 528
> Van Nuys, CA 91408
> (818) 989-7841
> (800) 736-9805

Gam-Anon Family Groups. International organization for family members and friends of compulsive gamblers. Also sponsors Gam-a-teen groups. Founded in 1960. About 400 groups.

> Gam-Anon Family Groups
> P.O. Box 157
> Whitestone, NY 11357
> (718) 352-1671

Gamblers Anonymous. International organization of men and women recovering from compulsive gambling. Founded in 1957. About 1,200 chapters.

> Gamblers Anonymous
> P.O. Box 17173
> Los Angeles, CA 90017
> (213) 386-8789

International Doctors in Alcoholics Anonymous.   Organization whose members are mostly medical doctors who are alcoholic. Founded in 1949.

> International Doctors in Alcoholics Anonymous
> P.O. Box 199
> Augusta, MO 63332
> (314) 781-1317

JACS (Jewish Alcoholics, Chemically Dependent Persons and Significant Others) Foundation.   National organization for alcoholic and chemically dependent Jews, families, and communities. A bridge group to the 12-step programs. Founded in 1980. About 20 chapters.

> JACS
> 426 W. 58th Street
> New York, NY 10019
> (212) 473-4197

Nar-Anon.   International organization based on Twelve Steps of AA. Founded in 1967 for family and friends of drug addicts.

> Nar-Anon Family Group Headquarters
> P.O. Box 2562
> Palos Verdes Peninsula, CA 90274-0119
> (310) 547-5800

Narcotics Anonymous.   International organization based on the Twelve Steps of AA. Men and women meet together in community meetings to support one another in recovery from drug addiction. Founded in 1953. More than 24,000 groups.

> Narcotics Anonymous World Services, Inc.
> P.O. Box 9999
> Van Nuys, CA 91409
> (818) 773-9999

Overcomers Outreach, Inc.   A national group in the Christian community for people who could benefit from secular 12-step groups. Includes alcoholics, drug addicts, compulsive overeaters, gamblers, sexual addicts, codependents, adult children of alcoholics, etc. Founded in 1985. About 1,000 groups.

> Overcomers Outreach, Inc.
> 2290 W. Whittier Boulevard, Suite A/D
> La Habra, CA 90631
> (213) 697-3994

Overeaters Anonymous.   International organization for those suffering from compulsive eating disorders. Also sponsors groups for teens. Founded in 1960. About 10,000 chapters.

> Overeaters Anonymous
> P.O. Box 92870
> Los Angeles, CA 90009
> (310) 618-8835

Pill Addicts Anonymous.   International organization for recovery from addiction to prescribed and over-the-counter mood-changing pills and drugs. Founded in 1979.

> General Service Board of Pill Addicts Anonymous
> P.O. Box 278
> Reading, PA 19603
> (215) 372-1128

Rational Recovery Systems.   International nonspiritual mutual-aid groups for individuals with chemical dependence problems. An alternative to 12-step programs. Membership groups use professional advisers. Founded in 1986. About 350 groups.

> Rational Recovery Systems
> P.O. Box 800
> Lotus, CA 95651
> (916) 621-4374

Tough Love International. International mutual-aid group for parents, children, and communities to support parents in taking a stand to help adolescent children take responsibility for their own behavior. Founded in 1979. About 650 groups.

Tough Love International
P.O. Box 1069
Doylestown, PA 18901
(800) 333-1069

Women for Sobriety. International organization founded in 1976 to meet the special needs of women in recovery from alcoholism. More than 350 groups.

Women for Sobriety
Box 618
Quakertown, PA 18951-0618
(215) 536-8026

Appendix 2

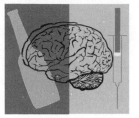

Resources

The following organizations offer a wide variety of material on addiction and recovery, including general information, books, articles, pamphlets, catalogs, films, videotapes, and training materials. Write or call for further information.

Alcohol and Drug Problems Association of America
1555 Wilson Boulevard, Suite 300
Arlington, VA 22209
(703) 875-8684

Alcoholism and Substance Abuse Program Branch of the Indian Health Service
2401 12th Street, NW, Suite 4S
Albuquerque, NM 87102
(505) 766-2115

American Council for Drug Education (ACDE)
164 West 74th Street
New York, NY 10023
Orders: (800) 488-DRUG (3784)
Information: (212) 595-5810, ext. 7860

American Council on Alcohol Problems
3426 Bridgeland Drive
Bridgeton, MO 63044
(314) 739-5944

American Psychiatric Press, Inc.
1400 K Street, NW, 11th Floor
Washington, DC 20005
(202) 682-6000
(800) 368-5777

American Self-Help Clearinghouse
St. Clares-Riverside Medical Center
Denville, NJ 07834
(201) 625-7101

American Society of Addiction Medicine (ASAM)
4601 North Park Avenue, Suite 101
Chevy Chase, MD 20815
(301) 656-3920

Betty Ford Center
39000 Bob Hope Drive
Rancho Mirage, CA 92270
(619) 773-4100
(800) 854-9211

Center for Alcohol and Addiction Studies
Box G, Brown University
Providence, RI 02912
(401) 863-1109

Center for Science in the Public Interest (CSPI)
1875 Connecticut Avenue, NW, Suite 300
Washington, DC 20009
(202) 332-9110

Center for Substance Abuse Prevention (CSAP)
Substance Abuse and Mental Health Services Administration
5600 Fishers Lane, Rockwall II
Rockville, MD 20857
(301) 443-0373

Center on Addiction and Substance Abuse at Columbia University (CASA)
152 West 57th Street
New York, NY 10019
(212) 841-5200

Children of Alcoholics Foundation, Inc.
555 Madison Avenue, 4th Floor
New York, NY 10022
(212) 754-0656

Coalition on Advertising and Family Education
c/o Center for Science in the Public Interest (CSPI)
1875 Connecticut Avenue, NW, Suite 300
Washington, DC 20009
(202) 332-9110

Coalition on Alcohol and Drug Dependent Women and Their Children
c/o National Council on Alcoholism and Drug Dependence (NCADD)
1511 K Street, NW, Suite 926
Washington, DC 20005
(202) 737-8122
(800) NCA-CALL (622-2255)

CompCare Publishers
2415 Annapolis Lane
Minneapolis, MN 55441
(612) 559-4800
(800) 328-3330

**Employee Assistance
Professionals Association**
4601 North Fairfax Drive, Suite
1001
Arlington, VA 22203
(703) 522-6272

Entertainment Industries Council
4444 Riverside Drive, Suite 203
Burbank, CA 91505
(818) 841-9933

Hazelden Educational Materials
Pleasant Valley Road
Box 176
Center City, MN 55012-0176
(800) 328-9000

Hazelden Foundation
Box 11
Center City, MN 55012-0011
(800) 257-7800

Health Communications, Inc.
3201 South West 15th Street
Deerfield Beach, FL 33442
(800) 851-9100

**Hispanic Information and
Telecommunication Network**
449 Broadway, 3rd Floor
New York, NY 10013
(212) 966-5660

**Institute on Black Chemical
Abuse**
2616 Nicollet Avenue
Minneapolis, MN 55408
(612) 871-7878

**International Parents Resource
Institute for Drug Education,
Inc. (PRIDE)**
10 Park Place South
Suite 340
Atlanta, GA 30303
(404) 577-4500

The Johnson Institute
7205 Ohms Lane
Minneapolis, MN 55439-2159
(800) 231-5165

Just Say No International
International Headquarters
2101 Webster Street, Suite 1300
Oakland, CA 94612
(800) 258-2766

Legal Action Center
153 Waverly Place
New York, NY 10014
(212) 243-1313

**Marin Institute for the
Prevention of Alcohol and
Other Drug Problems**
24 Belvedere Street
San Rafael, CA 94901
(415) 456-5692

Mothers Against Drunk Driving (MADD)
511 East John Carpenter
Freeway, Suite 700
Irving, TX 75062-8187
(214) 744-6233

Multi-Cultural Training Resource Center
1540 Market Street, Suite 320
San Francisco, CA 94102
(415) 861-2142

National Asian Pacific American Families Against Substance Abuse, Inc. (NAPAFASA)
420 East Third Street
Suite 909
Los Angeles, CA 90013-1647
(213) 617-8277

National Association for Children of Alcoholics (NACoA)
11426 Rockville Pike, Suite 100
Rockville, MD 20852
(301) 468-0985

National Association of Addiction Treatment Providers (NAATP)
25201 Paseo De Alicia, Suite 100
Laguna Hills, CA 92653
(714) 837-3038

National Association of Alcoholism and Drug Abuse Counselors (NAADAC)
3717 Columbia Pike, Suite 300
Arlington, VA 22204
(800) 548-0497

National Association of Lesbian and Gay Alcoholism Professionals (NALGAP)
204 West 20th Street
New York, NY 10011
(212) 713-5074

National Association of State Alcohol and Drug Abuse Directors (NASADAD)
444 North Capitol Street, NW,
Suite 642
Washington, DC 20001
(202) 783-6868

National Black Alcoholism Council
1629 K Street, NW, Suite 802
Washington, DC 20006
(202) 296-2696

National Clearinghouse for Alcohol and Other Drug Information (NCADI)[1]
P.O. Box 2345
Rockville, MD 20852-2345
(800) 729-6686
(301) 468-2600

---

[1] The Clearinghouse provides free material and information on alcohol, tobacco, and other drug problem prevention and treatment, from The Center for Substance Abuse Prevention, Substance Abuse and Mental Health Services Administration, Public Health Service.

National Coalition of Hispanic
Health and Service
Organizations (COSSMHO)
1501 16th Street, NW
Washington, DC 20036
(202) 387-5000

National Coalition to Prevent
Impaired Driving
1730 Rhode Island Avenue, NW,
Suite 600
Washington, DC 20036
(202) 659-0054

National Council on
Alcoholism and Drug
Dependence (NCADD)
12 West 21st Street, 8th Floor
New York, NY 10010
(212) 206-6770
or
1511 K Street, NW, Suite 926
Washington, DC 20005
(202) 737-8122
(800) NCA-CALL (622-2255)

National Families in Action
2296 Henderson Mill Road,
Suite 300
Atlanta, GA 30345
(404) 934-6364

National Family Partnership
(NFP)
(Formerly National Federation of
Parents for Drug Free Youth)
National Office
11159-B South Towne Square
St. Louis, MO 63123
(314) 845-1933

National Federation of State
High School Associations
(TARGET)
11724 Plaza Circle
P.O. Box 20626
Kansas City, MO 64195
(816) 464-5400

National Highway Traffic
Safety Administration
400 7th Street, SW
Washington, DC 20590
(202) 366-9550

National Nurses Society on
Addiction (NNSA)
5700 Old Orchard Road
Skokie, IL 60077
(708) 966-5010

National Organization of
Student Assistance Programs
and Partners
4760 Walnut Street, Suite 106
Boulder, CO 80301
(800) 972-4636

National Organization on Fetal
Alcohol Syndrome
1815 H Street, NW, Suite 750
Washington, DC 20006
(202) 785-4585

National Resource Center for
the Prevention of Perinatal
Abuse of Alcohol and Other
Drugs
9300 Lee Highway
Fairfax, VA 22031
(703) 218-5600

National Safety Council
444 North Michigan Avenue
Chicago, IL 60611
(312) 527-4800

National Self-Help Clearinghouse
25 West 43rd Street, Room 620
New York, NY 10036
(212) 642-2944

Office of Minority Health Resource Center
P.O. Box 37337
Washington, DC 20013-7337
(800) 444-6472

Parkside Publishing Corporation
205 West Touhy Avenue
Park Ridge, IL 60068
(800) 221-6364

PRIDE
See International Parents
Resource Institute
for Drug Education, Inc.

Remove Intoxicated Drivers (RID)
P.O. Box 520
Schenectady, NY 12301
(518) 372-0034

Resource Center on Substance Abuse Prevention and Disability
1331 F Street, NW, Suite 800
Washington, DC 20004
(202) 783-2900

Rutgers University Center of Alcohol Studies
Smithers Hall, Busch Campus
Piscataway, NJ 08855-0969
(908) 932-4442

Serendipity House
P.O. Box 1012
Littleton, CO 80160
(800) 525-9563
(Materials with a religious orientation)

Solvent Abuse Information Foundation
750 17th Street, NW, Suite 250
Washington, DC 20006
(202) 332-7233

Substance Abuse Librarians and Information Specialists (SALIS)
c/o Alcohol Research Group
Library
2000 Hearst Avenue
Berkeley, CA 94709-2176
(510) 642-5208

Superintendent of Documents
U.S. Government Printing Office
Mail Stop; SSOP
Washington, DC 20402-9328
(202) 512-0000 (information)
(202) 783-3238 (order and inquiry desk)

Suzanne Somers Institute
340 South Farrell Drive, Suite A203
Palm Springs, CA 92262
(619) 325-0110

Texans' War on Drugs
313 East Anderson Lane
Chevy Chase III, #101
Austin, TX 78752
(512) 452-0141

The Trauma Foundation
Building One, Room 306
San Francisco General Hospital
San Francisco, CA 94110
(415) 821-8209

Index

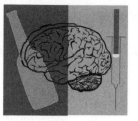

*Page numbers printed in **boldface** type refer to tables or figures.*

introduction of, 39
as synthetic depressants, 136
Behavior responsibility. *See also*
    Cognitive behavior therapy;
Criminal behavior
    in addiction, xx–xxi, 14–17, 398
        dangerous choices and,
            17–19
        conservative vs. liberal
            viewpoint on, 19–21
    shaping of, 116–118
Bensinger, DuPont, and
    Associates, Inc., xxix, xxxii
Benzodiazepine
    depression and, 153
    GABA system and, 137
    receptors of, 104
Betty Ford Center, xiii, 342, 359
    contact information on, 520
Bias, Len, 173–174
Bibliotherapy, 507–510
Blame
    uselessness of, xiv
    on the victim, 14–17
Blood alcohol concentration
    (BAC)
    driving restrictions and,
        143–148
    explanation of, 142–143, **144**
    state-dependent learning and,
        145–146
*Bridge to Recovery: An Introduction
    to 12-Step Programs, A*, 393
Buchman, Frank N. O., 367
Bush, George, 93–94
Butyl nitrite, 214

Caffeine, 167
CAGE test for alcoholism, 306
Calix Society, 380, 513

Canada, drug use trends in, 80–81
Cancer
    long-term alcohol abuse and,
        139
    marijuana as medicine and,
        162, 165
Cannabis. *See* Marijuana
Cardiovascular disease, 141
Carter, Jimmy, xxix, xxxiii
Case histories
    of 12-step programs, 46–50,
        281–282, 412–417
    of alcoholism, 223–226
    of children of affluence,
        317–319
    of cocaine addiction, 183–186
    of codependence, 132–133,
        280–282
    of college addiction, 319–320
    of competitive athletic
        training, 462–463
    of criminal behavior, 86–88
    of dishonesty, 132–133
    of genetic predisposition, 28–29
    of heroin addiction, 132–133,
        223–225
    of intervention and treatment,
        356–360
    of multigenerational
        codependence, 280–281
    of NA, 356–359
    of panic disorder comorbidity,
        180–182
    of parental dilemmas, 259–262
    of physician addiction, 463
    of prescription addiction,
        461–462
    of pseudoaddiction, 27–28
    of public figure, 262–267
    of self-medication, 130–133